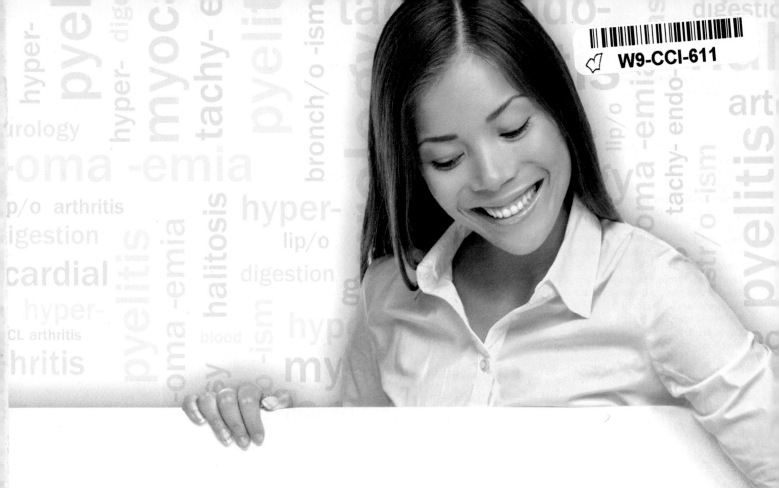

Second Edition

MEDICAL TERMINOLOGY

Complete!

Bruce Wingerd Edison State College / Fort Myers, Florida

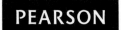

Boston   Columbus   Indianapolis   New York   San Francisco   Upper Saddle River
Amsterdam   Cape Town   Dubai   London   Madrid   Milan   Munich   Paris   Montreal   Toronto
Delhi   Mexico City   Sao Paulo   Sydney   Hong Kong   Seoul   Singapore   Taipei   Tokyo

Publisher: Julie Levin Alexander
Publisher's Assistant: Regina Bruno
Editor-in-Chief: Mark Cohen
Development Editors: Elena Mauceri and Sara Wilson
Associate Editor: Melissa Kerian
Director of Marketing: David Gesell
Executive Marketing Manager: Katrin Beacom
Marketing Coordinator: Michael Sirinides
Senior Managing Editor: Patrick Walsh
Project Manager: Christina Zingone-Luethje
Senior Operations Supervisor: Ilene Sanford
Operations Specialist: Lisa McDowell
Illustrator: Body Scientific International, LLC.
Senior Art Director: Maria Guglielmo
Cover and Interior Designer: Wanda España
Media Editor: Amy Peltier
Lead Media Project Manager: Lorena Cerisano
Full-Service Project Management: Patty Donovan
Composition: Laserwords
Printer/Binder: R.R. Donnelley / Willard
Cover Printer: Lehigh-Phoenix/Hagerstown
Text Font: 11/13 Gill Sans

Dedication

For Mala, who has shown so many
students how learning can be
made fun . . . including me.

Library of Congress Cataloging-in-Publication Data

Wingerd, Bruce D.
  Medical terminology complete! / Bruce Wingerd. — 2nd ed.
    p. ; cm.
  Includes index.
  ISBN-13: 978-0-13-284322-5
  ISBN-10: 0-13-284322-6
  I. Title.
  [DNLM: 1. Medicine—Programmed Instruction. 2. Terminology as Topic—Programmed Instruction.   W 18.2]
  LC Classification not assigned
  610.1'4—dc23
                                        2011045735

10 9 8 7 6 5 4 3 2 1

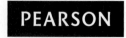

ISBN-13: 978-0-13-284322-5
ISBN-10: 0-13-284322-6

Welcome!

Welcome to *Medical Terminology Complete!* You have chosen an exciting time to begin a career as a healthcare professional. The healthcare industry is a dynamic field that is filled with opportunities for those who care about helping other people. Although many aspects of health care remain relatively constant, research breakthroughs occur each year to keep us moving forward in the war against human suffering. And you can be a part of this exciting process!

This book is designed to help you through the process of building a medical vocabulary. It teaches you the language by using a method known as programmed learning. With this approach, you read through the information at your own pace, one small box (or frame) at a time. Within most frames are blanks, which you fill in as you read. The answers to the blanks are provided in the left column, making it easy and quick to check your answer to make sure you are on the right track. By filling in the blanks as you read, you become an active learner, which improves your chance of successfully mastering medical terminology. You'll have the opportunity to learn thousands of medical terms, and our simple goal is to provide you with the tools and confidence to help you master this brand new vocabulary.

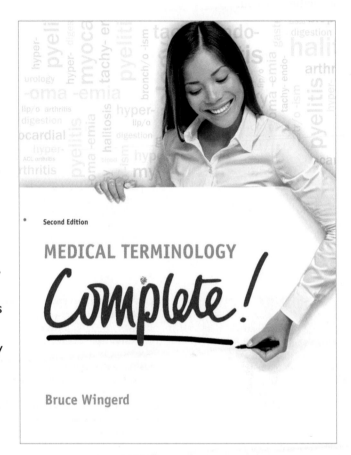

Second Edition

MEDICAL TERMINOLOGY

Complete!

Bruce Wingerd

You may be wondering about the title of this book: *Medical Terminology Complete!* Let us explain the two goals we had in mind as we developed this text.

1. To place a **complete** resource at your fingertips. With its interactive format and its wealth of clear definitions, vivid images, practical examples, and challenging exercises, it's all that you need to become proficient in speaking and understanding the language of medicine.

2. To allow you to **complete** the exercises on every page. This book features a programmed method that prompts you, the reader, to fill in the content as you read. This approach keeps your pen or pencil on every page, so you stay engaged and retain more.

Now please turn the page to get a glimpse of what makes this book an ideal guide to your exploration of medical terminology. ▶▶▶▶▶

Discover What Makes This Book Unique ▶▶▶▶▶

This section provides you with a snapshot of what makes this book special. Consider this your user's manual to the book and all the accompanying resources that are available to you.

Diseases and Disorders of the Male Reproductive System

Here are the word parts that specifically apply to the diseases and disorders of the male reproductive system that are covered in the following section. Note that the word parts are color-coded to help you identify them: prefixes are green, combining forms are red, and suffixes are blue.

Prefix	Definition
an-	without, absence of
hyper-	excessive, abnormally high, above
para-	alongside, abnormal

Combining Form	Definition
andr/o	male
balan/o	glans penis
crypt/o	hidden
epididym/o	epididymis
hydr/o	water
orchi/o, orchid/o	testis
prostat/o	prostate gland
varic/o	dilated vein

Suffix	Definition
-cele	hernia, swelling, or protrusion
-ism	condition or disease
-itis	inflammation
-pathy	disease
-plasia	formation, growth

Color-Coded Word Parts

Prefixes, word roots/combining vowels, and suffixes are each designated by a unique color—making it easier for you to visually recognize the distinctions between each word part, thereby aiding in your mastery of word building.

KEY TERMS A–Z

andropathy
an DROPP ah thee

12.17 A combining form that means "male" and the suffix meaning "disease" may be combined to form a general term for a disease afflicting only males, _____. This constructed term includes three word parts, which can be represented as andr/o/pathy.

anorchism
an OR kizm
an/orch/ism

12.18 The word root that means "testis" is *orch* or *orchid*. When the prefix meaning "without, absence of" is added along with the suffix *-ism*, the constructed term _____ is created. It means "condition of without testis" and refers to the absence of one or both testes. The constructed form of the term is written ____/_____/____. The term **anorchidism** may also be used with the same meaning.

balanitis
bal ah NYE tiss

12.19 Inflammation of the glans penis is a disorder called _____. It is a constructed term with two word parts, written balan/itis.

benign prostatic hyperplasia
bee NINE * pross TAT ik * HIGH per PLAY zee ah

12.20 Among many men older than 50 years, the prostate gland enlarges to constrict the urethra passing through it. Known as **benign prostatic hyperplasia**, symptoms include nocturia (nighttime urination) and a frequent need to void (Figure 12.4■). It is not a form of cancer and does not spread to other tissues, but its symptoms are uncomfortable. _____ _____ _____ is also called **benign prostatic hypertrophy**; both are abbreviated **BPH.**

Key Terms A–Z

The most important terms are listed in alphabetical order, helping you to easily review those important terms before an exam.

Programmed Instruction

This format allows you to learn actively but at your own pace, filling in blanks as you read. Answers appear in the left column, making it easy and quick to check your answer to make sure you are on the right track.

Medically Accurate Illustrations

Concepts come to life with vibrant, clear, consistent, and scientifically precise images.

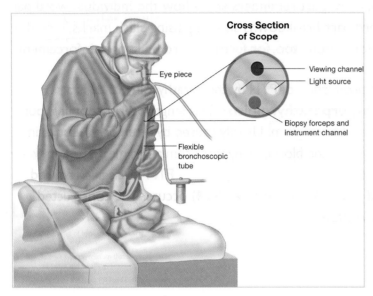

Cross Section of Scope

Eye piece

Viewing channel
Light source
Biopsy forceps and instrument channel
Flexible bronchoscopic tube

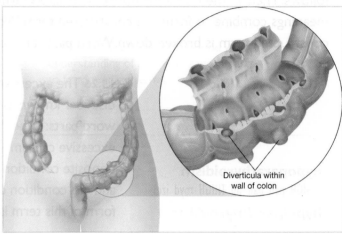

Diverticula within wall of colon

Image Labeling Frames

These frames provide you with opportunities to actively engage with the illustrations, helping to reinforce your knowledge of anatomy.

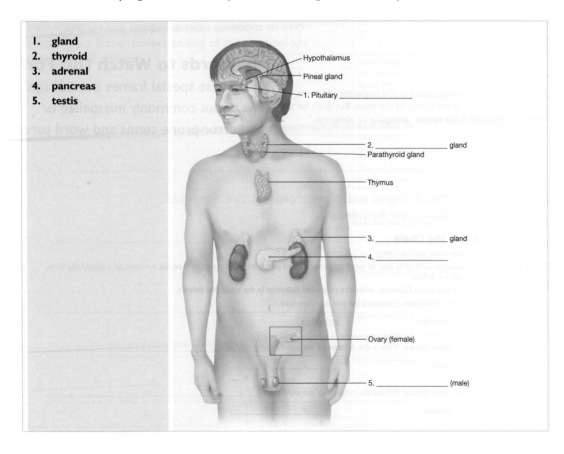

1. gland
2. thyroid
3. adrenal
4. pancreas
5. testis

Hypothalamus
Pineal gland
1. Pituitary _____

2. _____ gland
Parathyroid gland

Thymus

3. _____ gland
4. _____

Ovary (female)

5. _____ (male)

Online Learning ▶▶▶▶▶

The ultimate personalized learning tool is available at **www.pearsonhighered.com/mti.** This online course correlates with the textbook and is available for purchase separately or for a discount when packaged with the book. **Medical Terminology Interactive** is an immersive study experience that takes place within Pearson General Hospital—a virtual world of fun quizzes, word games, videos, and other self-study challenges. The system allows learners to track their own progress through the course and use a personalized study plan to achieve success.

    Medical Terminology Interactive saves instructors time by providing quality feedback, ongoing individualized assessments for students, and instructor resources all in one place. It offers instructors the flexibility to make technology an integral part of their course, or a supplementary resource for students.

    Visit **www.pearsonhighered.com/mti** to log in to the course or purchase access. Instructors seeking more information about discount bundle options or for a demonstration, please contact your Pearson sales representative.

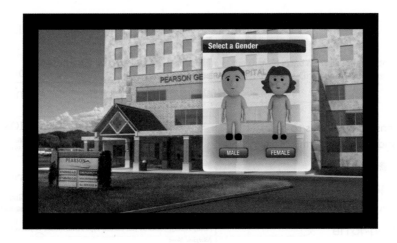

Comprehensive Instructional Package ▶▶▶▶▶

Perhaps the most gratifying part of an educator's work is the "aha" learning moment when the lightbulb goes on and a student truly understands a concept—when a connection is made. Along these lines, Pearson is pleased to help instructors foster more of these educational connections by providing a complete battery of resources to support teaching and learning. Qualified adopters are eligible to receive a wealth of materials designed to help instructors prepare, present, and assess. For more information, please contact your Pearson sales representative or visit **www.pearsonhighered.com/educator.**

Preface ▶▶▶▶▶

Medical Terminology Complete! presents the most current and accepted language of health care in a programmed learning approach. It has helped prepare thousands of students for careers in health professions by providing a self-guided tool for learning medical terminology. The book may be used as a text to support lectures or as an independent student workbook. The flexibility of its application is made possible by the book's text-like format combined with its self-guided learning program, self-assessment questions, and reinforcement exercises. To provide an optimum learning format, the text discussions are basic, clear, and concise. The programmed learning modules are simple and easy to follow, and the self-assessment questions and exercises provide reviews and clinical applications of the information at frequent intervals.

New to This Edition

Based on extensive feedback from students and instructors, we have revised *Medical Terminology Complete!* so that it provides for an even more valuable teaching and learning experience. Here are the enhancements we have made:

- Additional medical reports and case studies appear in every chapter.

- Material on the special senses of sight and hearing has been expanded and placed into its own chapter (14). This content was previously included within the Nervous System and Mental Health chapter of the first edition.

- The Key Terms Double Check activity has been removed from the student text and added to the instructor's manual.

- A robust online tool has been developed to support the text. Medical Terminology Interactive provides a fun, interactive study experience with a variety of games and activities to enhance learning.

- Many new images have been included throughout the book to help learners better visualize the concepts and meanings of selected terms.

The Programmed Approach

Each learning frame contains a clear and concise statement, usually describing a single medical term. This allows learners to focus on one term at a time. Each frame includes at least one blank space, which can be completed based on clues within the frame. The answer to the blank is provided in the left column. Students can either cover the answer column or can leave it uncovered. Either way, the kinesthetic component of filling in the blank provides another level of learning that ensures retention.

Each body systems chapter presents the most important terms (or "Key Terms") in the answer column with color-coded word parts, where applicable, as well as a phonetic

About the Author

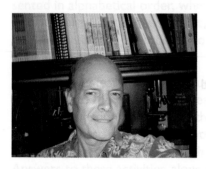

Bruce Wingerd is Professor of Biology at Edison State College in Fort Myers, Florida. Previously, he has held administrative/teaching positions at Broward College and at San Diego State University. His degrees are in the fields of zoology and physiology. Courses taught include medical terminology, human anatomy, advanced human anatomy, and anatomy and physiology. He has written numerous textbooks, lab manuals, and multimedia learning resources in medical terminology, human anatomy, anatomy and physiology, histology, and comparative mammalian anatomy. His goal in teaching and writing is to provide students with learning tools that will help them reach their potential through education. He enjoys counseling students in the health sciences, developing novel approaches to teaching and learning, and leading faculty in the drive for excellence in education.

About the Illustrators

Marcelo Oliver is president and founder of Body Scientific International, LLC. He holds an MFA degree in Medical and Biological Illustration from the University of Michigan. For more than 15 years, his passion has been to condense complex anatomical information into visual education tools for students, patients, and medical professionals.

Body Scientific's lead artists in this publication were medical illustrators Carol Hrejsa, Liana Bauman, and Katie Burgess. They each hold Master of Science degrees in Biomedical Visualization from the University of Illinois at Chicago. Their contribution was the creation and editing of clear, effective, vibrant, and medically accurate artwork throughout.

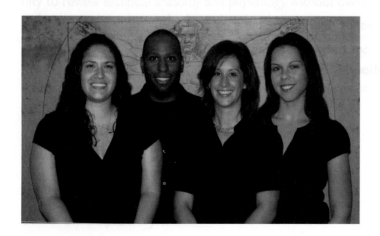

Acknowledgments ▶▶▶▶▶

This book is the product of collective hard work from a talented team focused on creating a unique learning tool.

Our team received direction from Editor in Chief Mark Cohen, who spearheaded the project from start to finish by providing the resources needed to attract a large body of peer reviewers and contributing his experience in identifying and applying effective ways of learning. Elena Mauceri of Dynamic WordWorks, Inc., provided expert daily management of the project, made important contributions to the content of each chapter, and established most of the compositional details of every page to maximize the learning benefits of the book. Elena's talented contributions to the final product are enormous. Working with Elena as Development Editor, Sara Wilson sacrificed many long hours with heart and soul while raising a young family, solving many technical problems and making numerous creative suggestions that are revealed in every page. Her seemingly tireless efforts and important contributions were nothing less than amazing. To each of these individuals, I express my sincere appreciation for their contributions.

Many other talented people worked hard to make this book a valuable teaching and learning resource. I extend to each of them my warmest gratitude:

Melissa Kerian, Managing Development Editor, who coordinated the development of a world-class teaching and learning package.

Rosalie Hawley, Editorial Assistant, who executed the complex process of managing our peer review program.

Marcelo Oliver and his team of medical illustrators at Body Scientific International, LLC, who created a dynamic, clear, and precise art program.

Christina Zingone-Luethje, Project Manager, who directed the flow of textual and visual content throughout the production of the book and ancillary materials.

Patty Donovan, Production Editor for Laserwords, who oversaw the copyediting and page composition processes.

A Commitment to Accuracy ▶▶▶▶▶

As a student embarking on a career in health care you probably already know how critically important it is to be precise in your work. Patients and coworkers will be counting on you to avoid errors on a daily basis. Likewise, we owe it to you—the reader—to ensure accuracy in this book. We have gone to great lengths to verify that the information provided in *Medical Terminology Complete!* is complete and correct. To this end, here are the steps we have taken:

1. **Editorial Review**—We have assembled a large team of developmental consultants (listed on the preceding pages) to critique every word and every image in this book. No fewer than 12 content experts have read each chapter for accuracy. In addition, some members of our developmental team were specifically assigned to focus on the precision of each illustration that appears in the book.

2. **Medical Illustrations**—A team of medically trained illustrators was hired to prepare each piece of art that graces the pages of this book. These illustrators have a higher level of scientific education than the artists for most textbooks, and they worked directly with the author and members of our development team to make sure that their work was clear, correct, and consistent with what is described in the text.

3. **Accurate Ancillaries**—The teaching and learning ancillaries are often as important to instruction as the textbook itself. Therefore, we took steps to ensure accuracy and consistency of these components by reviewing every ancillary component. The author and editorial team studied every PowerPoint slide and online course frame to ensure the context was correct and relevant to each lesson.

Although our intent and actions have been directed at creating an error-free text, we have established a process for correcting any mistakes that may have slipped past our editors. Pearson takes this issue seriously and therefore welcomes any and all feedback that you can provide along the lines of helping us enhance the accuracy of this text. If you identify any errors that need to be corrected in a subsequent printing, please send them to:

Pearson Health Editorial
Medical Terminology Corrections
One Lake Street
Upper Saddle River, NJ 07458

Thank you for helping Pearson reach its goal of providing the most accurate medical terminology textbooks available.

Contents ▶▶▶▶▶

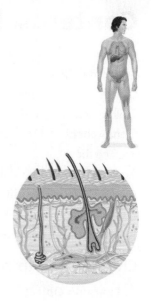
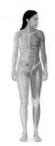
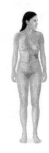

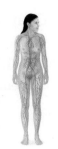

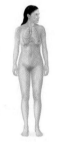

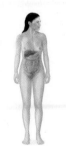

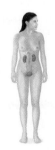

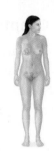

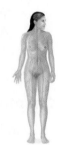

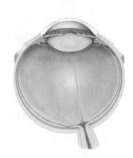

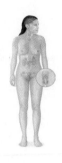

Introduction to Word Parts and Word Construction

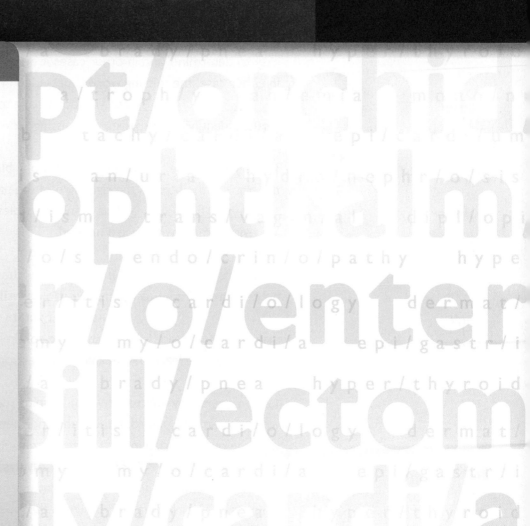

LEARNING OBJECTIVES

After completing this chapter, you will be able to:

1 Use the technique of programmed learning and frames.

2 Apply the phonetic pronunciation guides that are used in frames.

3 Recognize that medical terminology has both constructed and nonconstructed terms.

4 Identify each of the three word parts (word roots, prefixes, and suffixes) used to construct medical terms.

5 Identify the function of a combining vowel that is added to a word root to form a combining form.

6 Recognize that many medical terms are constructed from word parts and can be deconstructed into their word parts.

The Programmed Learning Approach ▶▶▶▶▶

frame

1.1 This textbook teaches you medical terminology by using the friendly technique of **programmed learning.** This technique has been used for many years to teach many subjects, such as math, world languages, and of course, medical terminology. It consists of blocks of information, known as frames, which contain one or more blanks. The blanks are provided for you to write in the missing word. In some cases, the missing word is easy to determine, and in other cases it becomes more of a challenge. In either case, the missing word is provided in the left margin of the _____, so you don't have to feel frustrated if you have trouble identifying or spelling the missing word correctly.

number

1.2 As you can see, each frame consists of a block of information with the blank in the box on the right side of the page. Note the frame _____. This number enables you to locate and flip back to a previous frame with ease if needed.

blank

1.3 The far left box in each frame contains the missing word. As you proceed from frame to frame, you should write the missing word in the _____. Try to work without looking at the answer first to make each frame a challenge. By doing so, the activity will engage your mind and help you to learn the meanings of the words.

spelling

1.4 Spelling is very important when learning medical terminology. By writing the missing word in the blank and then comparing your answer with the one provided in the far left margin, you will be practicing the _____ of the word. Always check your answer before moving to the next frame. Pay special attention to the "Did You Know?" and "Words to Watch Out For" boxes in this text. These will alert you to tricky spelling issues or terms that might easily be confused.

phonetic
phoh NET ik

1.5 In addition to spelling, correct pronunciation of medical terms is also important. To help you with pronunciation, the phonetic ("sounds like") form of the word is provided in parentheses whenever a new term is introduced, for example, _____ and pronunciation (proh NUN see AYE shun). You should say the new word aloud whenever possible, using the phonetic guide to assist you.

guides

1.6 In the phonetic _____ that appear in this text, note that the syllable with the most spoken emphasis is shown in all capital letters. Here are some examples:

- The term *cardiology* is pronounced kar dee ALL oh jee. Note that the middle syllable *ALL* carries the most emphasis.

- The term *gastrohepatic* is pronounced GAS troh heh PAT ik. Note that the long *o* sound in the second syllable is demonstrated when spelled phonetically as *oh,* and the short *e* sound is demonstrated when spelled *eh.*

- The term *osteopathic* is pronounced oss tee oh PATH ik. Note that the long *e* sound in the second syllable is shown as *tee.*

You can also refer to the student website for audio samples of the pronunciation of each medical term presented in this text. Spend time listening to the _____ of each term presented in each chapter. Doing so will help you complete the pronunciation exercise in this chapter, "Talking Shop."

pronunciation

PRACTICE: The Programmed Learning Approach

The Right Match

Match the term on the left with the correct definition on the right.

_____ 1. pronunciations

_____ 2. spelling

_____ 3. blank

_____ 4. programmed learning

_____ 5. Words to Watch Out For boxes

a. alert you to terms that might easily be confused

b. learning technique that consists of blocks of information, known as frames, which contain one or more blanks for the student to fill in

c. by comparing your filled-in answer with the one provided in the far left margin, you will be practicing this

d. as you proceed from frame to frame, you should write the missing word into this

e. you can also refer to the student website for audio samples of these

Talking Shop

In the blank, write the letter of the pronunciation that matches the term. The first one is completed for you as an example. Visit the student website to hear the correct pronunciation of these terms.

Term		Pronunciation	
_f_	1. cardiologist	a.	pee dee ah TRI shun
	2. lymphoma	b.	men IN goh seel
	3. pneumonia	c.	limm FOH mah
	4. fracture	d.	ep ih KAR dee um
	5. meningitis	e.	FRAK sher
	6. meningocele	f.	kar dee ALL oh jist
	7. epicardium	g.	NEFF roh lith EYE ah siss
	8. nephrolithiasis	h.	HEPP ah toh MEG ah lee
	9. psychologist	i.	bak ter ee YOO ree ah
	10. hepatomegaly	j.	noo MOH nee ah
	11. pediatrician	k.	sigh KALL oh jist
	12. bacteriuria	l.	MEN in JYE tis

Constructed and Nonconstructed Terms ▶▶▶▶▶

language

medical terminology

1.7 Medical terminology is a functional language. This _____ has rules of grammar, spelling, and pronunciation, just like any other language. Because medical terminology is the universal language of medicine, its terms must be understood by speakers of many languages in many parts of the world, especially in our age of globalization. For the purpose of learning the language of _____ _____, terms in this specialized language can be separated into two main categories: constructed terms and nonconstructed terms.

constructed terms

word

1.8 Many medical terms are **constructed terms,** which are made up of multiple word parts that are combined to form a new word. In most cases, the word parts are derived from Latin and Greek. The key to learning _____ _____ is to first learn the meaning of the various word parts. It may be helpful to think of constructed terms as if they were written in code. Once you have the key to a code, it becomes a fairly simple process to decode the messages or to use the code to form messages yourself. Similarly, once you learn the meanings of the individual _____ parts, you have the key to the medical terminology code. See Figure 1.1■.

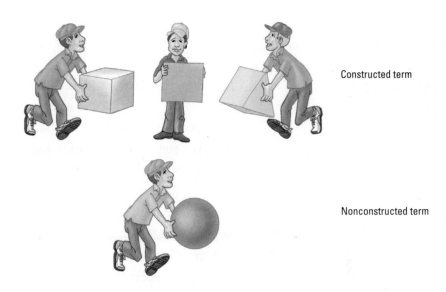

Constructed term

Nonconstructed term

Figure 1.1 ■
Medical terms are either constructed words, which are composed of more than one word part, or words you must memorize, which include terms that are a single Latin or Greek word part, eponyms, acronyms, abbreviations, and so on.

eponym

nonconstructed terms

1.9 The second group of medical terms is **nonconstructed terms,** terms that are not formed from individual word parts. Nonconstructed terms include eponyms, which are terms derived from the names of people. For example, *eustachian tube* is an _____ because it is derived from the name of Bartolommeo Eustachio, who first discovered this tube between the throat and the middle ear. Other forms of nonconstructed terms include acronyms, which are words derived from the first letters of words in a compound term, such as *LASIK* for *laser-assisted in situ keratomileusis;* words derived from languages other than Greek or Latin, such as *jaundice,* which is derived from the French word for yellow, *jaune;* and abbreviations, such as *Ab* for *antibody* and *bx* for *biopsy.* To learn _____ _____, you must commit them to memory.

PRACTICE: Constructed and Nonconstructed Terms

The Right Match

Match the term on the left with the correct definition on the right.

_____	1. nonconstructed terms	a. term derived from a person's name
_____	2. constructed terms	b. must be committed to memory
_____	3. medical terminology	c. made up of word parts
_____	4. eponym	d. the universal language of medicine

The Word Parts ▶▶▶▶▶

word parts	1.10 When a constructed term is formed, individual _____ _____ are assembled to create a term with a new meaning. This is very useful in medicine because new discoveries are made frequently, and the need to provide them with relevant names is important. The three primary types of word parts are prefixes, word roots, and suffixes.
prefix	1.11 A **prefix** is a word part that is affixed to the beginning of a word. Its purpose is to expand or enhance the meaning of the word. Let's look at an example of a prefix in action, using the word *construction*. In our sample word, *con-* is the prefix. It means "with, together, jointly." Notice the hyphen following the prefix. You will know that a word part is a _____ by the hyphen that immediately follows it (for example, *con-*).
word root	1.12 A **word root** is a word part that provides the primary meaning of the term. The _____ _____ provides the basis for the term and is the part to which other word parts are attached. Nearly all terms have a word root, and some have more than one. In our sample word *construction, struct* is the word root. It means "make, build."
suffix	1.13 A **suffix** is a word part that is affixed to the end of a word. The _____ often indicates the word's part of speech (noun, verb, adjective, adverb, etc.) or modifies the word's meaning. In our sample word *construction*, the suffix is *-ion.* It indicates that the word is a noun and it means "process." You will know that a word part is a suffix by the hyphen that immediately precedes it (for example, *-ion*).

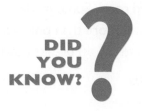

This text has a special color-coding system to help you recognize the individual word parts. Each time a word part is presented, it appears in a specific color:

- Prefixes are **green**
- Word roots and combining forms are **red**
- Suffixes are **blue**

---

three

1.14 To summarize using our example, the word *construction* is composed of _____ word parts (Figure 1.2■):

con- + struct + -ion

(prefix + word root + suffix)

We decipher the meaning of medical words by defining each of the word parts. First, we look at the meaning of the suffix, then we look at the meaning of the prefix. Finally, we define the word root. Then we combine the meanings of all the word parts in the way that makes the most sense. Thus, con- + struct + -ion means "process of building together."

Figure 1.2 ■
Most medical terms are formed by assembling word parts.

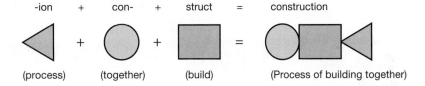

-ion	+	con-	+	struct	=	construction
(process)		(together)		(build)		(Process of building together)

word parts

1.15 The word *construction,* then, as we use it in medical terminology, refers to *building words out of word parts.* This is what we do every time we write and speak. This is also what we do when we use medical terminology by speaking and writing medical terms. Understanding how to build words out of _____ _____ is essential to understanding the meaning of medical terms. Equally important is understanding how to deconstruct or break down a medical term into its component word parts. That is exactly what we did when we deciphered the meaning of our sample word *construction.* We broke the word down into its prefix, word root, and suffix parts and then combined the definitions of the word parts to derive the meaning of the term.

word root

1.16 Not every medical term has all three word parts. Some medical terms lack a prefix, word root, or suffix, and some have more than one word root. For example, the term *gastroenteritis* (GAS troh en ter EYE tis) breaks down like so:

gastroenteritis

gastr + enter + -itis

(word root + word root + suffix)

gastr is a word root that means "stomach"

enter is a _____ _____ that means "small intestine" *-itis* is a suffix that means "inflammation"

Thus, the term *gastroenteritis* means "inflammation of the stomach and small intestine." Notice the letter *o* between the two word roots. You will learn about the importance of its use very soon (Frame 1.18).

suffix

1.17 Some medical terms are made simply of a prefix and a suffix. The term *aphasia* is an example.

aphasia

a- + -phasia

(prefix + suffix)

a- is a prefix that means "without or absence of"

-phasia is a _____ that means "speaking"

Thus, the term *aphasia* means "absence of speaking."

combining vowel

1.18 A fourth word part is the **combining vowel.** It is used when a word root requires a connecting vowel in order to add a suffix that begins with a consonant, or to add another word root, when forming a term. The _____ _____ does not add to or alter the meaning of the word root; it simply assists us in pronouncing a term. In most cases, the combining vowel is the letter *o,* and in some cases it is the letter *i* or *e.*

combining form

1.19 Generally, it is best to learn a word root with its combining vowel. This word root plus combining vowel form is called a **combining form.** Whenever possible, the combining forms are presented in this text to ease your building and deconstructing of medical terms, some of which are shown in Figure 1.3■. The method for writing a _____ _____ involves the use of a slash between the word root and the combining vowel, such as

cardi/o
(word root/combining vowel)

The combining vowel in _cardi/o_ is _o_.

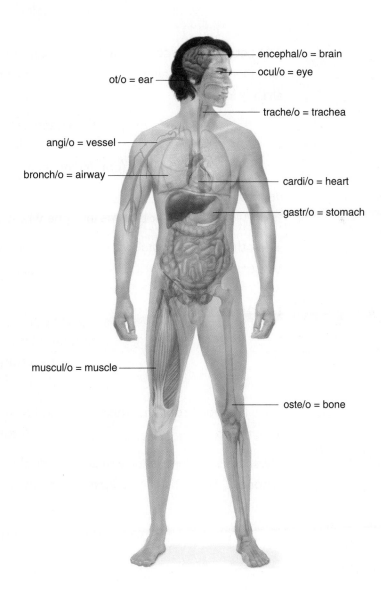

encephal/o = brain
ocul/o = eye
ot/o = ear
trache/o = trachea
angi/o = vessel
bronch/o = airway
cardi/o = heart
gastr/o = stomach
muscul/o = muscle
oste/o = bone

Figure 1.3 ■
The human body, with many of the common combining forms.

o

1.20 You learned from Frame 1.18 that the most common combining vowel is the letter _____. As practice, let's take a look at a medical term with which you may already be familiar:

cardiology

This term is made up of three word parts: a word root, a combining vowel, and a suffix. The combining form is *cardi/o* and the suffix is *-logy*. *Cardi/o* means "heart" and *-logy* means "study or science of." Thus, when we define the word parts of the term *cardiology* and then combine their definitions in a logical way, we know it means "the study or science of the heart." It may help to write the constructed form of the term, which is written with slashes separating each word part:

cardi/o/logy

1.21 Let's practice deconstructing medical terms and using word parts to decipher their meaning. Here are some more medical terms that you may already know.

dermatologist
dermat/o + -logist
(combining form + suffix)

combining form

dermat/o is a _____ _____ that means "skin" *-logist* is a suffix that means "one who studies"

Thus, the term *dermatologist* means "one who studies the skin." The constructed form is written dermat/o/logist.

1.22 Another example is:

tonsillectomy
tonsill + -ectomy
(word root + suffix)

tonsill is a word root that means "almond or tonsil"
-ectomy is a _____ that means "surgical excision, removal"

suffix

Thus, the term *tonsillectomy* means "surgical removal of tonsil (shaped like an almond)." The constructed form is written tonsill/ectomy.

1.23 Another example is:

microscopic

micro- + scop + -ic

(prefix + word root + suffix)

micro- is a prefix that means "small"

scop is a word root that means "viewing instrument"

-ic is a suffix that means "pertaining to"

Thus, the term *microscopic* means "pertaining to the viewing instrument for investigating small things," or "visible only by means of a microscope." The constructed form is written _____/_____/_____.

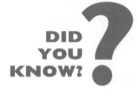

micro/scop/ic

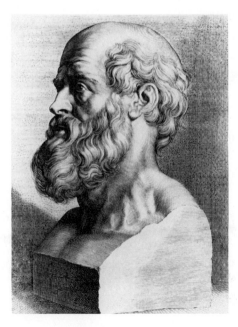

DID YOU KNOW?

▶▶▶▶▶ **The Origins of Medical Terms**

Just as Greek and Latin have played a critical role in the formation and meaning of words in many languages such as English, French, Italian, Spanish, Portuguese, and others, these two ancient languages have contributed to the development of the language of medicine and many related disciplines. The ancient Greeks are considered the fathers of modern medicine (Figure 1.4■). These early scholars explored and observed the human body and its functions, and they wrote about their discoveries using everyday words from their native language. The Romans advanced medicine with their own experiments and observations. They added Latin terms to the growing body of medical language.

Figure 1.4 ■
The Greek father of medicine, Hippocrates, who originated many medical terms.
Source: Courtesy of the National Library of Medicine.

continued

For example, the fallopian tube that connects the ovary with the uterus is known as a *salpinx* (plural, *salpinges*). This is an ancient Greek word meaning "trumpet." The organ in the female body was named for its trumpetlike shape. From this descriptive Greek word, we can build many medical terms such as *salpingitis* ("inflammation of the uterine tube"), *salpingoplasty* ("surgical repair of the uterine tube"), *salpingo-oophorectomy* ("surgical removal of the ovary and uterine tube"), and many others. See Table 1.1■ for examples of combining forms that are from Greek and Latin.

Sometimes the origins of medical terms relate to history, poetry, mythology, geography, physical objects, and ideas. For example, the medical term *psychology* has its origins in the meaning of the Greek word *psyche* ("mind, soul"). Further investigation leads to the Greek myth of a princess named Psyche who falls in love with the god of love, Eros. Knowing the myth of Psyche and Eros may help some students remember the meaning of the term *psyche* when they encounter it.

We will briefly explore the origins of medical terms in other "Did You Know?" features throughout the text. Look for these boxes to expand your understanding of medical terminology and provide a useful way to remember meanings.

Table 1.1 ■ Word Roots from Greek and Latin

Root	Origin	Definition	Medical Term Example
lith	*lithos*, Greek	stone	*cholelithiasis* condition of having gallstones
maxim	*maximus*, Latin	biggest, highest	*gluteus maximus* the biggest (outermost) gluteus muscle in the buttocks
derm	*derma*, Greek	skin	*dermatitis* inflammation of the skin
path	*pathos*, Greek	disease	*pathogen* disease-causing agent

PRACTICE: The Word Parts

The Right Match

Match the term on the left with the correct definition on the right.

_____ 1. prefix

_____ 2. word root

_____ 3. -*ectomy*

_____ 4. *o*

_____ 5. *cardi/o*

_____ 6. constructed term

a. the most common combining vowel

b. a combining form

c. a word part that is affixed to the beginning of a word

d. a term built from word parts

e. a word part that provides the primary meaning of the term

f. a suffix

Forming Words from Word Parts ▶▶▶▶▶

word parts	**1.24** You have learned that constructed medical terms are created from building blocks called word parts and include word roots, prefixes, suffixes, and combining forms. You will now learn how to form medical terms by using these _____ _____.
combining vowel	**1.25** One rule to remember when forming words from word parts is the proper use of the combining vowel. The combining vowel is not always used at the end of a word root to create a combining form. As a general rule, the _____ _____ is used to connect a word root with a suffix that begins with a consonant.
cardi/o/logy	**1.26** For example, let's use the word root for heart, *cardi*. As you know, *cardiology* means "study or science of the heart." The constructed form of this term is written _____/_____/_____. Notice that it contains the combining vowel *o* and the suffix begins with a consonant (*l*). Another term that includes the word root for heart is *carditis*, which means "inflammation of the heart." The constructed form of this term is written *card/itis*. Notice that the suffix begins with a vowel (*i*), and there is no combining vowel. If you wanted to change the suffix to -*plasty*, which means "surgical repair," to form the term that means "surgical repair of the heart," how would you write the new term? Because the suffix -*plasty* begins with a consonant (*p*), you would include the combining vowel (*o*) to form a new term, which is _____. The constructed form of this term is written *cardi/o/plasty*.
cardioplasty	
combining vowel **consonant**	**1.27** There are exceptions to this rule, so it is not absolute. You will learn these exceptions as you learn the material in this book. For now, just keep in mind that you need to include the _____ _____ when the suffix begins with a _____.
word roots *muscul/o/skelet/al*	**1.28** A second rule to remember when forming new constructed terms involves combining two word roots. Constructed medical terms use combining vowels to unite two _____ _____. For example, when describing an injury that involves both the muscular and skeletal systems, the two word roots (*muscul* and *skelet*) are united by placing the combining vowel between them. To make the term complete, the suffix -*al* is added to form the term *musculoskeletal*. Literally, the term means "pertaining to muscles and the skeleton," and its constructed form is written _____/_____/_____/_____.

cardiopulmonary

1.29 Another example of this use of combining vowels occurs when forming the term describing a condition of the heart and lungs. As you know, the word root for heart is *cardi*. The word root for lung is *pulmon*. The suffix *-ary* ("pertaining to") is added to form the term *pulmonary*. A combining vowel is added to unite the two word roots, creating the new term _____, which can be written as cardi/o/pulmon/ary.

epi/derm/is

1.30 A third rule to remember when forming constructed words from word parts occurs when prefixes are added to other word parts. Generally, a prefix requires no change when another word part unites with it to form a new term. For example, *epi-* is a prefix that means "upon, over, above, or on top." When it is combined with the word *dermis*, which means "skin," it forms the new term *epidermis* that means "on top of the skin." The constructed form of this new term is written _____/_____/_____. Notice that the prefix *epi-* did not change.

1.31 Finally, because most medical terms are composed of Latin or Greek word parts, changing a singular medical term into a plural form is handled differently than in most English-language words where an *s* is simply added to the end. Here are some helpful points:

vertebrae

- If the term ends in *a,* the plural is usually formed by adding an *e*. For example, the plural form of the term *vertebra* is _____.

diagnoses

- If the term ends in *is,* the plural form is usually formed by changing the *is* to *es*. For example, the plural form of *diagnosis* is _____.

- If the term ends in *itis,* the plural form is *itides*. For example, the plural form of *gastritis* is *gastritides*.

myocardia

- If the term ends in *on* or *um,* the plural form drops the *on* or *um* and adds *a*. For example, the plural form of *ganglion* is *ganglia* and *myocardium* is _____.

fibromata

- If the term ends in *ma,* the plural form is changed to *mata*. For example, the plural form of *fibroma* is _____.

episiotomies

- If the term ends in *y,* the plural form drops the *y* and adds the ending *ies*. For example, the plural form of *episiotomy* is _____.

fungi

- If the term ends in *us,* the plural form drops the *us* and adds the ending *i*. For example, the plural form of *fungus* is _____.

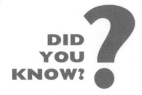

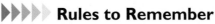

Rules to Remember

- A prefix comes before the word root or combining form.
- A suffix is a word ending and comes after the word root(s) or combining form(s).
- The word root or combining form provides the primary meaning of the term.
- The combining vowel for most word roots is *o*. The vowels *i* and *e* are also used as combining vowels for some word roots. If the combining form is to be joined with another word root or combining form that begins with a consonant, retain the combining vowel. When adding a suffix starting with a vowel to a combining form, drop the combining vowel.
- Prefixes do not require combining vowels to join with other word parts. Rarely, a prefix will drop its ending vowel to combine with another word part.
- Medical terms are deciphered by breaking them into word parts, then defining first the suffix, then the prefix, then the word root(s) or combining forms.

The following list of word parts includes prefixes, word roots/combining vowels (combining forms), and suffixes. These are provided for you to practice constructing and deconstructing medical terms in the exercises that follow. You will be asked to learn these terms and their definitions later in this text. For now, concentrate on practicing the principles of constructed medical terms that you learned in the previous frames.

Prefix	Definition
anti-	against, opposite of
brady-	slow
endo-	within
epi-	upon, over, above, on top
neo-	new
pre-	to come before

Word Root/ Combining Vowel	Definition
append/o, appendic/o	appendix
bi/o	life
cardi/o	heart
cerebr/o	brain, cerebrum
dermat/o	skin
electr/o	electricity
encephal/o	brain
gastr/o	stomach
hem/o	blood
hepat/o	liver
hyster/o	uterus
laryng/o	voice box, larynx
leuk/o	white
mamm/o	breast
mast/o	breast
ment/o	mind
nat/o	birth
neur/o	nerve
path/o	disease
proct/o	rectum or anus
psych/o	mind
rhin/o	nose
tonsill/o	almond, tonsil
vas/o	vessel

Suffix	Definition
-al	pertaining to
-ectomy	surgical excision, removal
-emia	condition of blood
-gram	a record or image
-ia	condition of
-iatry	treatment, specialty
-ic	pertaining to
-itis	inflammation
-logist	one who studies
-logy	study or science of
-pathy	disease
-philia	loving, affinity for
-plasty	surgical repair
-scope	instrument used for viewing
-tic	pertaining to

PRACTICE: Forming Words from Word Parts

The Right Match

Match the term on the left with the correct definition on the right.

_____ 1. combining vowel

_____ 2. -al

_____ 3. prefix

_____ 4. consonant

a. adding this word part to a word root requires no combining vowel

b. a suffix

c. if a suffix begins with this type of letter, use a combining vowel

d. used to connect a word root with another word root or a suffix

Break the Chain

Analyze these medical terms:

a) Separate each term into its word parts and label each word part using **p** = prefix, **r** = root, **cv** = combining vowel, and **s** = suffix.

b) For the Bonus Question, write the requested word part or definition in the blank that follows.

The first set has been completed for you as an example.

1. a) cardiology   _cardi/o/logy_
                             r   cv   s

    b) *Bonus Question:* What is the definition of the suffix?   _study or science of_ _____

2. a) appendicitis   _____/_____
                                        /

    b) *Bonus Question:* What is the definition of the suffix? _____

3. a) hepatitis   _____/_____
                                     /

    b) *Bonus Question:* What is the definition of the word root? _____

4. a) neonatology   _____/_____/_____/_____
                                       /   /   /

    b) *Bonus Question:* Does this term contain a word root? _____

5. a) mammoplasty   _____/_____/_____
                                       /   /

    b) *Bonus Question:* What is the definition of the suffix? _____

6. a) electrocardiogram   _____/_____/_____/_____/_____
                                             /   /   /   /

    b) *Bonus Question:* How many word roots/combining forms does this term have? _____

7. a) prenatal   _____/_____/_____
                                    /   /

    b) *Bonus Question:* What is the definition of the prefix? _____

Fill It In

Complete the following sentences with the correct plural endings. The first one is completed for you as an example.

1. The plural form of appendicitis is appendic_itides_.
2. In one day, the surgeon performed several mammoplast_____.
3. The pericardium of the heart includes two layers, the parietal and visceral pericardi_____.
4. The patient was diagnosed with multiple sarcoma tumors, or sarco_____.
5. The diseased heart was found to have many cardiopath_____.

Linkup

Link the word parts in the list to create the terms that match the definitions. You may use word parts more than once. Remember to add combining vowels when needed—and that some terms do not use any combining vowel. The first one is completed for you as an example.

Prefixes	Word Roots/ Combining Vowel	Suffixes
endo-	encephal/o	-ectomy
neo-	hyster/o	-gram
	mamm/o	-itis
	mast/o	-logist
	nat/o	-logy
	neur/o	-pathy
	path/o	-plasty
	rhin/o	-scope

	Definition	Term
1.	inflammation of the brain	_encephalitis_
2.	study or science of newborns	_____
3.	disease of the nerves	_____
4.	surgical removal of a breast	_____
5.	surgical repair of the nose	_____
6.	instrument for viewing within	_____
7.	X-ray image of a breast	_____
8.	one who studies disease	_____
9.	surgical removal of the uterus	_____

▶▶▶▶ Chapter Review

Word Building _____

Construct medical terms from the following meanings. (All are built from word parts. Refer to the word parts table on page 15 for word part meanings). The first question has been completed for you as an example.

1. disease within the nose   endorhino_pathy_____

2. surgical removal of the tonsils   tonsill_____

3. surgical repair of the fallopian tube   salpingo_____

4. inflammation of the skin   _____itis

5. study or science of the nose   _____logy

6. pertaining to the mind   _____al

7. disease of the nerves   _____pathy

8. inherited defect in blood coagulation   _____philia

9. inflammation of the larynx   laryng_____

10. study or science of the skin   dermato_____

11. instrument used for viewing the larynx   _____scope

12. study or science of life   _____logy

13. inflammation of within the heart   endo_____itis

14. condition of slow heart (beat)   _____cardia

15. pertaining to against life   anti_____

16. surgical repair of the skin   _____plasty

17. study or science of nerves   neuro_____

18. pertaining to the cerebrum   cerebr_____

19. surgical removal of the stomach   _____ectomy

20. inflammation of the brain   encephal_____

21. instrument used for viewing the uterus   hystero_____

22. surgical repair of the breast   mammo_____

23. surgical removal of the appendix   append_____

24. pertaining to the liver   _____ic

2

Understanding Suffixes

After completing this chapter, you will be able to:

1 Define and spell the suffixes often used in medical terminology.

2 Identify suffixes in medical terms.

3 Use suffixes to build medical terms that pertain to medical specialties, symptoms, and diseases.

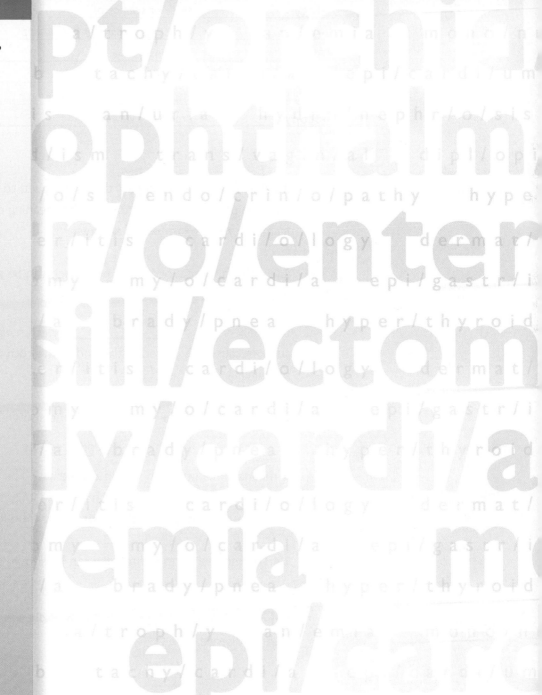

Getting Started With Suffixes ▶▶▶▶▶

Review the following list of common suffixes and their definitions. This will help you to recognize suffixes and their meanings.

Suffixes	Definition
-al	pertaining to
-ic	pertaining to
-itis	inflammation
-logy	study or science of
-meter	measure, measuring instrument
-ous	pertaining to
-pathy	disease
-scope	instrument used for viewing
-scopy	process of viewing

	2.1 A **suffix** is the word part that is attached to the end of the word root. Like the prefix, the suffix modifies the meaning of a term. The following frames contain examples of suffixes.
-al	**2.2** In the familiar word *abnormal,* which can be shown as: *ab/norm/al* the suffix is _____, which means "pertaining to." It is the suffix because it is placed at the end of the root and it modifies the word meaning.
-itis	**2.3** The medical term *endocarditis* can be shown as *endo/card/itis* It means "inflammation within the heart." The suffix is _____, which means "inflammation." It is a suffix because it is placed at the end of the root and it modifies the word meaning.
-pathy	**2.4** The medical term *arthropathy* can be shown as: *arthr/o/pathy* It means "disease of the joint." The suffix is _____, which means "disease."

-itis

2.5 The medical term *gastritis* can be shown as:

gastr/itis

It means "inflammation of the stomach." The suffix is
_____, and the word root *gastr* means "stomach."

Suffix Introduction

Complete the following frames to expand the suffixes you know.

pertaining to
pertaining to
pertaining to

2.6 The suffixes *-ic, -ous,* and *-al* all share the same meaning, which is "pertaining to." This can be seen in the terms:

hypodermic, which means "_____ _____ below the skin";

fibrous, which means "_____ _____ fiber"; and

intradermal, which means "_____ _____ within the skin."

inflammation

2.7 Because the suffix *-itis* means "inflammation," the term *esophagitis* means "_____ of the esophagus."

study or science of

2.8 Because the suffix *-logy* means the "study or science of," the term *cardiology* means "the _____ _____ _____ _____ the heart."

measures

2.9 Because the suffix *-meter* means "measure or measuring instrument," a thermometer is an instrument that _____ temperature.

disease

2.10 Because the suffix *-pathy* means "disease," the term *cardiopathy* means any "_____ of the heart."

viewing

2.11 The suffix *-scope* indicates the instrument that is used for viewing. A laparoscope is an instrument used for _____ the abdomen.

process

2.12 Because the suffix *-scopy* means "process of viewing," the term *laparoscopy* indicates a _____ in which an instrument (in this case, a laparoscope) is used to view the abdomen. (See Figure 2.1 ■.)

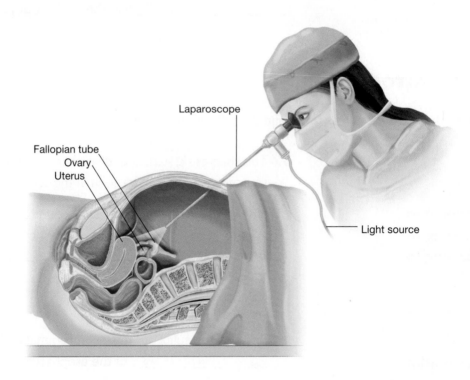

Figure 2.1 ■
A lighted endoscope specialized for insertion into the abdomen, called a laparoscope, is used to view reproductive organs. The laparoscope may also be outfitted with surgical devices for excision of structures.

PRACTICE: Suffix Introduction

The Right Match

Match the suffix on the left with the correct definition on the right.

_____	1. -meter	a.	disease
_____	2. -al	b.	pertaining to
_____	3. -scopy	c.	inflammation
_____	4. -itis	d.	pertaining to
_____	5. -logy	e.	process of viewing
_____	6. -ous	f.	study or science of
_____	7. -pathy	g.	measure, measuring instrument
_____	8. -scope	h.	pertaining to
_____	9. -ic	i.	instrument used for viewing

Suffix Linkup

Link the suffixes in the list to create the terms that match the definitions.

Suffix	Definition	Suffix	Definition
-scopy	*process of viewing*	**-logy**	*study or science of*
-meter	*measure, measuring instrument*	**-itis**	*inflammation*

Definition	**Term**

1. study or science of the heart — cardio*logy* _____

2. an instrument that measures temperature — thermo _____

3. a procedure in which an instrument (in this case, a laparoscope) is used to view the abdomen — laparo _____

4. inflammation of the stomach — gastr _____

Suffixes That Indicate an Action or State

Complete the following frames to learn about suffixes that indicate an action or state.

running	**2.13** In the term *syndrome*, the suffix *-drome*, which means "run or running," and the prefix *syn-*, which means "together," combine to literally mean "_____ together." The medical term is formally defined as a group of symptoms that together are characteristic or indicative of a specific disorder, condition, or disease.
-emesis	**2.14** In the term *hematemesis*, the word root *hemat*, which means "blood," is modified by the suffix _____, which means "vomiting." The term *hematemesis* means "vomiting of blood."
softening	**2.15** The suffix *-malacia* means "softening" as in the term *cardiomalacia*, which is the _____ or degeneration of heart tissue, usually from insufficient blood supply or tissue degeneration.
view	**2.16** In the term *biopsy*, the suffix *-opsy* means "view of"; the term is defined as the removal and examination (or _____) of tissue.
oxygen	**2.17** In the term *hypoxia*, the suffix *-oxia* means "condition of oxygen"; the term indicates that the level of _____ in the blood is below normal.

affinity for	**2.18** The suffixes *-phil* and *-philia* mean "loving or affinity for," as in the term *hemophilia*, which literally means "_____ _____ blood" and is a condition of uncontrolled blood loss.
swallowing	**2.19** The suffix *-phagia* means "eating or swallowing." In the term *dysphagia*, the prefix adds to the meaning of the term; together these word parts combine literally to mean "painful or difficult eating or swallowing." The term is defined as a difficulty in _____.
speaking	**2.20** The suffix *-phasia* means "speaking." In the term *aphasia*, the prefix *a-*, which means "without or absence of," adds to the meaning of the term; together these word parts combine to literally mean "without or absence of _____." The term is defined as an absence or impairment of speech.

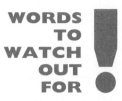

WORDS TO WATCH OUT FOR

▶▶▶▶▶ *-phagia* or *-phasia*?

Don't confuse the suffix *-phagia* with the suffix *-phasia*. Although they are spelled almost the same, their meanings are very different: *-phagia* means "eating or swallowing"; *-phasia* means "speaking."

growth	**2.21** The suffix *-physis* means "growth." In the term *hypophysis*, it combines with the prefix *hypo-*, which means "below," to literally mean "_____ below." The hypophysis is the pituitary gland, which is located below the brain.
paralysis	**2.22** In the term *quadriplegia*, the suffix *-plegia* means "paralysis." When it is combined with the prefix *quadri-*, the whole term means "_____ of four limbs."
tumor	**2.23** In the term *osteoma*, the suffix *-oma* means "tumor"; when combined with the word root *oste*, the combined word parts mean "_____ of bone."
standing still	**2.24** The suffix *-stasis* means "standing still." In the term *homeostasis*, the literal meaning of the word parts, "similar _____ _____," gives an idea of continual balance; the term is defined as the process of maintaining internal stability despite changes in the environment.

PRACTICE: Suffixes That Indicate an Action or State

The Right Match

Match the suffix on the left with the correct definition on the right.

_____ 1. -plegia		a.	tumor
_____ 2. -oma		b.	speaking
_____ 3. -emesis		c.	growth
_____ 4. -phasia		d.	condition of oxygen
_____ 5. -oxia		e.	paralysis
_____ 6. -physis		f.	softening
_____ 7. -malacia		g.	loving, affinity for
_____ 8. -philia		h.	vomiting

Suffix Linkup

Link the suffixes in the list to create the terms that match the definitions.

Suffix	Definition		Suffix	Definition
-drome	_run, running_		**-philia**	_loving, affinity for_
-opsy	_view of_		**-stasis**	_standing still_
-phagia	_eating or swallowing_			

Definition	**Term**
1. a group of symptoms that together are characteristic or indicative of a specific disorder, condition, or disease	syn_____
2. the removal and examination (or view) of tissue	bi_____
3. a condition of uncontrolled blood loss	hemo_____
4. a difficulty in swallowing	dys_____
5. the tendency of an organism or system to maintain internal stability	homeo_____

Suffixes That Indicate a Condition or Disease

Complete the following frames to learn about suffixes that indicate a condition or disease.

pain	**2.25** In the term _arthralgia,_ the suffix _-algia,_ which means "condition of pain," combines with the root _arthr_ to mean "_____ in a joint."
weakness	**2.26** The suffix _-asthenia,_ which means "weakness," makes the term _myasthenia_ mean the "_____ of muscle."

absence	**2.27** The suffix *-atresia* means "a closure or the absence of a normal body opening," so the term *hysteratresia* is the _____ of the uterine cavity.
hernia	**2.28** Because the suffix *-cele* means "hernia, swelling, or protrusion," a meningocele is a _____ of the meninges of the brain or spinal column that protrudes through an abnormal opening in the skull or spinal column. (See Figure 2.2■.)

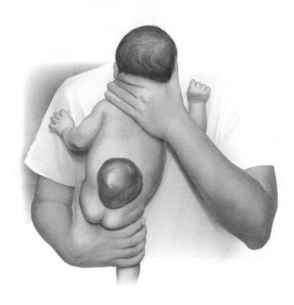

Figure 2.2 ■
Illustration of a child born with spina bifida, with a large meningocele.

pain	**2.29** Because the suffix *-dynia* means "pain," the term *tenodynia* means "_____ in a tendon."
condition	**2.30** The suffix *-ia* means "condition of," so the term *anorexia* means "a nervous _____ in which a person has no appetite."
condition	**2.31** The suffix *-osis* also means "condition of." In the term *adenosis,* the word root for gland is included to form the meaning "_____ of a gland."
condition	**2.32** Another suffix with the meaning "condition or disease" is *-ism.* Thus, the term *embolism* means "a _____ in which a blood vessel is blocked by an embolus, or clot."
inflammation	**2.33** The suffix *-itis* means "inflammation." Adding this ending to the word root that means "stomach" forms the term *gastritis,* which means "_____ of the stomach."

tumor	**2.34** The suffix *-oma* means "tumor." Adding this suffix to the word root for fat, *lip*, forms the term *lipoma,* which means "_____ of fat tissue."
disease	**2.35** The suffix *-pathy* is very common and means "disease," as in the terms *neuropathy, gastropathy,* and *adenopathy.* In the latter, it makes the term mean "_____ of a gland."
abnormal reduction	**2.36** Because *-penia* means "deficiency or abnormal reduction in number," the term *calcipenia* means "an _____ _____ of calcium" in the tissues and fluids of the body.
fear	**2.37** The suffix *-phobia* is well known and means "fear"; hence, *hydrophobia* means "_____ of water."
growth	**2.38** Because *-plasia* means "formation, growth," *neoplasia* means "new formation or _____," referring to a tumor.
discharge	**2.39** Because *-rrhagia* means "abnormal discharge," the term *rhinorrhagia* means "abnormal _____ of the nose."
discharge	**2.40** The suffix *-rrhea* means "discharge," so the term *seborrhea* is a _____ from the sebaceous glands.
rupture	**2.41** Because *-rrhexis* means "rupture," an *amniorrhexis* is a _____ of the membrane enclosing a fetus known as the amnion.
hard	**2.42** The suffix *-sclerosis* means "condition of hard." In the term *arteriosclerosis,* the artery walls are becoming _____ and lose their elasticity.
sudden involuntary	**2.43** The word *spasm* and the suffix *-spasm* both indicate a sudden, involuntary muscle contraction. Thus, the term *bronchospasm* indicates a _____ _____ contraction of the muscular lining of the bronchi.

PRACTICE: Suffixes That Indicate a Condition or Disease

Suffix Linkup

Link the suffixes in the list to create the terms that match the definitions.

Suffix	Definition
-asthenia	weakness
-cele	hernia, swelling, protrusion
-dynia	condition of pain
-ia	condition of
-itis	inflammation
-oma	tumor

Suffix	Definition
-penia	abnormal reduction in number, deficiency
-plasia	formation, growth
-rrhagia	abnormal discharge
-rrhea	discharge
-rrhexis	rupture

Definition	Term
1. a nosebleed	rhino_____
2. pain in a tendon	teno_____
3. rupture of the amnion	amnio_____
4. a tumor of fat tissue	lip_____
5. an abnormal reduction of calcium in the tissues and fluids of the body	calci_____
6. a nervous condition in which a person has no appetite	anorex_____
7. growth or formation of a tumor	neo_____
8. debility and weakness of muscle	my_____
9. a discharge from the sebaceous glands	sebo_____
10. hernia or swelling of the meninges of the brain or spinal column that protrudes through a hole in the skull or spinal column	meningo_____
11. inflammation of the stomach	gastr_____

The Right Match

Match the suffix on the left with the correct definition on the right.

_____	1. -spasm	a.	rupture
_____	2. -algia	b.	disease
_____	3. -rrhexis	c.	sudden, involuntary muscle contraction
_____	4. -ism	d.	formation, or growth
_____	5. -oma	e.	condition of pain
_____	6. -sclerosis	f.	fear
_____	7. -pathy	g.	condition of hard
_____	8. -dynia	h.	condition or disease
_____	9. -plasia	i.	abnormal discharge
_____	10. -rrhagia	j.	tumor
_____	11. -phobia	k.	condition of pain

Suffixes That Indicate Location, Number, or a Quality

Complete the following frames to learn about suffixes that indicate location, number, or a quality.

toward	**2.44** Because the suffix -*ad* means "toward," the term *cephalad* means "_____ the head."
blood	**2.45** The suffixes -*emia* and -*hemia* mean "condition of blood." The prefix *poly-* means "excessive, over, many," and the root *cyt* means "cell." These word parts combine in the term *polycythemia*, which is a condition in which there is an overproduction of red _____ cells.
fistulae	**2.46** The suffix -*a* indicates that the term is singular; the suffix -*ae* indicates the plural form, as in the singular form *fistula* versus its plural form _____.

2.47 There are numerous suffixes that mean "pertaining to." They are

- *-ac*
- *-al*
- *-ar*
- *-ary*
- *-ic*
- *-ous*

Here are some examples of terms using these suffixes:

- *cardiac,* which means "pertaining to the heart"
- *cervical,* which means "pertaining to the cervix"
- *ocular,* which means "pertaining to the eyes"
- *pulmonary,* which means "_____ _____ the lungs"
- *cephalic,* which means "pertaining to the head"
- *nervous,* which means "pertaining to the nerves"

pertaining to

PRACTICE: Suffixes That Indicate Location, Number, or a Quality

The Right Match

Match the suffix on the left with the correct definition on the right.

_____ 1. -ad	a.	singular
_____ 2. -emia	b.	plural
_____ 3. -a	c.	pertaining to
_____ 4. -ac	d.	toward
_____ 5. -ae	e.	condition of blood

Suffix Linkup

Link the suffixes in the list to create the terms that match the definitions. You may use them more than once.

Suffix	Definition
-a	singular
-ac	pertaining to
-ad	toward
-al	pertaining to
-ar	pertaining to
-ary	pertaining to
-hemia	condition of blood
-ic	pertaining to
-ous	pertaining to

Definition

1. pertaining to the heart
2. pertaining to the cervix
3. pertaining to the eyes
4. pertaining to the lungs
5. pertaining to bacteria
6. pertaining to the head
7. pertaining to the nerves
8. toward the head
9. a condition in which there is an overproduction of red blood cells

Term

cardi_____

cervic_____

ocul_____

pulmon_____

bacteri_____

cephal_____

nerv_____

cephal_____

polycyt_____

Suffixes That Indicate a Medical Specialty

Complete the following frames to learn about suffixes that indicate a medical specialty.

treatment	**2.48** Because the suffix *-iatry* means "treatment, or specialty," the term *podiatry* refers to the field of health care involving the diagnosis and _____ of diseases of the feet.
studies	**2.49** The suffix *-logist* means "one who studies," so the term *audiologist* describes a specialist who _____ about and practices in evaluating and rehabilitating communication disorders that are caused by hearing disorders.

study	**2.50** Similarly, the suffix *-logy* means "study or science of "; hence the term *pathology* is the _____ of diseases and the structural and functional changes they cause.
practice	**2.51** The suffix *-practic* comes from the Greek word *praktikos,* which means "a practice." The suffix means "practice"; hence the term *chiropractic* is the healthcare _____ involving the diagnosis and treatment of musculoskeletal disorders by manipulation of the spinal column and other body structures.

PRACTICE: Suffixes That Indicate a Medical Specialty

The Right Match

Match the suffix on the left with the correct definition on the right.

_____ 1. -iatry   a. practice

_____ 2. -logist   b. study or science of

_____ 3. -logy   c. treatment, specialty

_____ 4. -practic   d. one who studies

Suffix Linkup

Link the suffixes in the list to create the terms that match the definitions.

Suffix	Definition
-iatry	*treatment, specialty*
-logist	*one who studies*
-logy	*study or science of*
-practic	*practice*

Definition   **Term**

1.   a specialist who studies and practices evaluating and rehabilitating   audio_____
     communication disorders that are caused by hearing disorders

2.   the study of diseases and the structural and functional changes   patho_____
     caused by them

3.   the healthcare profession involving the practice (diagnosis and treatment)   chiro_____
     of musculoskeletal disorders by manipulation of the spinal
     column and other body structures

4.   the healthcare field involving the diagnosis and treatment of diseases of the feet   pod_____

Suffixes That Indicate a Procedure or Treatment

Complete the following frames to learn about suffixes that indicate a procedure or treatment.

puncture	**2.52** The suffix *-centesis* means "surgical puncture"; so the term *thoracocentesis* describes a medical procedure in which a surgical _____ is made into the chest cavity to remove fluid.
broken apart	**2.53** The suffixes *-clasia*, *-clasis*, and *-clast* all mean to "break apart." So the term *osteoclasis* describes a surgical procedure in which a bone is artificially fractured (or _____ _____) to correct deformity.
fusion	**2.54** An arthrodesis is a procedure that involves the surgical fixation or fusion of two or more joints using either bone grafts or metal rods. The suffix *-desis* means "surgical fixation or _____."
excision	**2.55** The suffix *-ectomy* means "surgical _____," or "removal." For example, a chondrectomy is the excision of cartilage, and a thyroidectomy is the excision of the thyroid gland in the neck. (See Figure 2.3■.)

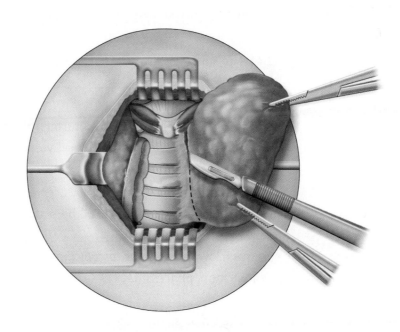

Figure 2.3 ■
Thyroidectomy. A portion of the thyroid gland is undergoing removal in a thyroidectomy procedure.

recording	**2.56** The suffixes *-gram*, *-graph*, and *-graphy* are closely related: *-gram* means "a record or image," *-graph* means "an instrument for recording," and *-graphy* is a "recording process." When the combining form *angi/o* is added to these suffixes, the resulting terms are: ■ *angiogram,* a record or X-ray image of arteries ■ *angiograph,* an instrument for _____ arteries using radioactive dye injected into the artery ■ *angiography,* the process of recording an angiogram
measuring	**2.57** Because the suffix *-meter* means "measure, measuring instrument," a thermometer is an instrument used for _____ temperature.
measurement	**2.58** Similarly, the suffix *-metry* means "measurement, process of measuring." Hence, urinometry is the _____ or process of measuring the specific gravity of urine.
fixation	**2.59** The suffix *-pexy* means "surgical fixation, suspension." The term *mastopexy* means "a surgical _____ or lifting of the breasts."
protective	**2.60** The suffix *-phylaxis* means "protection" as in the term *prophylaxis,* which means "_____ treatment to prevent disease."
surgical repair	**2.61** The suffix *-plasty* means "surgical repair," so the term *gastroplasty* means "a _____ _____ of the stomach."
suturing	**2.62** Because *-rrhaphy* means "suturing," the term *angiorrhaphy* means "the _____ of a blood vessel."
instrument **viewing**	**2.63** The suffixes *-scope* and *-scopy* are very similar: *-scope* means "a viewing instrument," and *-scopy* means "the process of viewing." So the term *gastroscope* means "an _____ for examining and treating the stomach," whereas a *gastroscopy* indicates the _____, or examination, process itself.
surgical	**2.64** The suffix *-stomy* means "surgical creation of an opening," so the term *gastrostomy* means "the _____ creation of an opening into the stomach."

cutting instrument	**2.65** The suffixes *-tome* and *-tomy* are closely related. The suffix *-tome* is a cutting instrument, and *-tomy* is an incision. So the craniotome is the _____ _____ used during a craniotomy.
crush	**2.66** The suffix *-tripsy* means "surgical crushing," as in the term *lithotripsy*, which means "to _____ unwanted stones" that may form in the kidneys or gallbladder.
process	**2.67** The suffix *-ion* means "process," as in the term *ovulation*, which is the _____ of ovulating.

PRACTICE: Suffixes That Indicate a Procedure or Treatment

The Right Match

Match the suffix on the left with the correct definition on the right.

_____ 1. -centesis
_____ 2. -graphy
_____ 3. -clast
_____ 4. -tomy
_____ 5. -metry
_____ 6. -desis
_____ 7. -stomy
_____ 8. -scopy
_____ 9. -pexy
_____ 10. -rrhaphy
_____ 11. -ectomy
_____ 12. -plasty

a. measurement, process of measuring
b. surgical creation of an opening
c. fusion
d. process of viewing
e. suturing
f. recording process
g. break apart
h. incision
i. surgical puncture
j. excision or surgical removal
k. surgical repair
l. surgical fixation, suspension

Suffix Linkup

Link the suffixes in the list to create the terms that match the definitions. You may use them more than once.

Suffix	Definition
-centesis	surgical puncture
-clasis	break apart
-desis	surgical fixation, fusion
-gram	a record or image
-graphy	recording process
-ion	process
-meter	measure, measuring instrument
-pexy	surgical fixation, suspension
-phylaxis	protection
-plasty	surgical repair
-scope	instrument used for viewing
-tome	cutting instrument
-tomy	incision, to cut
-tripsy	surgical crushing

Definition		**Term**
1.	a medical procedure in which a surgical puncture is made into the chest cavity to remove fluid	thoraco_____
2.	a surgical procedure in which a joint is artificially fractured (or broken apart) to correct deformity	osteo_____
3.	to surgically crush or pulverize kidney stones or gallstones	litho_____
4.	the cutting instrument used during a craniotomy	cranio_____
5.	a procedure that involves the surgical fixation or fusion of two or more joints using either bone grafts or metal rods	arthro_____
6.	the image or recording or X-ray of arteries	angio_____
7.	the process of recording an angiogram	angio_____
8.	an instrument used for measuring temperature	thermo_____
9.	the process of ovulating	ovulat_____
10.	a surgical fixation or lifting of the breasts	masto_____
11.	protective treatment against disease	pro_____
12.	surgical repair of the stomach	gastro_____
13.	an instrument for examining and treating the stomach	gastro_____
14.	a procedure of cutting into the cranium with a craniotome	cranio_____

▶▶▶▶ **Chapter Review**

Word Building

Construct medical terms from the following meanings. The first question has been completed for you as an example.

1. disease of the joint
    arthro*pathy*

2. pertaining to the nerves
    nerv_____

3. group of symptoms that together are characteristic
    or indicative of a specific disorder, condition, or disease
    syn_____

4. surgical procedure in which a bone is artificially fractured
    (or broken apart) to correct deformity
    osteo_____

5. benign tumor made of fat tissue
    lip_____

6. condition of uncontrolled blood loss
    hemo_____

7. specialist who studies about and practices in evaluating
    and rehabilitating communication disorders
    that are caused by hearing disorders
    audio_____

8. study of diseases and the structural and functional
    changes they cause
    patho_____

9. vomiting of blood
    hemat_____

10. painful or difficult eating or swallowing
    dys_____

11. protective treatment against disease
    pro_____

12. surgical puncture into the chest cavity to remove fluid
    thoraco_____

13. healthcare field involving the diagnosis and treatment
    of diseases of the feet
    pod_____

14. softening or degeneration of heart tissue
    cardio_____

15. to surgically crush unwanted stones that may
    form in the kidneys or gallbladder
    litho_____

16. pain in a tendon
    teno_____

17. surgical repair of the stomach
    gastro_____

18. nervous condition in which a person has no appetite
    anorex_____

19. hernia of the meninges of the brain or spinal column
    that protrudes through a hole in the skull
    or spinal column
    meningo_____

20. level of oxygen in the blood is below normal
    hyp_____

21. instrument for examining and treating the stomach
    gastro_____

22. pertaining to the cervix
    cervic_____

23. healthcare practice (diagnosis and treatment) of
    musculoskeletal and nervous system disorders by manipulation
    of the spinal column and other body structures
    chiro_____

24. procedure that involves the surgical fixation or fusion of two or more joints using either bone grafts or metal rods

arthro_____

25. removal and examination (or view) of tissue

bi_____

26. debility and weakness of muscle

my_____

27. instrument that measures temperature

thermo_____

28. inflammation of the esophagus

esophag_____

29. process of using an instrument to view the abdomen

laparo_____

30. without or absence of speaking

a_____

31. literally, "growth below"

hypo_____

32. paralysis of four limbs

quadri_____

33. pain in a joint

arthr_____

34. abnormal reduction of calcium

calci_____

35. new formation or growth

neo_____

36. condition of profuse bleeding of the nose (nosebleed)

rhino_____

37. record or X-ray image of arteries

angio_____

38. process of recording an angiogram

angio_____

39. pertaining to below the skin

hypoderm_____

40. process of maintaining internal stability despite changes in the environment

homeo_____

41. absence of the uterine cavity

hyster_____

42. condition of a gland

aden_____

43. condition in which a blood vessel is blocked by a clot

embol_____

44. discharge from the sebaceous glands

sebo_____

45. condition of hardening of the artery walls

arterio_____

46. sudden, involuntary contraction of the bronchi

broncho_____

47. toward the head

cephal_____

48. plural form of *fistula*

fistul_____

MEDICAL TERMINOLOGY INTERACTIVE

Medical Terminology Interactive is a premium online homework management system that includes a host of features to help you study. Registered users will find:

- Fun games and activities built within a virtual hospital
- Powerful tools that track and analyze your results—allowing you to create a personalized learning experience
- Videos, flashcards, and audio pronunciations to help enrich your progress
- Streaming video lesson presentations and self-paced learning modules

www.pearsonhighered.com/mti

Understanding Prefixes

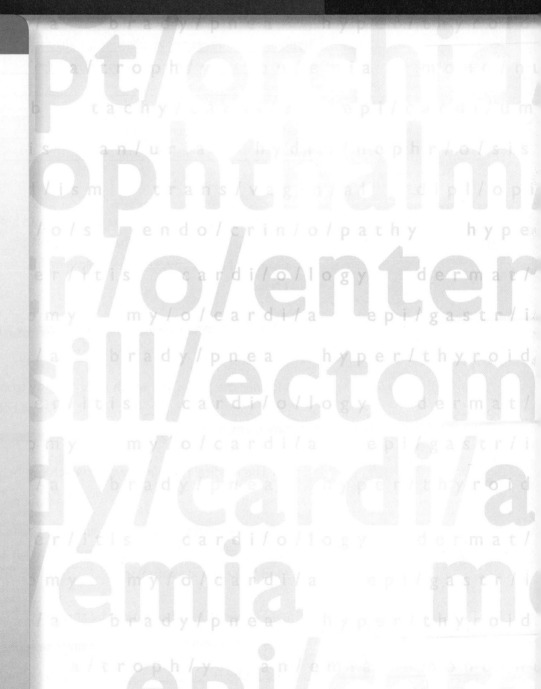

LEARNING OBJECTIVES

After completing this chapter, you will be able to:

1. Define and spell the prefixes commonly used in medical terminology.

2. Identify prefixes in medical terms.

3. Use prefixes to build medical terms.

Getting Started with Prefixes ▶▶▶▶▶

Review the following list of some prefixes and their definitions. This will help you become more familiar with prefixes.

Prefixes	Definition
a-	without, absence of
ab-	away from
bi-	two
endo-	within
hyper-	excessive, abnormally high, above
hypo-	deficient, abnormally low, below
intra-	within
post-	to follow after
pre-	to come before
sub-	under, beneath, below

fix	**3.1** A **prefix** is the word part that is placed before the root to modify its meaning. The word *prefix* literally means "to _____ at the beginning of a word." The following frames contain some examples of prefixes.
prefix	**3.2** The familiar word *abnormal,* which can be shown as: *ab/norm/al* includes the prefix *ab-*, which means "away from." It is the _____ because it is placed before the root to modify the word's meaning.
intra-	**3.3** The medical term *intravenous,* which can be shown as: *intra/ven/ous* means "pertaining to within a vein." The prefix is _____, which means "within." It is the prefix because it is placed before the root to modify the word's meaning.
hyper-	**3.4** The word *hypertension* can be shown as: *hyper/tens/ion* The prefix is _____, which means "excessive, abnormally high, or above."

Prefix Introduction

Complete the following frames to expand the prefixes you know.

convulsions	**3.5** The prefix *anti-* means "against or opposite of" as in the term *anticonvulsive*, which is a type of drug used to stop _____.
a-	**3.6** The one-letter prefix that means "without or absence of" is _____. An example of its use is found in the term *aphasia*, which means "absence of speech."
together	**3.7** The prefix *con-* means "with, together, or jointly." For example, when twins are conjoined the *con-* prefix indicates that the twins are joined _____.
conception	**3.8** *Contra-* means "counter or against" as in the term *contraception*, which literally means "against _____."

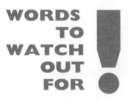
WORDS TO WATCH OUT FOR ▶▶▶▶▶ *contra-* **or** *con-***?**

Don't confuse the prefix *contra-* with the prefix *con-*. Their meanings are very different. *Contra-* means "counter or against"; the prefix *con-* means "with, together, or jointly."

changed	**3.9** *Meta-* means "after or change" as in the term *metabolism*, which is the process by which foods are _____ into energy for use by the body.

PRACTICE: Prefix Introduction

The Right Match

Match the prefix on the left with the correct definition on the right.

_____	1. meta-	a.	against or opposite
_____	2. a-	b.	after or change
_____	3. contra-	c.	without or absence of
_____	4. con-	d.	counter or against
_____	5. anti-	e.	with, together, or jointly

Prefix Linkup

Link the prefixes in the list to create the terms that match the definitions.

Prefix	Definition
a-	without or absence of
con-	with, together, or jointly
contra-	counter or against
meta-	after or change

Definition

1. prevention of conception

2. the process by which foods are changed into energy for use by the body

3. when twins are joined together

4. the absence of speech

Term

_____ *contra*ception

_____ bolism

_____ joined

_____ phasia

Prefixes That Indicate Number or Quantity

Complete the following frames to learn about prefixes that indicate number or quantity.

both	**3.10** The prefix *ambi-* means "both"; the term *ambidextrous* is the ability to use _____ hands equally.
bifocal	**3.11** The prefix *bi-* means "two." For example, _____ means "pertaining to two focal points," as in eyeglasses that correct for both near vision and far vision.
two	**3.12** The term *bicuspid* means "having _____ points."
second	**3.13** Another way to say "two" is "second." Therefore, a woman who has given birth for the _____ time is bipara.
double	**3.14** The prefix *di-* means "double." Therefore, diplegia is _____ plegia, or paralysis of double (two) limbs.
double	**3.15** The prefix *dipl-* also means "double." In the term *diplopia*, the prefix *dipl-* indicates that a person with the condition perceives a single object as two images; it is also called _____ vision.

one	**3.16** Because the prefix *hemi-* means "half," hemiplegia is a paralysis of half the body; in other words, on _____ side of the body.
one	**3.17** The prefix *mono-* means "one." Monoplegia means "paralysis of _____ limb or muscle/muscle group."
many	**3.18** The prefix *multi-* means "many, more than once, or numerous." A multipolar neuron is a nerve cell that includes _____ branches, called dendrites, at one end of the cell.
once	**3.19** When a woman's chart indicates *multipara,* it means that she has given birth multiple times, or more than _____.
never	**3.20** The terms *nullipara* and *nulligravida* share the prefix *nulli-,* which means "none." Nullipara means "the condition of never having given birth or no births"; nulligravida means "_____ having been pregnant or no pregnancies."
all	**3.21** Because the prefix *pan-* means "all," the term *pandemic* refers to a disease occurring over a wide geographic area. Also, pansinusitis is inflammation of _____ paranasal sinuses on one or both sides of the nose.
poly-	**3.22** The term *polyphagia* includes the prefix _____. The prefix means "excessive, over, or many." The term means "excessive eating."
excessive	**3.23** Polydipsia is _____ thirst.
excessive	**3.24** Polyuria is the _____ excretion of urine.
many	**3.25** Polyarteritis is the inflammation of _____ medium and small arteries where they branch.
first	**3.26** The prefix *primi-* means "first." A woman who has given birth for the _____ time is a primipara.
primi-	**3.27** A woman who is pregnant for the first time is a _____ gravida.

four	**3.28** The terms *quadriplegia* and *tetraplegia* both mean "paralysis of four limbs." Therefore, *quadri-* and *tetra-* are both prefixes that mean _____.
partially	**3.29** The prefix *semi-* means "half or partial." The term *semiconscious* means "_____ conscious."
three	**3.30** The prefix *tri-* means "three," as in *tricycle*. The term *tripara* means "a woman who has given birth _____ times."
three	**3.31** The tricuspid valve consists of _____ cusps, which are membranous flaps that control blood flow between the right atrium and the right ventricle of the heart.
one	**3.32** The prefix *uni-* means "one," similar to *mono-*. Therefore, a unipara woman has given birth to _____ child.

PRACTICE: Prefixes That Indicate Number or Quantity

The Right Match

Match the prefix on the left with the correct definition on the right.

_____ 1. di-

_____ 2. ambi-

_____ 3. quad-

_____ 4. hemi-

_____ 5. bi-

_____ 6. primi-

_____ 7. tri-

_____ 8. pan-

_____ 9. semi-

_____ 10. uni-

_____ 11. multi-

_____ 12. poly-

_____ 13. mono-

_____ 14. nulli-

a. excessive, over, or many

b. half

c. first

d. half or partial

e. two

f. double

g. both

h. four

i. one

j. one

k. null or none

l. all

m. many, more than once, or numerous

n. three

Prefix Linkup

Link the prefixes in the list to create the terms that match the definitions. You may use them more than once.

Prefix	Definition
ambi-	both
mono-	one
nulli-	none
poly-	excessive, over, or many
quadri-	four
tetra-	four
tri-	three

Definition   **Term**

1.   paralysis of one limb or muscle/muscle group   _____plegia

2.   never having been pregnant or no pregnancies   _____gravida

3.   the ability to use both hands equally   _____dextrous

4.   excessive eating   _____phagia

5.   the valve that consists of three cusps that control blood flow   _____cuspid
     between the right atrium and the right ventricle

6.   a condition of paralysis of all limbs   _____plegia

Prefixes That Indicate Location or Timing

Complete the following frames to learn about prefixes that indicate location or timing.

away	**3.33** The prefix *ab-* means "away from," so the term *abduction* means "_____ from the midline of the body."
toward	**3.34** The prefix *ad-* means "toward," so the term *adduction* means "_____ the midline of the body."
anatomy	**3.35** The prefix *ana-* means "up, toward"; the word root *tom* means "to cut"; and the suffix *-y* means "process of." So the term _____ means "process of cutting up."
before	**3.36** The terms *prenatal* and *antenatal* share the root *nat*, which means "birth." Both terms mean "before birth," so both prefixes, *pre-* and *ante-*, have the same meaning, which is "_____" or "to come before."

through	**3.37** The term *dialysis* literally means "to loosen through" because the prefix *dia-* means "_____," and the suffix *-lysis* means "to loosen." The term *dialysis* refers to the procedure that removes uric acid and urea from circulating blood.
apart **away**	**3.38** The prefix *dis-* means "apart or away." In the term *dislocation,* the prefix indicates that the dislocated part is _____ or _____ from its normal position in the body.
outside	**3.39** *Ec-* and *ecto-* mean "outside or out." An ectopic pregnancy is one in which the fertilized egg implants somewhere _____ the uterus.
within	**3.40** The prefix *endo-* means "within." Thus, the term *endogastric* means "_____ the stomach." (See Figure 3.1 ■.)

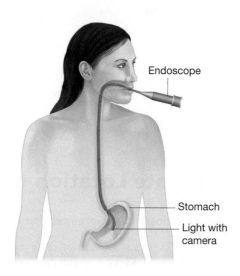

Endoscope

Stomach

Light with camera

Figure 3.1 ■
Endogastric procedure using an endoscope to observe the internal stomach lining.

over	**3.41** The prefixes *ep-* and *epi-* mean "upon, over, above, or on top." The epidermis is the outermost layer of skin because it is _____ the dermis layer.
inward	**3.42** Esotropia is a condition where the eye deviates _____ because the prefix *eso-* means "inward."
away from	**3.43** The prefixes *ex-* and *exo-* mean "outside or away from," so in the condition exotropia, the eye deviates _____ _____ its normal position.

extra-	**3.44** The common prefix shared by the terms *extracellular, extracorporeal,* and *extrauterine* is _____, which means "outside."
below	**3.45** *Infer-* has the meaning "below," as in the term *inferior.* The term *inferior* indicates a position _____ another point of reference.
between	**3.46** Because the prefix *inter-* means "between," the term *intervertebral* indicates a position _____ the vertebrae.
intra-	**3.47** The terms *intracellular* and *intrauterine* share the prefix _____, which also means "within."
within	**3.48** Because *intra-* means "within," the term *intradermal* means "_____ the layers of the skin."
abnormal	**3.49** The prefix *para-* means "alongside or abnormal." In the term *paracusis,* it indicates _____ hearing or a disorder in hearing.
around	**3.50** The prefix *peri-* means "around." In the term *pericardium,* this prefix indicates that the membrane called the pericardium covers the area _____ the heart.
after	**3.51** The prefix *post-* means "to follow after," thus the term *postpartum* means "to follow _____ birth."
after	**3.52** The terms *postnatal* and *postpartum* share the prefix *post-,* which means "to follow after." Both terms mean "to follow _____ birth."

hypo-	**3.53** The prefixes *sub-* and *hypo-* both mean "below." To build a term that means "below the skin," add the prefix _____ to the word root for skin, *dermis*. The resulting term is *hypodermis*. An alternate term for the area below the skin attaches the prefix *sub-* to another word for skin, *cutaneous*. The resulting term is _____. (See Figure 3.2■.)
subcutaneous	

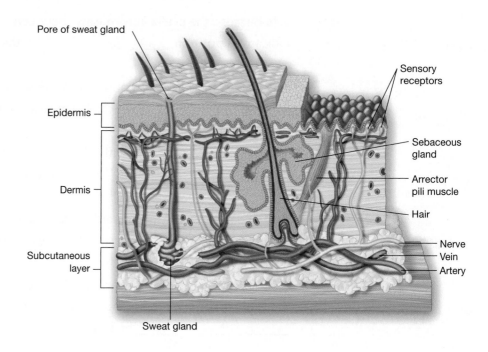

Figure 3.2 ■
Skin layers. The epidermis is on top of the dermis, and the hypodermis (or subcutaneous layer) is below the dermis.

above	**3.54** The prefixes *super-* and *supra-* share the meaning "above"; in the term *superior* it indicates a position _____ another point of reference.
together	**3.55** The prefixes *sym-* and *syn-* also share a meaning. In this case they mean "together or joined." For example, a syndrome is a group of symptoms or signs that occur _____.

PRACTICE: Prefixes That Indicate Location or Timing

The Right Match

Match the prefix on the left with the correct definition on the right.

_____ 1. ab-		a.	to come before
_____ 2. dia-		b.	up or toward
_____ 3. ad-		c.	apart or away
_____ 4. endo-		d.	outside
_____ 5. ante-		e.	away from
_____ 6. extra-		f.	outside or away from
_____ 7. ep-, epi-		g.	toward
_____ 8. ana-		h.	within
_____ 9. infer-		i.	inward
_____ 10. ec-, ecto-		j.	through
_____ 11. para-		k.	upon, over, above, or on top
_____ 12. dis-		l.	to follow after
_____ 13. peri-		m.	between
_____ 14. ex-, exo-		n.	alongside or abnormal
_____ 15. inter-		o.	below
_____ 16. eso-		p.	around
_____ 17. sub-		q.	outside or out
_____ 18. post-		r.	before
_____ 19. pre-		s.	together or joined
_____ 20. super-, supra-		t.	under, beneath, below
_____ 21. sym-, syn-		u.	above

Prefix Linkup

Link the prefixes in the list to create the terms that match the definitions. You may use them more than once.

Prefix	Definition
ab-	away from
ana-	up, toward
ante-	before
dia-	through
ecto-	outside, out
exo-	outside, away from
infer-	below
para-	alongside, abnormal
pre-	to come before
sub-	under, beneath, below
syn-	together, joined

Definition / Term

1. to cut up   _____tomy

2. away from the midline of the body   _____duction

3. a pregnancy in which the fertilized egg implants somewhere outside the uterus   _____pic

4. a procedure that removes uric acid and urea from circulating blood   _____lysis

5. a condition in which the eye deviates away from its normal position   _____tropia

6. a position below another point of reference   _____ior

7. a disorder in hearing   _____cusis

8. below the skin   _____cutaneous

9. a group of symptoms or signs that occur together   _____drome

10. before birth   _____natal

Prefixes That Indicate a Specific Quality about a Term

Complete the following frames to learn about prefixes that indicate a specific quality about a term.

without	**3.56** Because the prefix *a-* means "without or absence of," the term *aseptic* means "sterile," or "pertaining to _____ living pathogenic organisms."
a-	**3.57** Similarly, *asymptomatic* means "pertaining to not having symptoms," because the prefix _____ means "without."
without	**3.58** The prefix *an-* also means "without or absence of." Thus, the term *anoxia* means "_____ oxygen."
slow	**3.59** Because *brady-* means "slow," the term *bradycardia* means "condition of _____ heart."
slowing	**3.60** The term *bradykinesia* combines *brady-* with the root *kines* to mean "condition of _____ or decreasing movement."
around	**3.61** The term *circumference* contains the prefix *circum-*, which means "around." The term *circumcision* literally translates as a "cut _____." Circumcision is a surgery to remove the foreskin around the penis.
dys-	**3.62** The term *dyslexia* has the prefix _____ which means "bad, abnormal, painful, or difficult." It is a learning disability involving impaired reading, spelling, and writing ability.
good	**3.63** The prefix *eu-* means "normal or good." It is a prefix in the terms *euthanasia*, and *eupepsia*, where it alters the meaning of the root to include the meaning of "normal or _____."
different	**3.64** *Heter-* and *hetero-* both mean "different." In medicine, tropia is an abnormal deviation of the eye. Adding the prefix *hetero-* adds to the meaning of the term to indicate the eyes are oriented in _____ directions.
hyper-	**3.65** The terms *hyperacidity, hyperemesis, hyperkinesia,* and *hyperthermia* share the common prefix _____, which means "excessive, abnormally high, or above."

excessive	**3.66** Hyperthyroidism is a condition of _____ levels of thyroid hormones in the body.
low	**3.67** The prefix *hypo-* means "deficient, abnormally low, or below." Hypothyroidism is a condition of abnormally _____ levels of thyroid hormones in the body, causing high blood calcium, reduced energy, and weight gain.
hyper-	**3.68** The prefix *hypo-* has a meaning that is the opposite of the prefix _____.
abnormally	**3.69** In the term *hypocalcemia, hypo-* indicates that the levels of calcium in the blood are _____ low.
low	**3.70** The term *hypothermia* means a "state of abnormally _____ body temperature."
large	**3.71** The prefix *macro-* means "large." The word root *cephal* means "head," and the suffix *-y* means "process of," so the term *macrocephaly* means "process of _____ head."
bad	**3.72** The prefix *mal-* means "bad," so the term *malabsorption* literally means "_____ absorption."
large	**3.73** The prefix *mega-* is familiar to many people and is in common use today. It shares the meaning "large or great" with the prefix *megalo-* . So the term *megalocyte* literally means "_____ cell."
small	**3.74** The prefix *micro-* means "small." Microcephaly means "process of _____ head."
neo-	**3.75** The term *neonate* refers to a newborn, specifically a baby within the first 28 days of life. The prefix _____ means "new," and the root *nat* means "birth."
false	**3.76** The prefix *pseudo-* means "false," as in the term *pseudocyesis,* which means "_____ pregnancy."
rapid	**3.77** The prefix *tachy-* means "rapid, fast." Tachycardia is an abnormally _____ heart rate that is usually defined as more than 100 beats per minute at rest in adults.

through **across** **crossing** **across**	**3.78** The prefix *trans-* means "through, across, or beyond," as in *transvaginal,* which means "_____ or _____ the vagina," *transexual,* which means to "go through the process of _____ over to another gender," and *transverse,* which means to "lie _____ or in a crosswise direction."
beyond normal	**3.79** The prefix *ultra-* means "beyond normal," as in *ultrasound,* which is a noninvasive diagnostic procedure that provides images of internal structures by bouncing inaudible, or _____ _____, sound waves through the body (Figure 3.3■).

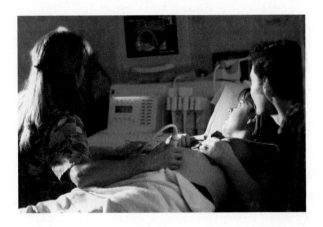

Figure 3.3 ■
Ultrasound imaging. In this noninvasive procedure, inaudible sound waves are bounced through the body, detected by a sensor, and interpreted by a computer to reveal internal structures, such as a fetus within the uterus.
Source: Photodisc/Thinkstock.

PRACTICE: Prefixes That Indicate a Specific Quality about a Term

Prefix Linkup

Link the prefixes in the list to create the terms that match the definitions. You may use them more than once.

Prefix	Definition
a-	without or absence of
brady-	slow
circum-	around
dys-	bad, abnormal, painful, or difficult
hyper-	excessive, abnormally high, above
mal-	bad
megalo-	large, great
neo-	new
pseudo-	false
trans-	through, across, or beyond
ultra-	beyond normal

Definition

1. false pregnancy

2. sterile, having no living pathogenic organisms

3. a newborn; specifically, a baby within the first 28 days of life

4. abnormally slow heart rate

5. a surgery to remove the foreskin around the penis

6. a person who goes through the process of crossing over to another gender

7. a learning disability involving impaired reading, spelling, and writing ability

8. a condition of excess levels of thyroid hormones in the body

9. bad absorption

10. large cell

11. a diagnostic procedure that provides images of internal structures by bouncing sound waves through the body

Term

_____cyesis

_____septic

_____nate

_____cardia

_____cision

_____sexual

_____lexia

_____thyroidism

_____absorption

_____cyte

_____sound

The Right Match

Match the prefix on the left with the correct definition on the right.

_____	1. a-, an-	a.	bad
_____	2. hypo-	b.	slow
_____	3. neo-	c.	small
_____	4. tachy-	d.	false
_____	5. trans-	e.	around
_____	6. dys-	f.	normal or good
_____	7. macro-	g.	deficient, abnormally low, below
_____	8. hyper-	h.	without or absence of
_____	9. circum-	i.	different
_____	10. brady-	j.	rapid, fast
_____	11. micro-	k.	bad, abnormal, painful, or difficult
_____	12. eu-	l.	large or great
_____	13. mal-	m.	large
_____	14. pseudo-	n.	through, across, or beyond
_____	15. heter-, hetero-	o.	new
_____	16. mega-, megalo-	p.	excessive, abnormally high, above

▷▷▷▷▷ Chapter Review

Word Building

Construct medical terms from the following meanings. The first question has been completed for you as an example.

1. excessive or abnormally high sensitivity to painful stimuli   _____*hyper*algesia

2. a substance that stops convulsions   _____convulsive

3. process by which foods are changed into energy for use by the body   _____bolism

4. condition of seeing a single object as two images   _____opia

5. paralysis of half the body   _____plegia

6. has given birth more than once   _____para

7. has never given birth   _____para

8. a disease that is highly prevalent   _____demic

9. paralysis of corresponding parts on both sides of the body   _____plegia

10. inflammation of many medium and small arteries   _____arteritis

11. having given birth for the first time   _____para

12. toward the midline of the body   _____duction

13. procedure that removes uric acid and urea from blood   _____lysis

14. body part that is apart or away from its normal position   _____located

15. pregnancy in which the fertilized egg implants somewhere outside the uterus   _____pic

16. within the layers of the skin   _____dermal

17. membrane that covers around the heart   _____cardium

18. a group of symptoms or signs occurring together   _____drome

19. pertaining to not having symptoms   _____symptomatic

20. a state of sterility, having no living pathogens   _____sepsis

21. slowing or decreasing movement   _____kinesia

22. removal of the foreskin around the penis   _____cision

23. "normal" or "good" death   _____thanasia

24. abnormally low levels of calcium in the blood   _____calcemia

25. false pregnancy   _____cyesis

26. rapid heart rate greater than 100 beats per minute   _____cardia

27. twins that are joined together   _____joined

28. literally, "against conception"   _____ception

29. ability to use both hands equally   _____dextrous

30. pertaining to two focal points   _____focal

31. paralysis of one limb or muscle/muscle group   _____plegia

32. paralysis of four limbs   _____plegia

33. partially conscious   _____conscious

34. a woman who has given birth three times   _____para

35. a woman who has given birth to one child   _____para

36. away from the midline of the body   _____duction

37. process of cutting up   _____tomy

38. before birth   _____natal

39. within the stomach   _____gastric

40. layer of skin that is over the dermis layer   _____dermis

41. condition in which the eye deviates inward   _____tropia

42. condition in which the eye deviates away from its normal position   _____tropia

43. outside the cellular area   _____cellular

44. position below another point of reference   _____ferior

45. position between the vertebrae   _____vertebral

46. abnormal hearing or a disorder in hearing   _____cusis

47. to follow after birth   _____partum

48. area below the skin   _____cutaneous

49. position above another point of reference   _____ior

50. without, or absence of, oxygen   _____oxia

51. learning disability that involves impaired reading, spelling, and writing ability   _____lexia

52. eyes oriented in different directions   _____tropia

53. literally, "process of large head"   _____cephaly

54. literally, "bad absorption"   _____absorption

CHAPTER

4 The Human Body in Health and Disease

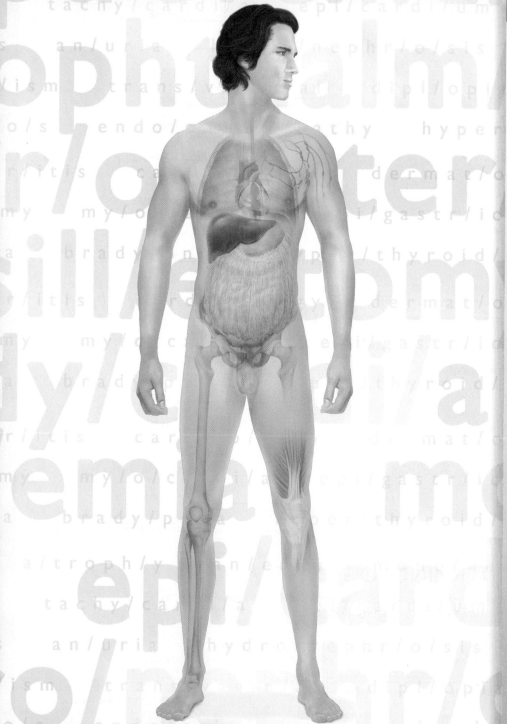

LEARNING OBJECTIVES

After completing this chapter, you will be able to:

1 Define and spell the word parts used to create terms for the human body.

2 Identify the building blocks, organ systems, and cavities of the body.

3 Identify the anatomical planes, regions, and directional terms used to describe areas of the body.

4 Break down and define the important terms associated with the anatomy and physiology of the human body.

5 Define the introductory terms associated with medical terminology.

6 Identify the five major diagnostic imaging procedures.

disease	**4.1** A study of medical terminology includes learning about the human body in a healthy state to understand the mechanisms of _____ and its terminology better. In this chapter, you will learn some basics about body organization and some general principles of function, which are necessary for understanding many of the medical terms that you will encounter later in the book.

Organization of the Body ▶▶▶▶▶

As a first step in learning the terminology of the human body, in this section you will explore how the body is organized and many of the terms that are used to describe its organization.

Combining Form	Definition	Combining Form	Definition
abdomin/o	abdomen	infer/o	below
anter/o	front	inguin/o	groin
brachi/o	arm	later/o	side
cardi/o	heart	lumb/o	loin, lower back
caud/o	tail	medi/o	middle
cephal/o	head	organ/o	tool
cervic/o	neck	pelv/o	bowl, basin
chondr/i	gristle, cartilage	physi/o	nature
cran/o, crani/o	skull	pleur/o	pleura, rib
cyt/o	cell	poster/o	back
dist/o	distant	proxim/o	near
dors/o	back	super/o	above
femor/o	thigh	thorac/o	chest, thorax
gastr/o	stomach	tom/o	to cut
glute/o	buttock	umbilic/o	navel, umbilicus
hom/o, home/o	same	ventr/o	belly
ili/o	flank, hip, groin		

Anatomy and Physiology Introduction

Complete the following frames to learn the basics of anatomy and physiology.

anatomy ann AH toe mee **structure**	**4.2** The study of body structure is called **anatomy**. The term is constructed from three word parts, as shown when it is written as ana/tom/y. The prefix *ana-* means "up, toward," the word root *tom* means "cut," and the suffix *-y* means "process of." Thus, _____ literally means "the process of cutting up." The word was first used by the ancient Greeks, who used cadaver dissection to explore body structure. Today, we use the term to describe the study of body _____, which includes the identification of body components and their locations relative to one another.

physiology fiz ee OL oh jee **functions**	**4.3** The combining form *physi/o* means "nature," and the suffix *-logy* means "study or science of." Combining these word parts forms the term _____, which literally means "study of nature." Thus, physiology refers to the study of the nature of living things. It is concerned with body _____ and seeks answers to the question, "How does it work?"
physiology **homeostasis** HOE mee oh STAY siss	**4.4** The functions of the body perform work to keep the body alive and as healthy as possible. Many body functions respond to a change, like a cold breeze or exposure to a virus, by making internal adjustments in the body. The goal of these functions is to keep the internal body in a constant, stable state despite changes in the world around us. The process of maintaining internal stability is a central concept of human _____ and is called **homeostasis**. This word is composed of three word parts, as shown when it is written as home/o/stasis. The combining form *home/o* means "sameness, unchanging" and *-stasis* is a suffix that means "standing still." Thus, _____ means "maintaining internal stability."
cell **tissues** **organs** **systems**	**4.5** The structure of the body may be described in terms of building blocks, in which small, simple blocks combine to form larger, more complex blocks until the ultimate structure, the whole body, is assembled. Notice in Figure 4.1■ that the simplest building block of the body is known as the **atom**. The atom is the simplest organized substance known, although it too is composed of smaller particles. Atoms may bind together to form **molecules**, which in turn combine to form large, nonliving structures such as parts of cells called **organelles**. These structures are assembled to form the next level of complexity, the living **cell**. The _____ is the most basic form of life in the body. Cells may be arranged into similar groups to form the next level, the **tissues**. There are four main categories of _____: epithelial tissue, connective tissue, muscle tissue, and nervous tissue. Two or more different tissues combine to form an **organ**, which maintains a certain shape and performs a general function. For example, the stomach, the brain, and the pancreas are all _____. Organs are associated with other organs with a common goal of performing a general function, such as digestion, transportation of oxygen, or maintaining the water balance in the body. A group of organs sharing a general function is called a **system**. There are 11 _____ of the body, which are summarized and illustrated in Table 4.1■, along with the organs they contain.

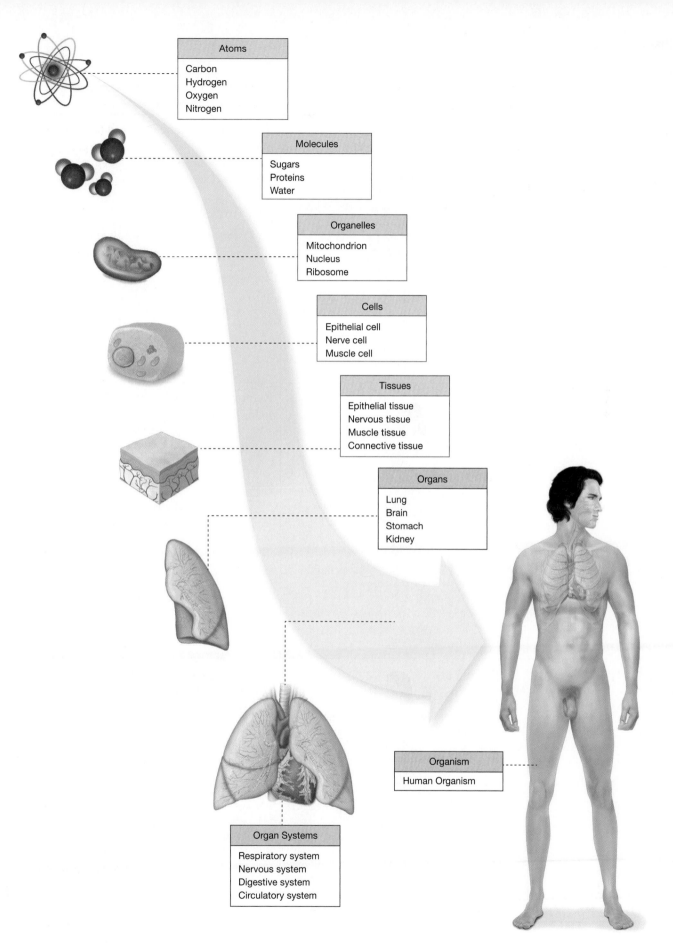

Atoms
Carbon
Hydrogen
Oxygen
Nitrogen

Molecules
Sugars
Proteins
Water

Organelles
Mitochondrion
Nucleus
Ribosome

Cells
Epithelial cell
Nerve cell
Muscle cell

Tissues
Epithelial tissue
Nervous tissue
Muscle tissue
Connective tissue

Organs
Lung
Brain
Stomach
Kidney

Organism
Human Organism

Organ Systems
Respiratory system
Nervous system
Digestive system
Circulatory system

Figure 4.1 ■
Building blocks of the body. Complexity increases in the direction of the arrow.

Table 4.1 ■ Systems of the Body

System	Major Organs	General Function
Cardiovascular	 Major arteries (in red) — Heart — Major veins (in blue)	Transport substances to and from body cells
Lymphatic	 Tonsils, Thymus, Lymphatic vessels, Spleen, Lymph nodes	Remove unwanted substances and recycle fluid to the blood
Respiratory	 Pharynx, Nose, Trachea, Larynx, Right lung, Bronchi, Left lung	Exchange gases between the external environment and blood

Table 4.1 ■ Systems of the Body

System	Major Organs	General Function
Digestive		Prepare foods for absorption into the bloodstream, and eliminate solid wastes from the body
Urinary		Remove nitrogenous wastes and excess water and salts from the bloodstream
Female Reproductive		Provide for creation of new individuals

(continued)

Table 4.1 ■ Systems of the Body (continued)

System	Major Organs	General Function
Male Reproductive	Vas deferens—Prostate Testis—Urethra Penis	Provide for creation of new individuals
Nervous	Brain— Spinal cord— Nerves	Control homeostasis by sensing changes in the environment, processing information, and initiating body responses
Endocrine	Pituitary gland— Thyroid gland—Thymus Adrenal glands— Pancreas— Ovary (female) Testis (male)	Control homeostasis by releasing hormones into the bloodstream, which alter body functions

Table 4.1 ■ Systems of the Body

System	Major Organs	General Function
Musculoskeletal	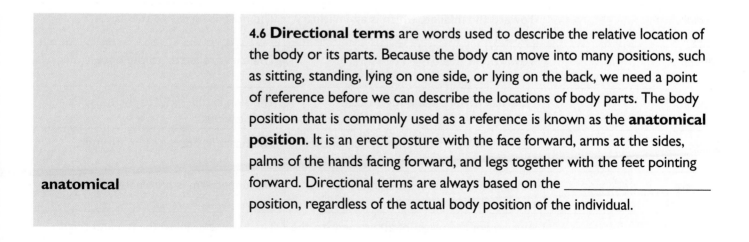	Muscles produce movement of body parts; bones and joints support and protect soft body parts, allow movement by forming attachments to muscles, store minerals, and form blood cells
Integumentary		Protect body from fluid loss, injury, and infection

anatomical

4.6 Directional terms are words used to describe the relative location of the body or its parts. Because the body can move into many positions, such as sitting, standing, lying on one side, or lying on the back, we need a point of reference before we can describe the locations of body parts. The body position that is commonly used as a reference is known as the **anatomical position**. It is an erect posture with the face forward, arms at the sides, palms of the hands facing forward, and legs together with the feet pointing forward. Directional terms are always based on the _____ position, regardless of the actual body position of the individual.

pertaining to	**4.7** The most commonly used directional terms are constructed from word parts, and each includes one word root and one suffix. The suffixes are either *-ior* or *-al*, both with the same meaning of "_____ _____." The word roots include *super*, which means "above"; *infer*, which means "below"; *anter*, which means "front"; *poster*, which means "back"; *medi*, which means "middle"; *later*, which means "side"; *proxim*, which means "near"; *dist*, which means "distant"; *ventr*, which means "belly"; *dors*, which means "back";
superior	and *caud*, which means "tail." Thus, the term _____ means "pertaining to above" and refers to a body part located above, or toward the head end, relative to another body part. For example, you would say that the nose is superior to the chest. Also, the term *dorsal* means "pertaining to the back." For example, you would say that the shoulder
dorsal	blades are _____ to the chest. Because posterior also means "pertaining to the back," *dorsal* and *posterior* are interchangeable
anterior	terms. This is also true of *ventral* and _____. Table 4.2■ provides a summary of the directional terms and additional examples of how they are used.

Table 4.2 ■ Directional Terms

Term	Definition	Example
Superior super/ior	Toward the head end or upper part of the body	The head is *superior* to the neck.
Inferior infer/ior	Away from the head end or toward the lower part of the body	The neck is *inferior* to the head.
Anterior (ventral) anter/ior	Toward the front or belly side	The eyes are on the *anterior* side of the head.
Posterior (dorsal) poster/ior	Toward the back	The vertebral column (or backbone) extends down the *posterior* (*dorsal*) side.
Medial medi/al	Toward the midline, which is an imaginary vertical line down the middle of the body	The nose is *medial* to the ears.
Lateral later/al	Toward the side	The ears are *lateral* to the nose.
Superficial super/ficial	External, toward the body surface	The skin is *superficial* to the muscles and body cavities.
Deep	Internal, inward from the surface of the body	The heart lies *deep* to the rib cage.
Proximal proxim/al	Toward the origin of attachment to the trunk	The upper arm is *proximal* to the wrist.
Distal dist/al	Away from the origin of attachment to the trunk	The knee is *distal* to the hip and thigh.

WORDS TO WATCH OUT FOR

▶▶▶▶▶ **When to Drop the Combining Vowel**

Remember the rule from Chapter 1: When a combining form is joined with a word part that begins with a vowel, the combining vowel is dropped, as in all of the directional terms that appear in Table 4.2.

anatomical planes

sagittal

4.8 A **plane** is an imaginary flat field that is used as a point of reference for viewing three-dimensional objects. Anatomical planes divide the body into imaginary sections that are useful in describing the location of body parts relative to one another. Three major _____ _____ are in common use. A **frontal** or **coronal plane** is a vertical plane passing through the body from side to side, dividing the body into anterior and posterior portions. A **sagittal** (SAJ ih tal) **plane** is a vertical plane dividing the body into right and left portions. A _____ plane dividing the body down the center into equal portions is called midsagittal, and one dividing the body into unequal portions is known as parasagittal. Finally, a **transverse plane** is a horizontal plane dividing the body into superior and inferior portions. The three major anatomical planes are shown in Figure 4.2■.

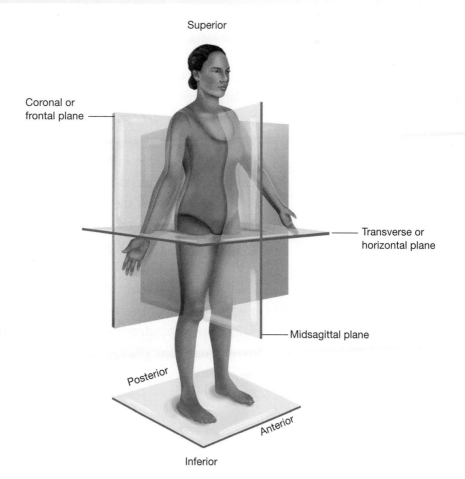

Figure 4.2 ■
Body planes.

regions

4.9 The **regions** of the body are areas that have been named to give medical health workers the ability to communicate possible problems that may be revealed during a physical examination. The most commonly used names of _____ are constructed from one word root and one suffix, similar to directional terms (see Frame 4.7). For example, the **thoracic** region is the area of the chest. The term is constructed from the word root *thorac*, which means "chest, thorax," and the suffix *-ic*, which means "pertaining to." Also, the **abdominal** region is the area of the abdomen; the word root *abdomin* means "abdomen," and the suffix *-al* means "pertaining to." The regions are further described in Table 4.3■.

Table 4.3 ■ Regions of the Body

Major Body Regions	Subdivisions
Head	Face, cranium
Neck	Anterior neck, posterior neck
Upper appendages	Shoulder, axilla (armpit), brachium (upper arm), elbow, antebrachium (forearm), carpus (wrist), manus (hand), digits (fingers)
Trunk	Thorax, abdomen, pelvis, back
Lower appendages	Gluteus (buttock), femorus (thigh), knee, crus (leg), tarsus (ankle), pes (foot), digits (toes)

abdominal
ab DOMM ih nahl

hypogastric
HIGH poh GASS trik

4.10 To aid healthcare professionals in pinpointing problems associated with the large region of the abdomen with accuracy, the _____ region is further divided into smaller regions. The name of each abdominal region is a constructed term descriptive of its location. The regions are illustrated in Figure 4.3a■ and include the **epigastric** (epi/gastr/ic, which means "on top of the stomach"), _____ (hypo/gastr/ic, which means "below the stomach"), **hypochondriac** (hypo/chondr/i/ac, which means "below the cartilage" of the ribs), **iliac** (ili/ac, which means "pertaining to the hip or groin"), **lumbar** (lumb/ar, which means "pertaining to the loin"), and **umbilical** (umbilic/al, which means "pertaining to the navel"). A second set of abdominal divisions is also shown, in Figure 4.3b■, in which the abdomen is divided into four quadrants. The quadrants are the **right upper quadrant (RUQ)**, **left upper quadrant (LUQ)**, **right lower quadrant (RLQ)**, and **left lower quadrant (LLQ)**. The quadrants are in common clinical use.

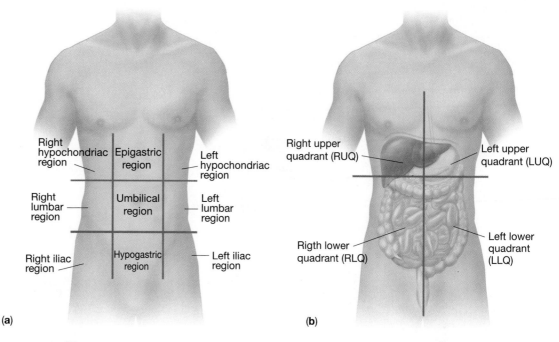

Figure 4.3 ■

The abdomen and abdominal regions. (a) Abdominal regions are mapped according to imaginary lines, as shown. (b) The abdomen may also be divided into four quadrants. The organs are shown superimposed.

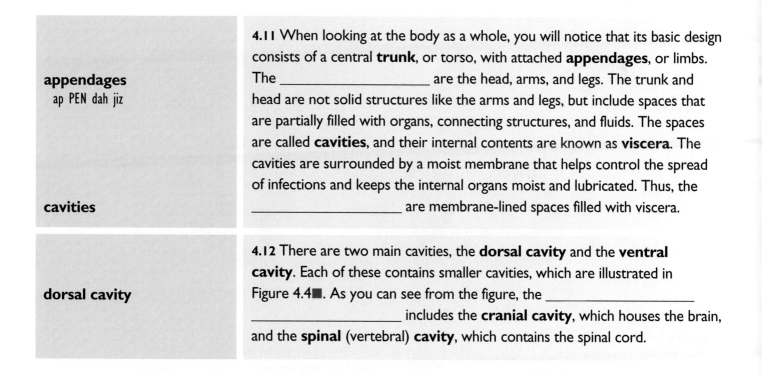

appendages
ap PEN dah jiz

cavities

4.11 When looking at the body as a whole, you will notice that its basic design consists of a central **trunk**, or torso, with attached **appendages**, or limbs. The _____ are the head, arms, and legs. The trunk and head are not solid structures like the arms and legs, but include spaces that are partially filled with organs, connecting structures, and fluids. The spaces are called **cavities**, and their internal contents are known as **viscera**. The cavities are surrounded by a moist membrane that helps control the spread of infections and keeps the internal organs moist and lubricated. Thus, the _____ are membrane-lined spaces filled with viscera.

dorsal cavity

4.12 There are two main cavities, the **dorsal cavity** and the **ventral cavity**. Each of these contains smaller cavities, which are illustrated in Figure 4.4■. As you can see from the figure, the _____ _____ includes the **cranial cavity**, which houses the brain, and the **spinal** (vertebral) **cavity**, which contains the spinal cord.

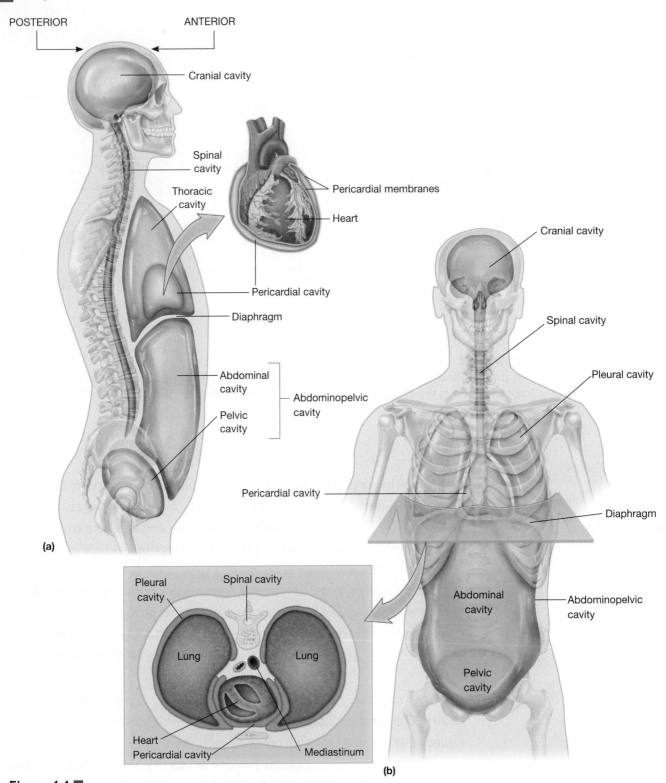

Figure 4.4 ■

Body cavities. (a) Lateral view of a sagittal section through the body. The insert shows the heart surrounded by the pericardial membranes. (b) Anterior view of a frontal section through the body. The insert is a transverse section through the thoracic cavity.

ventral cavity	**4.13** The _____ _____ in the anterior part of the body is much larger than the dorsal cavity. A muscular partition called the **diaphragm** (DYE ah fram) divides the ventral cavity into an upper and lower cavity. The cavity that is superior to the diaphragm is the **thoracic cavity**, and
inferior	the cavity _____ to the diaphragm is the **abdominopelvic cavity**. You learned in Frame 4.9 that the term *thoracic* is composed of two word parts and is written thorac/ic. The term *abdominopelvic* contains four word parts and is written abdomin/o/pelv/ic. As the names suggest,
abdominopelvic cavity	the thoracic cavity lies within the chest, and the _____ _____ lies within the abdominal and pelvic areas.
pericardial cavity	**4.14** The thoracic cavity contains several smaller cavities. The **pericardial cavity** lies along the midline of the thoracic cavity. The term *pericardial* consists of three word parts, peri/cardi/al, and literally means "pertaining to around the heart." Thus, the _____ _____ contains the heart. The other cavities within the thoracic cavity are the two **pleural cavities**. The term *pleural* is written pleur/al and contains two word parts, *pleur*, which means "pleura, rib," and *-al*, which means "pertaining to."
mediastinum mee dee ah STY num	**4.15** In addition to the pericardial cavity and the two pleural cavities, the thoracic cavity includes a potential space in the area between the two lungs. Because it lies along the midline and is deep to the breastbone or sternum, it is called the **mediastinum**. The _____ contains the heart, the large blood vessels located above the heart, and a gland called the thymus gland.
abdominal **pelvic**	**4.16** As you have learned, the abdominopelvic cavity is the large cavity of the abdominal and pelvic regions. It contains an upper and lower area, which are not divided by a partition. The upper area is the **abdominal cavity**, which contains the liver, stomach, pancreas, spleen, and most of the small and large intestines. Recall that _____ literally means "pertaining to the abdomen." At the level of the iliac crest (the tips of the hip bones), the **pelvic cavity** begins and continues to the base of the abdominopelvic cavity. The pelvic cavity contains the urinary bladder, internal reproductive organs, and parts of the small and large intestines. The word _____ may be separated into its two word parts, pelv/ic, and literally means "pertaining to a bowl or basin," describing this bowl-shaped cavity very accurately.

PRACTICE: Anatomy and Physiology Introduction

The Right Match

Match the combining form on the left with the correct definition on the right.

_____	1. abdomin/o	a.	skull
_____	2. anter/o	b.	neck
_____	3. brachi/o	c.	tail
_____	4. caud/o	d.	back
_____	5. cephal/o	e.	distant
_____	6. cervic/o	f.	front
_____	7. cran/o, crani/o	g.	abdomen
_____	8. cyt/o	h.	arm
_____	9. dist/o	i.	cell
_____	10. dors/o	j.	head
_____	11. femor/o	k.	below
_____	12. gastr/o	l.	groin
_____	13. glute/o	m.	loin, lower back
_____	14. hom/o, home/o	n.	tool
_____	15. ili/o	o.	stomach
_____	16. infer/o	p.	middle
_____	17. inguin/o	q.	flank, hip, groin
_____	18. lumb/o	r.	buttock
_____	19. medi/o	s.	thigh
_____	20. organ/o	t.	same
_____	21. pelv/o	u.	to cut
_____	22. physi/o	v.	chest, thorax
_____	23. poster/o	w.	navel
_____	24. proxim/o	x.	nature
_____	25. super/o	y.	belly
_____	26. thorac/o	z.	back
_____	27. tom/o	aa.	bowl or basin
_____	28. ventr/o	ab.	above
_____	29. umbilic/o	ac.	near

Word Root Linkup

Link the word roots in the list to create the terms that match the definitions. You may use them more than once.

Word Root	Definition
abdomin	abdomen
cardi	heart
chondr	gristle, cartilage
pelv	bowl, basin
physi	nature

Definition

Term

1. refers to the study of the nature of living things

_____/o/logy

2. the area of the abdomen

_____/al

3. below the cartilage

hypo/_____/i/ac

4. pertaining to around the heart

peri/_____/al

5. literally means "pertaining to a bowl or basin," describing this bowl-shaped cavity very accurately

_____/ic

Medical Terms Introduction ▶▶▶▶▶

As a second step in learning the terminology of the human body, in this section you will explore introductory medical terms and diagnostic procedures. Here are two combining forms that you will see in this section.

Combining Form	Definition
chron/o	time
path/o	disease

Complete the following frames to learn the basic medical terms and diagnostic procedures.

homeostasis **disease** dih ZEEZ	4.17 The body's goal is to keep itself alive and healthy. Each system performs functions that endeavor to keep the body in a constant, stable state by adjusting to changes. As you learned in Frame 4.4, this is the process of maintaining homeostasis. When body functions fail to maintain_____, a condition of instability results that is called **disease**. In general, the term _____ refers to a state of the body in which homeostasis has faltered due to any cause.

pathology
path AHL oh jee

4.18 The study of disease is a field of medicine called **pathology**. This term is derived from the Greek word for suffering or disease, *pathos*, creating the combining form *path/o*. The term is completed by adding the suffix *-logy*, which means "study or science of." A **pathologist** is a physician who specializes in _____, or the study of disease.

diagnosis
DYE ag NO sis

4.19 When examining a patient who is complaining of an illness, the healthcare professional must first identify the illness before it can be treated. Identification of the illness is called a **diagnosis**. This is a constructed word containing the word parts *dia-*, which means "through," and *-gnosis*, which means "knowledge." The _____ must be established before a treatment program can be made.

symptoms
SIMP tumz

4.20 To make a diagnosis, a healthcare professional listens to the patient to learn about clues that might suggest the nature of the illness. Experiences of the patient resulting from a disease are called **symptoms**. They are usually sensations—such as pain, heat, cold, or pressure—but can also be the loss of sensations, such as numbness or loss of appetite. Other _____ include dizziness, loss of balance, and mental confusion.

sign

4.21 Before a diagnosis can be made, a healthcare professional often examines the patient for physical signs of disease. A **sign** is a finding that can be discovered by an objective examination. For example, a thermometer inserted into the mouth or ear canal will indicate the presence of an elevated body temperature, or **fever,** which is a common _____ of an infectious disease. A clinical term for fever is **febrile** (FEH bril).

acute
ah KYOOT

4.22 As part of a diagnosis, a disease is commonly classified as having either an expected brief duration or a long duration. The term **acute** describes a disease of short duration, often with a sharp or severe effect. For example, a head cold is usually an _____ disease because of its short duration. The medical term for a head cold is **coryza** (kor EYE zah). Some acute diseases can be life threatening, so keep in mind that the term does not imply a mild disease.

2

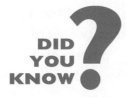

Acute

The term *acute* is derived from the Latin word *acutus,* which means "sharp." It describes how a symptom or sign that is of short duration strikes quickly, such as would result from a stinging stab from a sharp instrument.

chronic
KRON ik

4.23 A term frequently used to describe diseases that are of long duration is **chronic**. Derived from the Greek word for time, *kronos,* _____ diseases usually develop slowly and last for many years. An example of a chronic disease is the skin condition **psoriasis** (soh RYE ah siss), which lasts a lifetime.

infection
in FEKK shun

4.24 Diseases may also be classified on the basis of their cause or origin. One of the most common forms of disease is **infection**, in which parasitic organisms such as bacteria, viruses, and fungi attack body cells. The presence of _____ results in the development of **infectious disease**.

trauma
TRAW mah

4.25 Disease may also be caused by physical injury or **trauma**. For example, a fractured bone is a common _____ arising from an automobile collision. It is a disease because it upsets homeostasis of the affected bone. Disease resulting from trauma is called **traumatic disease**.

prognosis
prog NOH sis

4.26 Once a reliable diagnosis is made, the healthcare professional may predict the probable course of the disease and its probable outcome. This prediction is called a **prognosis**. Similar to the term *diagnosis,* _____ is a constructed word containing the word parts *pro-*, which means "before," and *-gnosis*, which means "knowledge."

diagnostic imaging

4.27 As you may suspect, making an accurate diagnosis is an essential part of medicine. As a result of improving technologies, making a diagnosis has become efficient and reliable. The most important improvements have been in the way instruments are able to observe the internal structure and functions of the body without the need for open surgical procedures. These noninvasive procedures are called **diagnostic imaging**. The five major types of _____ _____ are endoscopy, CT scan, PET scan, MRI, and ultrasound.

endoscopy

end AH skoh pee

4.28 The use of a long, flexible tube that can be inserted into a patient is called **endoscopy**. This constructed term includes two word parts: *endo-*, which means "within," and *-scopy*, which means "process of viewing." During the _____, a healthcare professional may observe the internal cavities and organs of the patient with the attachment of a camera at the far end of the tube (Figure 4.5■). The tube may also contain surgical attachments, enabling a surgeon to manipulate internal body parts while viewing a monitor.

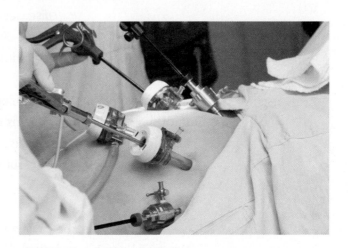

Figure 4.5 ■
Endoscopy. This is a minimally invasive surgical procedure because it reduces the amount of tissue to cut by making small openings for the insertion of specialized instruments, rather than making large openings.
Source: Reflekta/Shutterstock

CT scan

4.29 A **CT (CAT) scan** is a diagnostic procedure that combines multiple X-rays and computer enhancement to produce three-dimensional images of internal body structures (Figure 4.6■). The term _____ _____ is an acronym for **computed tomography scanning.** As a result of the computer enhancement, cross-sectional images or "slices" of body regions are produced. CT scans are useful when cross-sectional images of organs in the chest or abdomen, muscles, and joints are needed. Speed and relatively low cost make CT scans the standard for evaluation of trauma to most areas of the body.

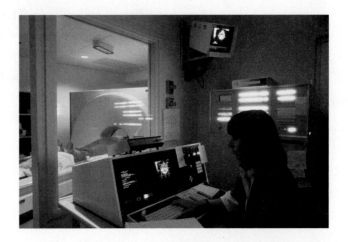

Figure 4.6 ■
CT scan. The patient is undergoing the scan in the procedure room while the radiologic technician is monitoring the instrument behind the glass wall. The CT scan image is visible on the monitor.
Source: Linda Bartlett/National Cancer Institute.

PET scan

4.30 A **PET scan** is a procedure that detects the journey of a radioactive-labeled substance, such as glucose (sugar), through the body. The PET scan instrument contains scanners that respond to radiolabeled glucose, and computers that create an image to track the pathway of the glucose as it is metabolized by body cells. As a result, the _____ _____ reveals areas of the body that have an unusually high metabolic rate, such as tumors (Figure 4.7■). The term *PET* is an acronym for **positron emission tomography**.

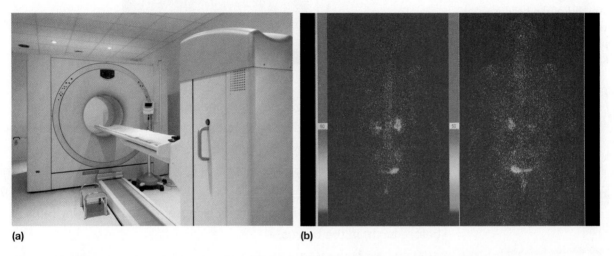

(a)   (b)

Figure 4.7 ■
PET scan. (a) Photograph of a PET scan instrument. The patient lies on the table while it is pushed through the doughnut-shaped scanner. *Source: © Grieze/Dreamstime.com*
(b) A PET scan image, such as the one shown on the monitor screen in the PET scan viewing room, reveals metabolically active tissues in the body with red colors whereas blue, white, and gray colors are metabolically inactive. It is a useful tool for diagnosing cancer because cancer cells are metabolically active. *Source: ballemans/Shutterstock*

MRI

4.31 Among all the diagnostic imaging techniques available, the **MRI** has generated the most excitement in the medical community because it offers the clearest, most complete images of internal anatomy. The term *MRI* is an acronym for **magnetic resonance imaging**. The instrument includes magnets that respond to hydrogen atoms in the body by sending signals to a computer, which analyzes the information to produce three-dimensional images (Figure 4.8■). The _____ can be used to diagnose many forms of cancer, joint disease, and trauma.

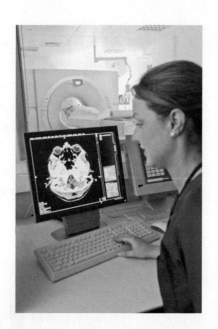

Figure 4.8 ■
MRI. The patient enters the MRI
instrument through the "doughnut"
opening. An MRI of the head is visible
on the monitor.
*Source: Jupiterimages/Polka Dot/
Thinkstock.*

ultrasound imaging

4.32 Ultrasound imaging, or **sonography**, involves the pulsation of
harmless sound waves through a body region. As the waves travel through
tissues of varying density, they produce echoes that can be detected by a
probe and interpreted by a computer (Figure 4.9■). Because of its harmless
nature, _____ _____ has proven useful
in prenatal care by providing an early glimpse of the developing fetus (a child
before birth) in the uterus.

Figure 4.9 ■
Ultrasound imaging. The use of sound
waves produces a computer-enhanced
image of the pregnancy status on
the monitor, giving the parents an
exciting early view of their child and
healthcare professionals a valuable
tool for mapping the progress of the
pregnancy.
Source: Photodisc/Thinkstock.

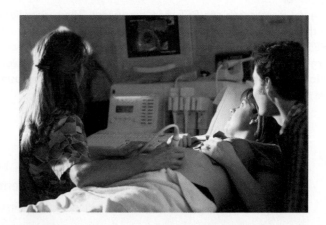

MEDICAL TERMINOLOGY INTERACTIVE

*MyMedicalTerminologyLab is a premium online homework management system that
includes a host of features to help you study. Registered users will find:*

- Fun games and activities built within a virtual hospital
- Powerful tools that track and analyze your results—allowing you to create a personalized
  learning experience
- Videos, flashcards, and audio pronunciations to help enrich your progress
- Streaming video lesson presentations and self-paced learning modules

www.pearsonhighered.com/mti

▶▶▶▶ Chapter Review

Word Building

Construct medical terms from the following meanings. (Some are built from word parts, some are not.) The first question has been completed for you as an example.

1. identification of an illness   dia/*gnosis*_____

2. maintaining internal stability   home/o/_____

3. common synonym of CAT scan   _____ scan

4. of long duration   _____/ic

5. the study of disease   _____/o/logy

6. a disease of short duration   _____ (do this one on your own!)

7. divides the body into superior and inferior portions   _____ plane

8. body cavity inferior to the diaphragm   _____/_____/ic cavity

9. procedure using a long flexible tube   _____/scopy

10. term for a finding following an objective examination   _____

11. formed from similarly grouped cells   _____

12. area of the chest   _____/ic region

13. MRI   magnetic _____ imaging

14. on top of the stomach   _____/ _____/ic

15. pertaining to the lung   _____/al

16. divides the body vertically into right and left portions   _____ plane

17. pertaining to the navel   _____/al

18. a common cause of disease   _____

19. study of body structure   _____/tom/y

20. study of nature   _____o/logy

21. pertaining to the back   _____/al

22. pertaining to the belly   _____/al

23. pertaining to above   _____/ior

24. pertaining to the front   _____/ior

25. pertaining to the middle   medi/ _____

26. pertaining to below   _____infer/_____

27. region of below the stomach   _____/gastr/ic

28. region of the loin   lumb/_____

29. cavity that contains the heart   _____/cardi/al

30. cavity that contains the urinary bladder, internal reproductive organs, and parts of the small and large intestines   _____/ic

5 The Integumentary System

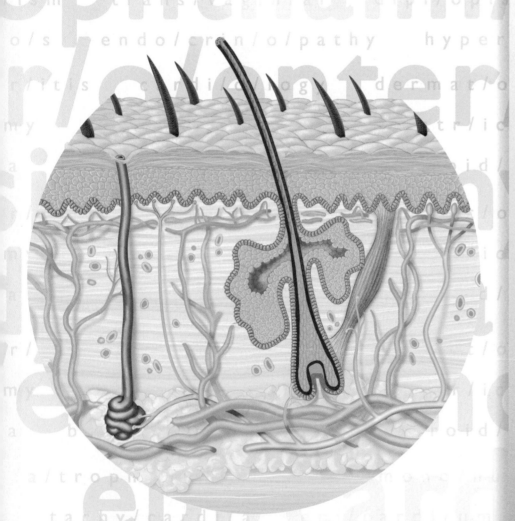

LEARNING OBJECTIVES

After completing this chapter, you will be able to:

1 Define the word parts used to create medical terms of the integumentary system.

2 Break down and define common medical terms used for symptoms, diseases, disorders, procedures, treatments, and devices associated with the integumentary system.

3 Build medical terms from the word parts associated with the integumentary system.

4 Pronounce and spell common medical terms associated with the integumentary system.

Anatomy and Physiology Terms ▶▶▶▶▶

Review the combining forms that specifically apply to the anatomy and physiology of the integumentary system. Note that the combining forms are colored red to help you identify them when you see them again later in the chapter.

Combining Form	Definition	Combining Form	Definition
aden/o	gland	follicul/o	little follicle
aut/o	self	kerat/o	hard
cutane/o	skin	onych/o	nail
cyan/o	blue	seb/o	sebum, oil
derm/o, dermat/o	skin		

integumentary
IN teg yoo MEN tar ee

epidermis

5.1 The _____ system forms the entire surface area of the body. It is dominated by the largest organ of the body, the **skin.** The skin is composed of two distinct layers: an inner, deep layer composed of connective tissue known as the **dermis,** and an outer layer of epithelium called the **epidermis.** The term *dermis* means "skin," and the term _____ means "on top of skin." The integumentary system also includes smaller accessory organs embedded within the skin, such as **hair follicles, nails, sebaceous glands, sweat glands,** and **sensory receptors.**

protection

regulate

sensation

5.2 The primary function of the integumentary system is protection. _____ is provided against outside temperature changes, dehydration, and infectious microorganisms that may cause disease. In addition, the sweat glands, blood vessels, and a layer of fat help the skin to _____ internal body temperature, while receptors in your skin provide the ability to detect changes in the environment, giving the skin the added function of _____.

5.3 In the next section, you will review anatomy terms by completing the illustration labels. Use the anatomy terms that appear in the left column to fill in the corresponding blanks in Figures 5.1■ and 5.2■.

1. epidermis
2. sebaceous gland
3. hair
4. root

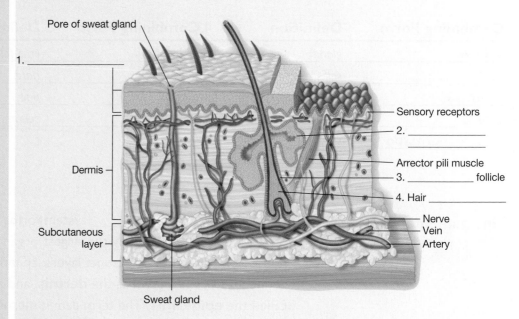

Figure 5.1 ■

Anatomy of the skin. Illustration of a section of skin showing key structures.

5. body
6. cuticle
7. nail
8. root

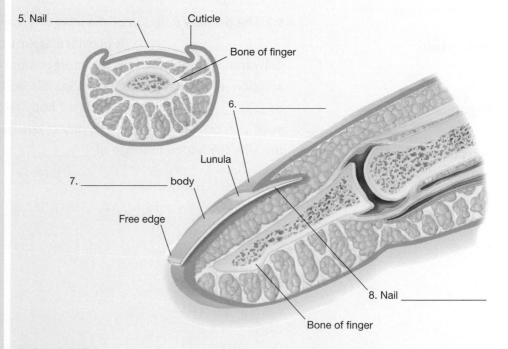

Figure 5.2 ■

Nail structure, side view and cross-sectional view.

Medical Terms of the Integumentary System ▶▶▶▶▶

organ

skin

protection

5.4 The integumentary system can experience many types of challenges to its homeostasis. As the outermost organ of the body, the skin is more exposed to the extremes of the external environment than any other _____, subjecting it to temperature fluctuations, physical injury, and invasion by unwanted microorganisms. Many types of inherited and acquired diseases may also afflict the _____.
In many cases, it is the first part of the body to display signs and symptoms of an internal disorder because it is the body part with which we are most familiar—we often see, feel, and touch our skin throughout the day. The _____ that it provides to your overall health is significant: A loss of skin can lead to severe consequences due to dehydration and infection, even death.

dermat/o/logy

5.5 The medical field that specializes in the health and disease of the integumentary system is known as **dermatology** (derm ah TOL oh jee). This term is a constructed word, written _____/_____/_____, using the combining form that means "skin," *dermat/o*, to carry the primary meaning. A physician specializing in dermatology is commonly known as a **dermatologist** (derm ah TOL oh jist).

integumentary

5.6 In the following sections, we will review the prefixes, combining forms, and suffixes that combine to build the medical terms of the _____ system.

Signs and Symptoms of the Integumentary System

KEY TERMS A–Z

abrasion
ah BRAY zhun

5.7 A common injury to the skin caused by scraping produces a superficial wound called an **abrasion.** Practice spelling this term: _____.

abscess
AB sess

5.8 An **abscess** is a localized elevation of the skin containing a cavity, which is a sign of a local infection. The _____ cavity contains a mixture of bacteria, white blood cells, damaged tissue, and fluids collectively known as **pus** and is surrounded by inflamed tissue. Several words may be used to describe the production of pus. They are **suppuration** (suhp ah RAY shun), **purulence** (PEWR yoo lens), and **pyogenesis** (PIE oh JENN eh SISS).

cellulite SELL yoo light	**5.9 Cellulite** is a local uneven surface of the skin and is a sign of subcutaneous fat deposition. _____ is relatively common in women on the thighs and buttocks.
cicatrix SIK ah trix	**5.10** An injury to the skin resulting in a break through the epidermis and into the dermis or deeper layers of skin requires the process of healing. During this process, epidermal cells migrate to the wound and produce new cells while cells within the dermis produce additional protein fibers. If the wound is too large for the epidermal cells to close the breakage, additional protein fibers (collagen) will be produced to seal the wound. In this case, the wound becomes closed by the formation of **scar tissue.** A clinical term for scar is **cicatrix.** _____ is a Latin word that means "scar." The plural form is **cicatrices** (sik ah TRYE sees).
comedo KOM ee doh	**5.11** The clinical term for pimple is **comedo.** It is a local elevation of the skin arising from the buildup of oil from sebaceous (oil) glands. Bacteria feed on the oil, attracting the movement of white blood cells and their products and resulting in the localized inflammation. In Latin, the word _____ means "glutton," referring to the fact that the lesion is caused by the action of "gluttonous" bacteria. The plural form is **comedones** (KOM ee DOH neez).
contusion kon TOO zhun	**5.12** Commonly known as a bruise, a **contusion** (kon TOO zhun) is a discoloration and swelling of the skin that is symptomatic of an injury, such as a blow to the body. A _____ is a common symptom following a physical trauma, such as an automobile accident.
cyanosis sigh ah NO siss	**5.13** The combining form for the color blue is _cyan/o_. Adding the ending _-osis_, which means "condition of," produces the term _____. It is a blue tinge of color to an area of the skin and is a sign of a cardiovascular disturbance. Cyanosis is usually apparent most clearly in the lips and fingertips.
cyst sist	**5.14** Derived from the Greek word _kystis_ that means "bladder," a **cyst** is a closed sac or pouch on the surface of the skin that is filled with liquid or semisolid material. Notice that the _c_ in the term _____ sounds like an _s_.
edema eh DEE mah	**5.15** An injury often leads to inflammation, which includes swelling. Swelling occurs when fluid accumulates in a confined space, such as beneath the skin. The clinical term for fluid accumulation is **edema.** Caused by the leakage of fluid across capillary walls, _____ is a common sign of injury and infection.

erythema
air ih THEE mah

5.16 The Greek word that means "blush" is *erythema*. We use the same word for any redness of the skin. It is a common sign of injury or infection. The correct spelling is the same as the original Greek word; it is spelled _____.

fissure
FISH er

5.17 The clinical term for a narrow break or slit in the skin is **fissure**. It is derived from the Latin word for a split or crack, *fissura*, and is illustrated in Figure 5.3■ with other signs of skin disease. Write the correct spelling of this term: _____.

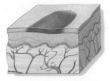
A macule is a discolored spot on the skin; freckle

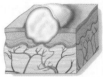
A pustule is a small, elevated, circumscribed lesion of the skin that is filled with pus; whitehead

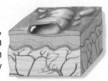
A wheal is a localized, evanescent elevation of the skin that is often accompanied by itching; urticaria

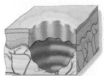
An erosion or ulcer is an eating or gnawing away of tissue; decubitus ulcer

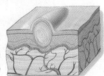
A papule is a solid, circumscribed, elevated area on the skin; pimple

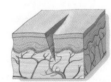
A fissure is a crack-like sore or slit that extends through the epidermis into the dermis; athlete's foot

Figure 5.3 ■
Common skin signs. Each of the illustrations depicts a section through skin.

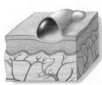
A vesicle is a small fluid-filled sac; blister. A bulla is a large vesicle.

furuncle
FOO rung kl

5.18 If an abscess is associated with a hair follicle, the local swelling on the skin is called a **furuncle.** A photograph of a _____ is provided in Figure 5.4■.

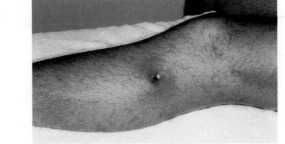

Figure 5.4 ■
Furuncle.
Source: Courtesy of Jason L. Smith, MD.

induration
in doo RAY shun

5.19 A local hard area on the skin, or perhaps elsewhere in the body, is known as an **induration.** This word is derived from the Latin word *induratio,* which means "the process of becoming firm or hard." An _____ is usually a sign of an excessive deposit of collagen or calcium.

jaundice
JAWN diss

5.20 The French word for yellow is *jaune.* It is the origin of the clinical term for an abnormal yellow coloration of the skin and eyes, **jaundice.** In most cases, _____ is a sign of liver or gallbladder disease. The yellowing results from an abnormal release of bile pigments by the liver.

keloid
KEE loyd

5.21 You have learned that a cicatrix may be formed when skin is torn (see Frame 5.10). An overgrowth of scar tissue that forms an elevated lesion on the skin is known as a **keloid.** This large scar, or _____, is often discolored, which sets it apart from adjacent, normal skin (Figure 5.5■).

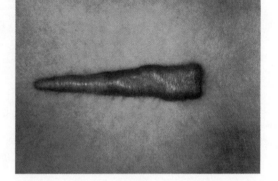

Figure 5.5 ■
Keloid.
Source: Courtesy of Jason L. Smith, MD.

laceration
LASS err AY shun

5.22 A **laceration** is the common result of an injury caused by a tear or perhaps a cut by a sharp object with an irregular surface. A _____ penetrating the dermis and extending for more than one inch often requires stitching with sutures to close the wound.

macule
MAK yool

5.23 A discolored flat spot on the skin surface, such as a freckle, is clinically called a **macule.** A _____ is a sign of sun damage to the skin, and the tendency to develop them is genetically determined. A macule is illustrated in Figure 5.3.

nevus
NEE vus

5.24 Similar to a macule but darker in color, a **nevus** is a pigmented spot that is commonly called a mole (Figure 5.6■). It is actually a sign of a benign tumor, and if its edges become irregular or the color changes, the _____ should be examined as a suspect malignancy known as a **melanoma** (see Frame 5.51).

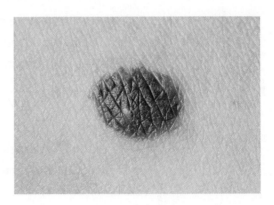

Figure 5.6 ■
Nevus.
Source: Courtesy of Jason L. Smith, MD.

pallor
PAL or

5.25 Pallor is an abnormally pale color of the skin. Derived from the Latin word *pallor* that means "paleness," _____ is a sign of an internal condition causing a decreased flow of blood to the skin.

papule
PAP yool

5.26 A **papule** is a general term describing any small, solid elevation on the skin (see Figure 5.3). An example of a _____ is a comedo, or pimple.

petechia
peh TEE kee ah

5.27 A **petechia** is a sign of a circulatory disorder. It occurs when a small blood vessel supplying the dermis of the skin ruptures. In people with light skin color, a _____ is observable as a small red dot on the skin.

pruritus
proo RYE tuss

5.28 The symptom of itchy skin is known as **pruritus.** As you might suspect, _____ means "an itching" in Latin.

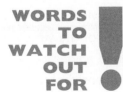 **WORDS TO WATCH OUT FOR** 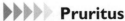 ▶▶▶▶▶ **Pruritus**

You might think at first glance that *pruritus* ("an itching") is a constructed term that uses the suffix *-itis*, meaning "inflammation." This isn't the case, however. Make a note of the spelling of this nonconstructed Latin term. The correct spelling of prurit**us** has a *u* near the end.

purpura
PER pew rah

5.29 The Greeks used the word *porphyra* to name a shellfish that releases a purple dye. In time, it was changed to name the color purple. Dermatologists use a form of the word, **purpura**, for a symptom of purple-red skin discoloration. _____ is usually the result of a hemorrhage (broken blood vessel) that spreads blood through the skin.

pustule
PUS tyool

5.30 You learned from Frame 5.8 that pus is a fluid containing bacteria, white blood cells, and their products. A general term for an elevated area of the skin filled with pus is **pustule**. An example of a _____ is a whitehead with pus. A pustule is illustrated in Figure 5.3.

ulcer
ULL ser

5.31 An **ulcer** is an erosion through the skin or mucous membrane (see Figure 5.3). The term is derived from the Latin word that means "a sore," *ulcus*. A common form of ulcer arises from lack of movement when lying supine for an extended period of time. It is called a **decubitus** (dee KYOO bih tus) _____.

urticaria
er tih KARE ree ah

5.32 A common allergic skin reaction to medications, foods, infection, or injury produces small fluid-filled skin elevations, known as **urticaria** (Figure 5.7■). Also known as hives, _____ may be accompanied by pruritus (see Frame 5.28).

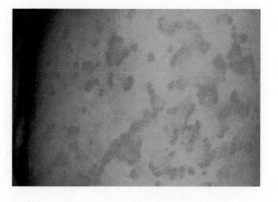

Figure 5.7 ■
Urticaria. Urticaria, or hives, is an allergic reaction resulting in small skin vesicles (Frame 5.34).
Source: Courtesy of Jason L. Smith, MD.

verruca
ver ROO kah

5.33 A wart is a sign of infection by a papilloma virus. The wart, or **verruca**, is an effort by the skin to rid itself of the virus and is observed as a skin elevation with a thickened epidermis. A _____ can be treated with antiviral medication.

vesicle VESS ih kl	**5.34** A **vesicle** is a small elevation of the epidermis that is filled with fluid (see Figure 5.3). A blister is an example of a _____ that results from injury to the skin.
wheal WEEL	**5.35** A temporary, itchy elevation of the skin, often with a white center and red perimeter, is called a **wheal**. A _____ is a symptom of an allergic reaction of the skin and is illustrated in Figure 5.3.

PRACTICE: Signs and Symptoms of the Integumentary System

The Right Match

Match the term on the left with the correct definition on the right.

_____ 1. cellulite

_____ 2. abscess

_____ 3. cicatrix

_____ 4. abrasion

_____ 5. jaundice

_____ 6. nevus

_____ 7. pruritus

_____ 8. ulcer

_____ 9. cyst

_____ 10. erythema

_____ 11. furuncle

_____ 12. pustule

_____ 13. verruca

_____ 14. wheal

_____ 15. comedo

_____ 16. vesicle

_____ 17. urticaria

_____ 18. pallor

_____ 19. papule

_____ 20. keloid

_____ 21. macule

a. localized skin swelling that is a sign of inflammation

b. abnormal yellow coloration of the skin

c. a local uneven surface of the skin caused by fat deposition

d. an erosion through the skin or mucous membrane

e. itchy skin

f. clinical term for scar

g. a pigmented spot on the skin; a mole

h. scraping injury to the skin

i. a wart

j. elevated area of the skin filled with pus

k. temporary, itchy elevation of the skin

l. redness of the skin

m. abscess associated with a hair follicle

n. a closed sac or pouch filled with liquid or semisolid material

o. any small, solid elevation on the skin

p. a discolored flat spot on the skin, such as a freckle

q. an overgrowth of scar tissue

r. small fluid-filled skin elevations caused by an allergic reaction

s. abnormally pale skin color

t. a small elevation of the epidermis that is filled with fluid

u. pimple

Diseases and Disorders of the Integumentary System

Review some of the word parts that specifically apply to the diseases and disorders of the integumentary system that are covered in the following section. Note that the word parts are color coded to help you identify them: prefixes are green, combining forms are red, and suffixes are blue.

Prefix	Definition	Combining Form	Definition	Suffix	Definition
ec-	outside, out	actin/o	radiation	-a	singular
par-	alongside, abnormal	aden/o	gland	-ia	condition of
		albin/o	white	-ic	pertaining to
		carcin/o	cancer	-ism	condition or disease
		cellul/o	little cell	-itis	inflammation
		chym/o	juice	-malacia	softening
		crypt/o	hidden	-oma	tumor
		derm/o, dermat/o	skin	-osis	condition of
		follicul/o	little follicle	-pathy	disease
		hidr/o	sweat	-rrhea	discharge
		kerat/o	hard		
		leuk/o	white		
		melan/o	black		
		myc/o	fungus		
		onych/o	nail		
		pedicul/o	body louse		
		scler/o	hard		
		trich/o	hair		
		xer/o	dry		

KEY TERMS A–Z

acne
AK nee

5.36 **Acne** is an uncomfortable condition of the skin resulting from bacterial infection of sebaceous glands and ducts (Figure 5.8■). The skin disease known as _____ is characterized by the presence of numerous open comedones (blackheads) and closed comedones (whiteheads) in affected parts of the face, and also often involves the neck, back, and chest. Acne is the most common skin disease of adolescence, due to the rapid growth of sebaceous glands during this period of life.

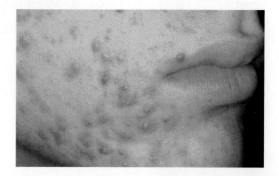

Figure 5.8 ■
Acne.
Source: Courtesy of Jason L. Smith, MD.

actinic keratosis
ak TIN ik * kair ah TOH siss

5.37 Actinic keratosis is a precancerous condition of the skin caused by exposure to sunlight. It forms skin lesions resulting from overgrowths of the epidermis, usually with scaly surfaces. The term _____ _____ is a constructed word, actin/ic kerat/osis, in which *actinic* is Greek for "pertaining to light rays" and *keratosis* means "a condition of keratin." In general, any form of keratosis produces a sign of scaly skin.

albinism
AL bin izm

5.38 A genetic condition characterized by the reduction of the pigment melanin in the skin is known as **albinism.** The term _____ uses the combining form *albin/o*, which is derived from the Latin word for white, *albus*. It is a constructed word, albin/ism, which means "a condition or disease of white." The term **albino** refers to the person affected with albinism.

alopecia
al oh PEE she ah

5.39 A loss or lack of scalp hair is a clinical sign known as baldness, or **alopecia.** Alopecia may be a sign of an infection of the scalp, high fevers, drug reactions, or emotional stress. The common appearance of _____ in men, often called **male-pattern baldness,** is the result of a genetically controlled factor that prevents the development of hair follicles in certain areas of the scalp.

burn

5.40 A **burn** is an injury to the skin caused by excessive exposure to fire, electricity, chemicals, or sunlight. The level of injury caused by the _____ is determined by the amount of surface area damaged, called **total body surface area (TBSA),** and the **depth** of the damage. A burn becomes life threatening when a large TBSA has become damaged, exposing the body to infection and exposure. In the past, burn depth classified burns into first-degree, second-degree, third-degree, and fourth-degree categories. More recently, burn depth is recorded as **partial thickness, full thickness,** and **deep.** These classifications are illustrated in Figure 5.9■.

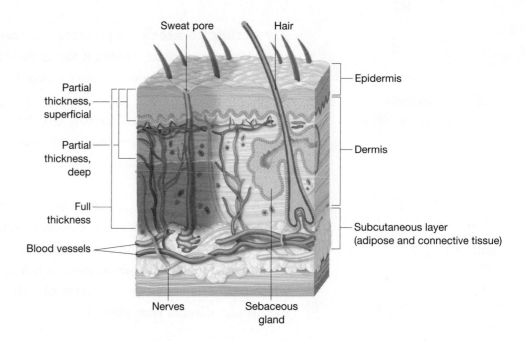

Figure 5.9 ■
Classification of burn injury by
depth in skin.

carbuncle
KAR bung kl

5.41 A **carbuncle** is a skin infection composed of a cluster of boils
(Figure 5.10■). The most common source of infection is *Staphylococci*
bacteria, or "staph." The term _____ is derived from
the Latin word *carbo,* which means "live coal" and refers to the hot pain
associated with this disease.

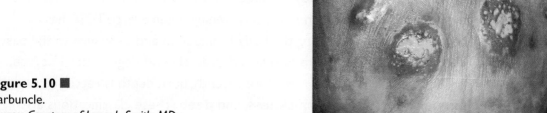

Figure 5.10 ■
Carbuncle.
Source: Courtesy of Jason L. Smith, MD.

carcinoma
kar sih NOH mah

5.42 Remember that the combining form *carcin/o* means "cancer."
When you add the suffix that means "tumor," it forms the word
_____. Several forms of cancer, or carcinoma, affect
the skin. **Basal cell carcinoma** (Figure 5.11■) and **squamous cell
carcinoma** are tumors arising from the epidermis that usually remain
localized, although the lesions do spread and can become serious if they
are not treated. Squamous cell carcinomas, in particular, can be dangerous.
The third major form of skin cancer is **melanoma,** which will be
described later in Frame 5.51.

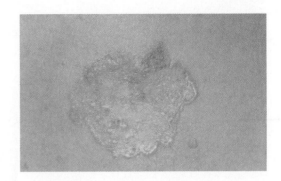

Figure 5.11 ■
Basal cell carcinoma.
Source: Courtesy of Jason L. Smith, MD.

cellulitis
sell you LYE tiss

5.43 Cellulitis is an inflammation of the connective tissue in the dermis (Figure 5.12■). It is caused by an infection that spreads from the skin surface or hair follicles to the dermis and sometimes the subcutaneous tissue. It is usually bacterial in origin. The term _____ is a constructed word, cellul/itis, which literally means "inflammation of little cells." The related term used for follicle infection, **folliculitis** (foh LIK yoo LYE tiss), is also a constructed word. It means "inflammation of little follicles."

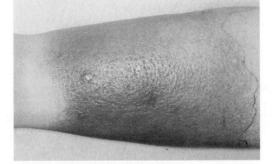

Figure 5.12 ■
Cellulitis.
Source: Courtesy of Jason L. Smith, MD.

dermatitis
der mah TYE tiss

5.44 Dermatitis is a generalized inflammation of the skin, involving edema (Frame 5.15) of the dermis (Figure 5.13■). In addition to swelling, symptoms may include pruritus (Frame 5.28), urticaria (Frame 5.32), vesicles (Frame 5.34), and wheals (Frame 5.35), or some combination of these. The major types of _____ include **contact dermatitis,** caused by physical contact with a triggering substance such as poison ivy; **seborrheic** (SEB or EE ik) **dermatitis,** which is an inherited form characterized by excessive sebum production; and **actinic dermatitis,** caused by sunlight exposure. **Eczema** (EK zeh mah) is a superficial form of dermatitis, with flakiness of the epidermis as the primary sign. Dermatitis is a constructed word, dermat/itis, which literally means "inflammation of the skin."

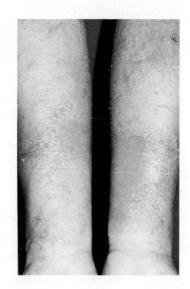

Figure 5.13 ■
Dermatitis.
Source: Courtesy of Jason L. Smith, MD.

ecchymosis
ek ih MOH siss

5.45 Ecchymosis is a condition of the skin caused by leaking blood vessels in the dermis, producing purplish patches of purpura (Frame 5.29) larger in size than petechiae (Frame 5.27). The term _____ is a constructed word, ec/chym/osis, which literally means "condition of leaking out."

herpes
HER peez

5.46 A skin eruption producing clusters of deep blisters is known as **herpes.** The vesicles (Frame 5.34) appear periodically, affecting the borders between mucous membranes and skin. There are several types of _____, all of which are caused by herpes simplex virus (HSV). The major types are **oral herpes,** caused by herpes virus type 1 (Figure 5.14■), **genital herpes,** caused by herpes virus type 2, and **shingles,** caused by the herpes zoster virus. Herpes is an infectious disease, transferable when the vesicles burst open and physical contact is made between the carrier and another person. In the absence of lesions, it may also be transferable by body fluid contact.

Figure 5.14 ■
Herpes. The blisters often last for several days to one week and form in response to periodic outbreaks of the virus.
Source: Courtesy of Jason L. Smith, MD.

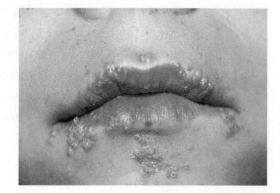

hidradenitis
high drad en EYE tiss

5.47 In the condition **hidradenitis,** the individual suffers from excessive perspiration. It is due to the inflammation of sweat glands, which can become worsened by bacterial infection. The word _____ is a constructed term, hidr/aden/itis, with two word roots: hidr, which means "sweat," and aden, which means "gland." Thus, the literal meaning of the term is "inflammation of sweat gland."

impetigo
imp eh TYE goh

5.48 Impetigo is a contagious skin infection (Figure 5.15■). Similar to oral herpes due to the development of small vesicles (Frame 5.34) usually forming around the lips, it is often caused by bacteria that enters a break in the skin (such as an animal or insect bite) and is characterized by the presence of golden crusts following the rupture of the vesicles. The term _____ is a Latin word meaning "scabby eruption."

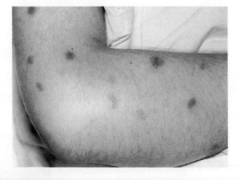

Figure 5.15 ■
Impetigo.
Source: Courtesy of Jason L. Smith, MD.

Kaposi's sarcoma
KAP oh seez * sar KOH mah

5.49 Kaposi's sarcoma is a form of skin cancer arising from the connective tissue of the dermis (Figure 5.16■). It is indicated by the presence of brown or purple patches on the skin and appears among some elderly patients. _____ _____ is also a common condition associated with HIV infection and AIDS.

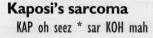

Figure 5.16 ■
Kaposi's sarcoma.
Source: Courtesy of Jason L. Smith, MD.

leukoderma
loo koh DER mah

5.50 As some people age, their skin becomes lighter in color due to reduced activity of the pigment-producing cells in the skin, the melanocytes. This condition is called **leukoderma.** The term _____ is a constructed word, leuk/o/derm/a, which literally means "white skin."

melanoma

mell ah NOH mah

5.51 The most life-threatening skin cancer is **malignant melanoma,** which is shown in Figure 5.17■. It arises from the cells normally providing the pigment **melanin** (MELL ah nin) to the skin, called **melanocytes** (mell AN oh sites). _____ is a constructed term, melan/oma, which literally means "black tumor." Once established in the skin, the tumor grows rapidly and metastasizes (goes elsewhere in the body). About one-half of cases arise from nevi (moles).

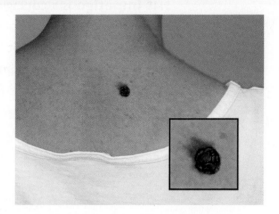

Figure 5.17 ■
Melanoma.

onychocryptosis

ON ih koh krip TOH siss

5.52 The combining form for nail is onych/o and is used in the construction of terms relating to nail diseases. In general, a disease of the nail is an **onychopathy** (ON ih KOHP a thee). In the nail condition called **onychocryptosis,** a nail becomes buried in the skin due to abnormal growth. It is commonly called an ingrown nail. The term _____ is a constructed word, onych/o/crypt/osis, and means "condition of hidden nail."

onychomalacia

ON ih koh mah LAY she ah

5.53 In the condition **onychomalacia,** a nail is abnormally soft. It is often a sign of calcium or vitamin D deficiency. The term _____ is a constructed word, onych/o/malacia, which means "softening of the nail."

onychomycosis

ON ih koh my KOH siss

5.54 The condition _____ is a fungal infection of one or more nails (Figure 5.18■). Notice that the word root for fungus, myc, is included in this constructed term, onych/o/myc/osis, to form its meaning into "condition of fungus of the nail."

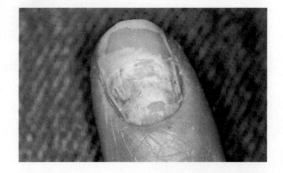

Figure 5.18 ■
Onychomycosis.
Source: Courtesy of Jason L. Smith, MD.

paronychia
pair oh NIK ee ah

5.55 In **paronychia,** the prefix *par-*, which means "alongside, abnormal," is included to build the term. Thus, the constructed word *par/onych/ia* means "condition of alongside the nail." As you might guess, _____ is an infection around the nail.

pediculosis
peh dik yoo LOH siss

5.56 The Latin word for a parasitic body louse is *pediculus*, which is the origin of the combining form of *pedicull/o*. When this combining form is combined with the suffix for "condition of," it forms the constructed word _____. Pediculosis occurs mostly on the scalp, where it is called head lice, but it may also be found in the pubic region (called pubic lice) and other parts of the body (called body lice). Pediculosis can be treated effectively with medicated shampoo.

psoriasis
soh RYE ah siss

5.57 Psoriasis is a painful, chronic disease of the skin characterized by the presence of red lesions covered with silvery epidermal scales (Figure 5.19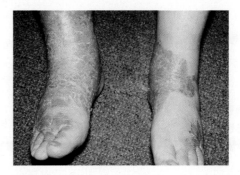). Believed to be an inherited inflammatory disease of the skin, _____ is a Greek word meaning "to itch" and is spelled exactly like the clinical term.

Figure 5.19 ■
Psoriasis.
Source: Courtesy of Jason L. Smith, MD.

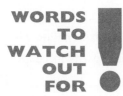
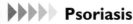

WORDS TO WATCH OUT FOR ❗

▶▶▶▶▶ **Psoriasis**

Psoriasis is a very commonly misspelled term. It is one of the medical terms that is spelled with a silent *p* (terms with the word root *psych* are the others). One way to remember to include the *p* is to think of the *p*atches of red lesions that characterize this condition.

scabies
SKAY bees

5.58 The condition **scabies** is a skin eruption caused by the female itch mite, which burrows into the skin to extract blood (Figure 5.20■). From the Latin word *scabere* that means "scratch," _____ produces the symptoms of dermatitis (Frame 5.44), such as erythema (Frame 5.16), swelling or edema (Frame 5.15), and pruritus (Frame 5.28).

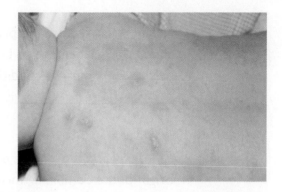

Figure 5.20 ■
Scabies.
Source: Courtesy of Jason L. Smith, MD.

scleroderma
  sklair oh DER mah

5.59 Scleroderma uses the combining form *scler/o*, which means "hard." It is an abnormal thickening or hardness of the skin, caused by overproduction of collagen in the dermis. The term _____ is a constructed word, *scler/o/derm/a*, which means "skin hardness."

systemic lupus erythematosus
  sis TEM ik * LOO pus *
  air ih them ah TOH siss

5.60 Systemic lupus erythematosus, abbreviated **SLE,** is a chronic, progressive disease of connective tissue in many organs including the skin. The early stages of _____ _____ _____, often commonly referred to as just **lupus,** are marked by red patches on the skin of the face and joint pain.

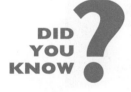 ▶▶▶▶▶ **Lupus**

DID YOU KNOW ?

The Latin word for wolf is *lupus.* The disease lupus was named by the appearance of the reddish face rash that reminded early physicians of a wolf.

tinea
  TIN ee ah

5.61 Tinea is a fungal infection of the skin. It is often called **ringworm** due to the ring-shaped pattern on the skin that forms in response to the fungi (Figure 5.21■). In fact, the term _____ is the Latin word for worm or larval moth. The three major forms of tinea are **tinea capitis,** which forms on the scalp and can lead to alopecia (Frame 5.39); **tinea pedis,** which forms on the feet and is also known as athlete's foot; and **tinea corporis,** which may occur elsewhere on the body.

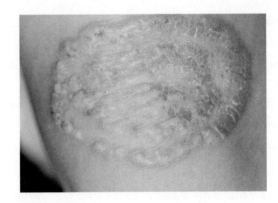

Figure 5.21 ■
Tinea. Although it is a fungal infection, tinea is often called ringworm.
Source: Courtesy of Jason L. Smith, MD.

trichomycosis
TRIK oh my KOH siss

5.62 A general term for a disease affecting the hair is **trichopathy** (trye KOH path ee), which combines the word root for hair (*trich*) and the suffix for disease (*-pathy*). The condition **trichomycosis** is a fungal infection of hair. In this constructed term, trich/o/myc/osis, the word roots for *hair* and *fungus* are combined to form the term _____.

xeroderma
zee roh DER mah

5.63 The combining form *xer/o* means "dry"; when this is combined with the word root that means "skin," it forms the word _____. Not surprisingly, the disease **xeroderma** is characterized by abnormally dry skin. It is caused by hyposecretion (abnormally low secretion) of the oil glands and is an inherited condition. It is a constructed term, xer/o/derm/a, which literally means "dry skin."

PRACTICE: Diseases and Disorders of the Integumentary System

The Right Match

Match the term on the left with the correct definition on the right.

_____ 1. tinea

_____ 2. acne

_____ 3. burn

_____ 4. herpes

_____ 5. alopecia

_____ 6. impetigo

_____ 7. scabies

_____ 8. psoriasis

a. results from bacterial infection of sebaceous glands and ducts

b. characterized by red lesions covered with silvery epidermal scales

c. baldness

d. contagious bacterial skin infection with a yellowish crust

e. caused by excessive exposure to fire, electricity, chemicals, or sunlight

f. skin eruption caused by the female itch mite

g. viral skin eruption that produces clusters of deep blisters

h. fungal infection of the skin

Break the Chain

Analyze these medical terms:

    a) Separate each term into its word parts; each word part is labeled for you (**p** = prefix, **r** = root, **cf** = combining form, and **s** = suffix).

    b) For the Bonus Question, write the requested word part or definition in the blank that follows.

The first set has been completed for you as an example.

1. a) dermatitis   *dermat/itis*
                                   r   s

    b) *Bonus Question:* What is the definition of the suffix?   *inflammation*

2. a) melanoma   _____/_____
                                  r   s

    b) *Bonus Question:* What is the definition of the suffix? _____

3. a) onychomycosis   _____/___/_____/_____
                                  cf   r   s

    b) *Bonus Question:* What is the definition of the *second* word root? _____

4. a) pediculosis   _____/_____
                                  r   s

    b) *Bonus Question:* What is the definition of the suffix? _____

5. a) scleroderma   _____/___/_____/_____
                                  cf   r   s

    b) *Bonus Question:* What is the definition of the combining form? _____

6. a) trichomycosis   _____/___/_____/_____
                                  cf   r   s

    b) *Bonus Question:* What is the definition of the combining form? _____

7. a) cellulitis   _____/_____
                                  r   s

    b) *Bonus Question:* What is the definition of the suffix? _____

8. a) leukoderma   _____/___/_____/_____
                                  cf   r   s

    b) *Bonus Question:* What is the definition of the *second* word root? _____

Treatments, Procedures, and Devices of the Integumentary System

Review some of the word parts that specifically apply to the treatments, procedures, and devices of the integumentary system that are covered in the following section. Note that the word parts are color coded to help you identify them: prefixes are green, combining forms are red, and suffixes are blue.

Combining Form	Definition	Suffix	Definition
abras/o	to rub away	-ectomy	surgical excision, removal
aut/o	self	-ion	process
derm/o, dermat/o	skin	-plasty	surgical repair
rhytid/o	wrinkle	-tome	cutting instrument

KEY TERMS A–Z

biopsy
BYE op see

5.64 A **biopsy** is a minor surgery involving the removal of tissue for evaluation. Abbreviated **bx** or **Bx**, a _____ is usually a necessary step toward making a diagnosis of a suspected tumor of the skin.

debridement
day breed MON

5.65 Wounds are often complicated by physical contact with a dirty object, including the ground. To clean the wound, a procedure called **debridement** is often used (Figure 5.22■). A French word meaning "unbridled," _____ involves excision of foreign matter and unwanted tissue.

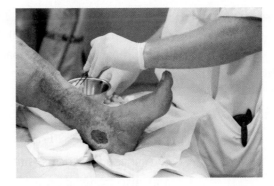

Figure 5.22 ■
Debridement, or wound cleansing.
Source: © ARNO MASSEE/SCIENCE PHOTO LIBRARY/Custom Medical Stock Photo

dermabrasion
DERM ah BRAY zhun

5.66 Remember that the combining form *derm/o* means "skin." When combined with the suffix that means "process" and the combining form that means "to rub away," *abras/o*, it forms the word _____. **Dermabrasion** is a form of **cosmetic surgery,** in which the skin is surgically changed to improve appearance. During dermabrasion, abrasives similar to sandpaper are used to remove unwanted scars and other elevations and may also be used to remove tattoos. Alternatives to dermabrasion include **chemical peels,** in which a chemical agent is used to remove the outer epidermal layers to treat acne, wrinkles, and sun-damaged skin.

dermatoautoplasty
DER mah toh AW toh PLASS tee

dermatome
DER mah tohm

5.67 Some burns and similar injuries cause extensive damage to a large area of skin, challenging the normal healing process. In these cases, the surgical procedure of **dermatoautoplasty** may be used to improve healing. This is a constructed term that can be written as dermat/o/aut/o/plasty. In this term, note the combining form that means "self," *aut/o*. This is because the surgery involves using the patient's own skin as a graft, usually after it has grown in a media solution. _____ is also called an **autograft.** Alternatively, a skin graft from another person may be used. This procedure is called **dermatoheteroplasty** (DER mah toh HETT er oh PLASS tee), or **allograft.** During both procedures, an instrument called a **dermatome** (DER mah tohm) is used to cut thin slices of skin for grafting. A _____ may also be used to excise (surgically remove) small skin lesions. Recall that the suffix *-tome* means "cutting instrument."

dermatoplasty
DER mah toh plass tee

5.68 The general term for a surgical procedure of the skin is **dermatoplasty.** This term uses the combining form that means "skin" with the suffix, *-plasty,* which means "surgical repair." In _____, skin tissue is transplanted to the body surface.

emollient
ee MALL ee ant

5.69 An _____ is a chemical agent that softens or smooths the skin. Topical and oral **antibiotics** (ahn tye bye OT iks) are used to manage infections, such as acne and carbuncles. **Retinoids** (RET ih noydz) may also be used to manage certain forms of acne because they cause the upper layers of the epidermis to slough away. Acne and related disorders may also be treated by **ultraviolet light therapy,** which causes a similar effect on the epidermis.

rhytidectomy

rit ih DEK toh mee

5.70 Plastic surgery is a popular form of skin treatment, which is used for skin repair following a major injury, correction of a congenital defect, or cosmetic improvement. Several of the terms related to plastic surgery use the combining form *rhytid/o*, which means "wrinkle." Plastic surgeries that are primarily cosmetic include **rhytidoplasty** (RIT ih doh PLASS tee), which is the surgical repair of skin wrinkles (Figure 5.23■); _____, during which wrinkles are surgically removed; and **liposuction** (LIE poh suk shun), which is the removal of subcutaneous fat (fat immediately deep to the skin) by insertion of a device that applies a vacuum to pull the fat tissue out of the body.

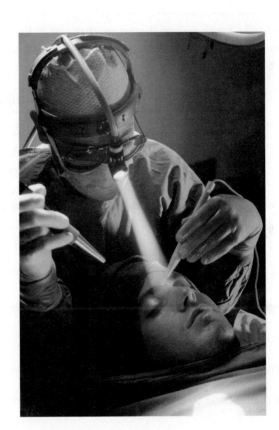

Figure 5.23 ■
Rhytidoplasty. This is a common form of plastic surgery in which the skin is pulled and sutured to decrease skin wrinkles.
Source: Kim Steele/Getty Images.

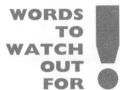

WORDS TO WATCH OUT FOR !

▶▶▶▶▶ **The *Y* in Rhytid**

It may be tempting to spell the term *rhytidectomy* with an *i* instead of a *y*. One way to remember to use a *y* is to think of the word *elderly*. As you've learned, the word root *rhytid* means "wrinkle." Elderly people commonly have wrinkles, and the word *elderly* ends with a *y*.

PRACTICE: Treatments, Procedures, and Devices of the Integumentary System

The Right Match

Match the term on the left with the correct definition on the right.

_____ 1. biopsy

_____ 2. emollient

_____ 3. debridement

_____ 4. cosmetic surgery

_____ 5. autograft

a. chemical agent that softens or smooths the skin

b. wound-cleaning procedure

c. surgically changing the skin to improve appearance

d. surgery that uses a patient's own skin as a graft

e. the removal of tissue for evaluation

Linkup

Link the word parts in the list to create the terms that match the definitions. You may use word parts more than once. Remember to add in combining vowels when needed—and that some terms do not use any combining vowel. The first one is completed for you as an example.

Combining Form	Suffix
abras/o	-ectomy
aut/o	-ion
derm/o, dermat/o	-plasty
rhytid/o	-tome

Definition

1. use of abrasives to remove unwanted scars and tattoos

2. the surgical repair of skin wrinkles

3. surgical repair of the skin

4. surgery that involves the use of the patient's own skin to improve healing

5. an instrument that is used to cut thin slices of skin for grafting

Term

dermabrasion _____

_____

_____

_____

_____

Abbreviations of the Integumentary System

The abbreviations that are associated with the integumentary system are summarized here. Study these abbreviations, and review them in the exercise that follows.

Abbreviation	Definition
BCC	basal cell carcinoma
bx, Bx	biopsy
SLE	systemic lupus erythematosus

Abbreviation	Definition
SqCCa	squamous cell carcinoma
TBSA	total body surface area

PRACTICE: Abbreviations

Fill in the blanks with the abbreviation or the complete medical term.

Abbreviation

1. _____

2. BCC

3. _____

4. SqCCa

5. _____

Medical Term

biopsy

_____

systemic lupus erythematosus

_____

total body surface area

▶▶▶▶ Chapter Review

Word Building _____

Construct medical terms from the following meanings. The first question has been completed for you as an example.

1. literally means "black tumor"   melan*oma*_____

2. inflammation of connective tissue   _____itis

3. disease of the nail   _____pathy

4. fungal infection of a nail   onycho_____

5. abnormally dry skin   _____derma

6. a skin wound caused by scraping   abras_____

7. an infection arising from a follicle   _____itis

8. disease that affects the hair   tricho_____

9. blisters that later form a yellowish crust   _____igo

10. a small, solid circumscribed skin elevation   nev_____

11. a discolored flat spot   _____ule

12. derived from the Latin word "to soften"   emoll_____

13. one who specializes in skin ailments   _____logist

14. overgrowth of scar tissue   kel_____

15. an ingrown nail   _____cryptosis

16. a precancerous condition caused by sunlight   actinic kerat_____

17. abnormally light skin   _____derma

►►►► Medical Report Exercises

Sally Garcia _____

Read the following medical report, then answer the questions that follow.

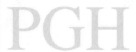

PEARSON GENERAL HOSPITAL

5500 University Avenue, Metropolis, TX
Phone: (211) 594-4000 • Fax: (211) 594-4001

Medical Consultation: Dermatology

Date: 11/20/2011

Patient: Sally Garcia

Patient Complaint: Itchy, painful rash on right upper arm.

History: 22-year-old Hispanic female has complained of itching, pain, and swelling of the right upper arm, for one month. Social History: During this time, she started work in a factory warehouse where she was exposed to dust and high humidity. She reports that chemicals are used in the workplace but does not now know what chemicals to which she was exposed.

Family History: Father, age 72, with melanoma; older brother with seborrheic dermatitis spreading to the scalp to contribute to alopecia.

Allergies: None

Physical Examination: All vital signs are normal. Skin shows generalized inflammation, including erythema and mild edema, of right upper arm spreading to shoulder and thorax with vesicular rash. There is some scarring occurring, and there is a 3 cm × 1 cm keloid located on the lateral aspect of the right arm.

Diagnosis: Contact dermatitis.

Treatment: Treat local skin rash with emollients and 2% cortisone ointment. Schedule follow-up appointment in two weeks. If inflammation persists, antibiotic ointment to be administered.

Jane K. Hernandez, M.D.
_____
Jane K. Hernandez, M.D.

Photo Source: Photoroller/Shutterstock

Comprehension Questions

1. What is the probable cause of the cicatrices on the skin? _____

_____

_____

2. If the symptom of pruritus returns after the initial treatment, how might the formation of new scar tissue be prevented? _____

_____

_____

3. Why do you think antibiotic therapy is included in the follow-up treatment if the condition persists? _____

_____

_____

Case Study Questions

The following case study provides further discussion regarding the patient in the medical report. Fill in the blanks with the correct terms. Choose your answers from the following list of terms. (Note that some terms may be used more than once.)

actinic keratosis	dermatitis	keloids	ulcers
biopsy	dermatology	pruritus	vesicles
cicatrices	emollients		

At the (a) _____ clinic where patients with skin ailments are referred, Sally Garcia, a patient

with an unusual skin condition, was observed. The skin condition included a generalized skin inflammation, or

(b) _____, which included abnormal redness, swelling, and pain. Skin damage caused by sunlight,

a precancerous condition known as (c) _____ _____, was ruled out as a

diagnosis, along with all known forms of skin cancer. Rather, an allergic agent was the likely cause. After several days

of general inflammation, fluid-filled skin elevations, or (d) _____, appeared. The elevations gave the

patient symptoms of itching or (e) _____. Scratching the elevations produced open sores, or

(f) _____, which upon healing left scars, or (g) _____. In some areas, the scar tissue

became overgrown, forming (h) _____. Treatment included the application of topical ointments, or

(i) _____, and antibiotic treatments were prescribed during a follow-up.

Patricia Velasquez

For a greater challenge, read the following medical report and answer the questions that follow.

PEARSON GENERAL HOSPITAL

PGH

5500 University Avenue, Metropolis, IL
Phone: (211) 594-4000 • Fax: (211) 594-4001

Medical Consultation: Dermatology

Date: 7/07/2011

Patient: Patricia Velasquez

Patient Complaint: Irritating and sometimes painful skin elevation on top of right shoulder.

History: 25-year-old female who spends a lot of time outdoors due to her interest in competitive swimming and diving.

Family History: Mother negative for skin disease. Father unknown.

Allergies: None

Physical Examination: All vital signs are normal. Nevus on the superior aspect of the right shoulder appears to be the source of irritation and pain with evidence of scratching. Appearance of nevus includes irregular border and elevated center with darker coloration.

Diagnosis: Melanoma

Treatment: Outpatient excision of nevus approved by patient. Performed after lidocaine injection and removal with #8 scalpel, and tissue sent to clinical lab stat for bx.

Robert M. O'Brady, M.D.

Robert M. O'Brady, M.D.

Photo Source: Andresr/Shutterstock

Comprehension Questions

1. What patient behaviors support the initial diagnosis? _____

   _____

   _____

2. What is a common word for nevus? _____

   _____

   _____

3. Do you think antibiotic therapy should be included in the treatment? _____

   _____

   _____

Case Study Questions

The following case study provides further discussion regarding the patient in the medical report. Recall the terms from this chapter to fill in the blanks with the correct terms.

Patricia Velasquez, a 25-year-old female, had trained for competitive swimming and diving since the age of 12 years. According to her mother, Patricia has had no prior medical concerns and was given the usual vaccinations as a young child. Several months before Patricia's visit to her personal physician, she had been complaining of a nagging irritation on the skin of her right shoulder. Because, at first, she believed the skin irritation to be a minor response to a new skin lotion, or (j) _____, she delayed consulting a physician. When her mother noticed the mole, or (k) _____, on Patricia's right shoulder had changed in shape and become darker, she decided to make an appointment. After a physical exam with otherwise negative findings, her personal physician observed the mole and referred her immediately to a skin specialist, or (l) _____. Upon observing the nevus, which had increased in size from 0.5 cm to 0.9 cm since her prior appointment only three weeks earlier, the skin specialist recorded the lesion as a possible form of skin cancer arising from pigment-producing skin cells, called (m) _____. He determined that an immediate course of action was necessary and asked for Patricia's approval to remove the suspected tumor as an outpatient treatment in his office. Patricia agreed, and the specialist performed the minor surgery within minutes. The specimen was sent to the lab for analysis as part of the biopsy procedure, abbreviated (n) _____. Because of the large incision necessary, a skin repair procedure, (o) _____, was performed to aid healing and prevent the formation of a scar, or (p) _____. Although the lab reported that the specimen was positive for melanoma, the specimen did not show evidence of metastasis, so no further cancer treatments were deemed necessary.

MEDICAL TERMINOLOGY INTERACTIVE

Medical Terminology Interactive is a premium online homework management system that includes a host of features to help you study. Registered users will find:

- Fun games and activities built within a virtual hospital
- Powerful tools that track and analyze your results—allowing you to create a personalized learning experience
- Videos, flashcards, and audio pronunciations to help enrich your progress
- Streaming video lesson presentations and self-paced learning modules

www.pearsonhighered.com/mti

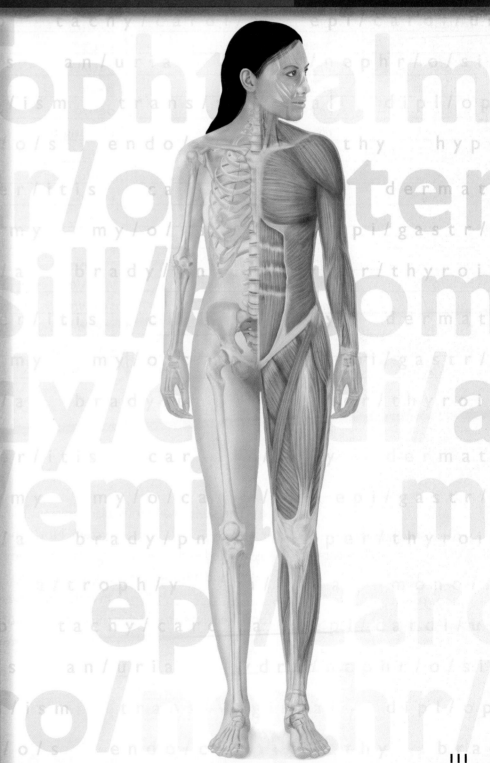

The Skeletal and Muscular Systems

6

LEARNING OBJECTIVES

After completing this chapter, you will be able to:

1. Define and spell the word parts used to create medical terms for the skeletal and muscular systems.

2. Break down and define common medical terms used for symptoms, diseases, disorders, procedures, treatments, and devices associated with the skeletal and muscular systems.

3. Build medical terms from word parts associated with the skeletal and muscular systems.

4. Pronounce and spell common medical terms associated with the skeletal and muscular systems.

Anatomy and Physiology Terms ▶▶▶▶▶

The following table provides the combining forms that specifically apply to the anatomy and physiology of the skeletal and muscular systems. Note that the combining forms are colored red to help you identify them when you see them again later in the chapter.

Combining Form	Definition	Combining Form	Definition
arthr/o	joint	orth/o	straight
articul/o	joint	ost/o, oste/o	bone
burs/o	purse or sac, bursa	pariet/o	wall
carp/o	wrist	patell/o	patella
chondr/o	gristle, cartilage	ped/o	child
condyl/o	knuckle of a joint	petr/o	stone
cost/o	rib	phalang/o	phalanges
cran/o, crani/o	skull, cranium	phys/o	growth
fasci/o	fascia	pub/o	pubis
femor/o	thigh, femur	radi/o	radius
fibr/o	fiber	sacr/o	sacred, sacrum
fibul/o	fibula	skelet/o	skeleton
ili/o	flank, hip, groin, ilium of the pelvis	spondyl/o	vertebra
ischi/o	haunch, hip joint, ischium	stern/o	chest, sternum
menisc/o	meniscus	synov/o, synovi/o	synovial
muscul/o	muscle	tars/o	tarsal bone
my/o, myos/o	muscle	ten/o, tendon/o	stretch, tendon
myel/o	bone marrow	vertebr/o	vertebra

musculoskeletal

MUS kyoo loh SKEHL eh tahl

movement

6.1 The skeletal and muscular systems are combined to form the _____ system. Notice how this constructed term is assembled with four word parts: muscul/o/skelet/al. As you know, the bones and muscles work together to support the body and produce body _____. In fact, nearly every one of the 206 bones in your body receives an attachment to one or more muscles.

muscle

bones

1. **compact bone**
2. **periosteum**
3. **diaphysis**
4. **epiphysis**

6.2 Each bone is an organ, composed of mainly connective tissue receiving blood vessels, lymphatics, and nerves. Bones function in the support of soft internal organs, the storage of mineral salts including calcium and phosphorus, and the production of blood cells within the red bone marrow, in addition to serving as an attachment site for muscles. Each _____ is an organ also, composed mainly of skeletal muscle tissue and connective tissue. As a muscle shortens in length by contraction, it pulls on the tendons connecting it to _____ to produce body movement. Muscle contraction also produces heat, assisting the body in regulating body temperature.

6.3 Use the anatomy terms that appear in the left column to fill in the corresponding blanks in Figures 6.1■ through 6.3■.

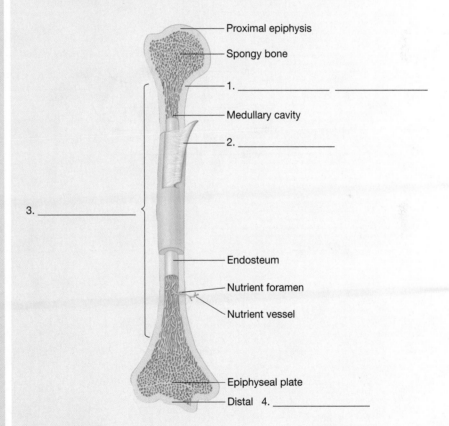

- Proximal epiphysis
- Spongy bone
1. _____ _____
- Medullary cavity
2. _____
3. _____
- Endosteum
- Nutrient foramen
- Nutrient vessel
- Epiphyseal plate
- Distal 4. _____

Figure 6.1 ■
Parts of a bone.

5. cranium
6. clavicle
7. humerus
8. sacrum
9. phalanges
10. femur

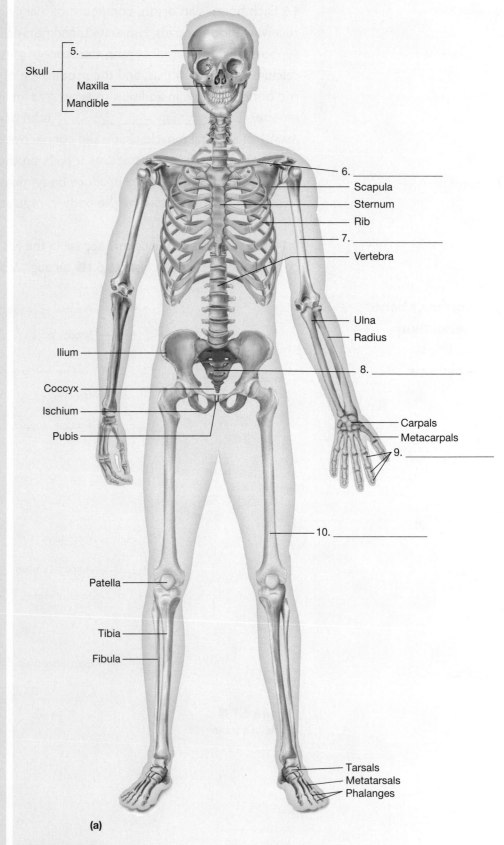

Skull
5. _____
Maxilla
Mandible

6. _____
Scapula
Sternum
Rib
7. _____
Vertebra

Ulna
Radius

Ilium
8. _____

Coccyx
Ischium
Pubis

Carpals
Metacarpals
9. _____

10. _____

Patella

Tibia
Fibula

Tarsals
Metatarsals
Phalanges

(a)

Figure 6.2 ■
The bones of the skeleton. The skeleton, anterior view.

11. **deltoid**
12. **gastrocnemius**
13. **sternocleidomastoid**
14. **biceps**
15. **rectus**

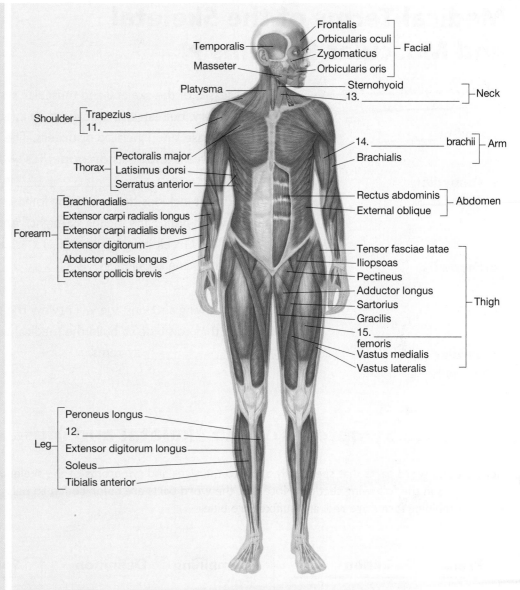

Figure 6.3 ■
The major muscles of the human body, anterior side.

Medical Terms of the Skeletal and Muscular Systems ▶▶▶▶▶

orthopedic
OR thoh PEE dik

orthopedist

6.4 The diseases of the skeletal and muscular systems are often the result of physical injury, but can also be caused by infections, tumor development, endocrine disease, and inherited disorders. The branch of medicine focusing on these diseases is known as **orthopedics**, which is commonly abbreviated to **ortho**. The term _____ is a constructed word, written orth/o/ped/ic. It includes the combining form *orth/o*, which is derived from the Greek word *orthos* and means "straight," and the word root *ped*, which is also from the Greek language and means "child." A physician specializing in this field of medicine is called an _____ (OR thoh PEE dist).

muscular
MUS kyoo lar

6.5 In the following sections, we will review the prefixes, combining forms, and suffixes that combine to build the medical terms of the skeletal and _____ systems.

Signs and Symptoms of the Skeletal and Muscular Systems

Here are the word parts that specifically apply to the signs and symptoms of the skeletal and muscular systems that are covered in the following section. Note that the word parts are color-coded to help you identify them: prefixes are green, combining forms are red, and suffixes are blue.

Prefix	Definition
a-	without, absence of
brady-	slow
dys-	bad, abnormal, painful, difficult
hyper-	excessive, abnormally high, above

Combining Form	Definition
arthr/o	joint
kinesi/o	motion
my/o	muscle
tax/o	reaction to a stimulus
ten/o	stretch, tendon
troph/o	development

Suffix	Definition
-a	singular
-algia	condition of pain
-dynia	condition of pain
-ia	condition of
-y	process of

KEY TERMS A–Z

arthralgia
ahr THRAL jee ah

6.6 Referring to the preceding word parts table, you'll see that the suffix *-algia* means "condition of pain." Add that to a combining form that means "joint," and it forms the word that means "condition of joint pain," or _____. This is often the first symptom of joint or bone disease. It is also a common complaint following injury to a joint. The constructed form of this word is arthr/algia.

ataxia
ah TAK see ah

6.7 The word root *tax* means "a reaction to a stimulus." By adding the prefix *a-* ("without"), the meaning of the term becomes negative. When the suffix *-ia* ("condition of") is added, it forms the word _____, which is the inability to coordinate muscles during a voluntary activity. Ataxia is a sign of a nervous system disorder that is often inherited. The constructed form of this word is a/tax/ia.

atrophy
AT roh fee

6.8 Stabilizing a broken limb by casting it in plaster is a common treatment for bone fractures. It prohibits movement of the limb to promote the healing process. Unfortunately, the lack of movement leads to a reduction in muscle strength due to disuse, a sign of reduced muscle size known as **atrophy**. The muscle reduction is reversible when healing is complete and muscle activity is restored. The term _____ also uses the prefix *a-* to make the meaning of the word root negative. The word root *troph* means "development" and *-y* means "process of." The three word parts that form the word can be written as a/troph/y.

bradykinesia
BRAD ee kih NEE see ah

6.9 An abnormally slow movement is a clinical sign of an underlying bone, muscle, or nervous disorder. It is known as _____, which literally means "condition of slow motion." This term is a constructed word that can be written as brady/kines/ia, in which *brady-* means "slow," *kinesi* is the word root that means "motion," and the suffix *-ia* means "condition of." (Note that the *i* in the word root is dropped when using a suffix that begins with an *i*.)

decalcification
DEE kal sih fih KAY shun

6.10 The abnormal reduction of calcium in bone is a clinical sign known as **decalcification**, which is often caused by a hormonal disorder upsetting the calcium balance between the bloodstream and bone. In many patients, _____ can be treated with a combination of hormonal therapy, a diet rich in calcium and vitamin D, and mild exercise.

dyskinesia
diss kih NEE see ah

6.11 Difficulty in movement is a common sign of a musculoskeletal disorder. Remember from the term *bradykinesia* that the word root *kinesi* means "motion," and the suffix *-ia* means "condition of." When the prefix *dys-* is added, it forms the word _____, which literally means "condition of bad, abnormal, painful, or difficult motion." The constructed form of this term can be written as dys/kines/ia.

dystrophy
DISS troh fee

6.12 A general term to describe a deformity arising during development is _____, which literally means "process of (-y) bad, abnormal, painful, or difficult (dys-) development (troph)." It is a constructed term that can be written as dys/troph/y. It is a sign of a congenital disease that occurs in different forms. For example, there are several types of muscular dystrophies, each of which appears during early childhood to produce musculoskeletal dysfunction.

hypertrophy
high PER troh fee

6.13 The sign of excessive muscle growth or development is known as _____. Although it is an abnormality, it is often induced by exercise enthusiasts by adding tension to weight-training activities. Muscular hypertrophy is produced by the addition of protein to muscle fibers, which is stimulated by strenuous muscle activity. The constructed form of this word is hyper/troph/y, in which hyper- means "excessive," troph means "development," and -y means "process of."

myalgia
my AL jee ah

6.14 During strenuous exercise, muscle cell activity may exceed the capacity of the cell to obtain and use oxygen during metabolism. When this occurs, the "oxygen debt" will cause the cell to metabolize without oxygen (called anaerobic respiration), resulting in the buildup of lactic acid in the muscle tissue. Because lactic acid causes muscle pain, a common symptom of strenuous exercise is _____, which literally means "condition of muscle (my) pain (-algia)." Its constructed form is my/algia. This form of myalgia is temporary, lasting about one day. Chronic forms of myalgia usually suggest an underlying musculoskeletal disease.

tenodynia
TEN oh DINN ee ah

6.15 Tendon pain, or **tenodynia**, is a common symptom of "weekend athletes": people who work inactive jobs during the workweek and become very active on their days off. The symptom of _____ usually indicates minor injury to one or more tendons, often lasting weeks or months. The suffix -dynia means "condition of pain," and ten/o means "stretch, tendon." The constructed form of this term is ten/o/dynia. Another suffix with the meaning of "condition of pain" is -algia. If tenodynia is intense, it may indicate tearing of the tendons that requires medical intervention.

PRACTICE: Signs and Symptoms of the Skeletal and Muscular Systems

Break the Chain

Analyze these medical terms:

a) Separate each term into its word parts; each word part is labeled for you (**p** = prefix, **r** = root, **cf** = combining form, and **s** = suffix).

b) For the Bonus Question, write the requested definition in the blank that follows.

The first set has been completed for you as an example.

1. a) arthralgia   *arthr/algia*
                                            r   s

    b) *Bonus Question:* What is the definition of the suffix? *condition of pain*

2. a) ataxia   _____/_____/_____
                                            p   r   s

    b) *Bonus Question:* What is the definition of the word root? _____

3. a) atrophy   _____/_____/_____
                                            p   r   s

    b) *Bonus Question:* What is the definition of the word root? _____

4. a) bradykinesia   _____/_____/_____
                                            p   r   s

    b) *Bonus Question:* What is the definition of the prefix? _____

5. a) dyskinesia   _____/_____/_____
                                            p   r   s

    b) *Bonus Question:* What is the definition of the word root? _____

6. a) dystrophy   _____/_____/_____
                                            p   r   s

    b) *Bonus Question:* What is the definition of the suffix? _____

7. a) hypertrophy   _____/_____/_____
                                            p   r   s

    b) *Bonus Question:* What is the definition of the prefix? _____

8. a) myalgia   _____/_____
                                            r   s

    b) *Bonus Question:* What is the definition of the word root? _____

9. a) tenodynia   _____/__/_____
                                            cf   s

    b) *Bonus Question:* What is the definition of the suffix? _____

Diseases and Disorders of the Skeletal and Muscular Systems

Here are the word parts that specifically apply to the diseases and disorders of the skeletal and muscular systems that are covered in the following section. Note that the word parts are color-coded to help you identify them: prefixes are green, combining forms are red, and suffixes are blue.

Prefix	Definition
a-	without, absence of
epi-	upon, over, above, on top
para-	alongside, abnormal
poly-	excessive, over, many
quadri-	four

Combining Form	Definition
ankyl/o	crooked
arthr/o	joint
burs/o	purse or sac, bursa
carcin/o	cancer
carp/o	wrist
chondr/o	gristle, cartilage
condyl/o	knuckle of a joint
fibr/o	fiber
kyph/o	hump
leuk/o	white
lith/o	stone
lord/o	bent forward
menisc/o	meniscus
my/o	muscle
myel/o	bone marrow
myos/o	muscle
ost/o, oste/o	bone
por/o	hole
sarc/o	flesh, meat
scoli/o	curved
spondyl/o	vertebra
synov/o, synovi/o	synovial
ten/o, tendon/o	stretch, tendon

Suffix	Definition
-algia	condition of pain
-asthenia	weakness
-cele	hernia, swelling, protrusion
-emia	condition of blood
-genesis	origin, cause
-itis	inflammation
-malacia	softening
-oma	tumor
-osis	condition of
-plasia	formation, growth
-plegia	paralysis
-ptosis	drooping

KEY TERMS A–Z

achondroplasia

ah kon droh PLAY zee ah

6.16 A **dwarf** is an individual with abnormally short limbs and stature. A disease that causes dwarfism is _____, which combines the prefix *a-* ("without, absence of"), the combining form *chondr/o* ("gristle, cartilage"), and the suffix *-plasia* ("formation, growth") to form the meaning "without cartilage formation." The constructed form of this term is a/chondr/o/plasia. It is genetically determined and involves the abnormal lack of growth of long bones. See Figure 6.4■.

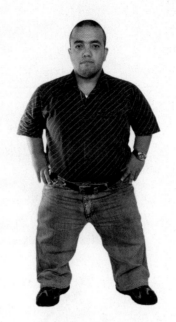

Figure 6.4 ■
Achondroplasia. The individual in this photograph has the reduced limb development that typifies this cause of dwarfism.
Source: © *itanistock/Alamy.*

ankylosis
an kill OH siss

6.17 In the disease that literally means "condition of crooked," _____, joints are abnormally stiff, and movement is difficult. Ankylosis is a condition that may follow another disease, such as arthritis, which may damage the joint structure. The constructed form of the term *ankylosis* is ankyl/osis.

arthritis
ahr THRYE tiss

6.18 The general disorder resulting in inflammation and degeneration of a joint is known as _____. It literally means "joint inflammation," which is easy to see in the constructed form of the term, arthr/itis, in which *arthr* means "joint," and the suffix *-itis* means "inflammation." There are two major forms of arthritis, each with a different cause. **Osteoarthritis (OA)** is a common condition as people age, in which the joint structures become worn over time and gradually replaced by bone. See Figure 6.5■. **Rheumatoid arthritis (RA)** is an autoimmune disease in which joint structures become eroded by the action of the body's own white blood cells.

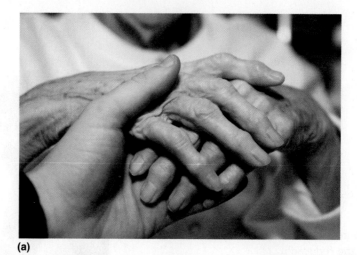
(a)

Figure 6.5 ■
Arthritis. (a) Photograph of osteoarthritis within the joints of the fingers.
Source: © painless/Fotolia
(b) Progressive changes of rheumatoid arthritis:
1. inflammation of synovial membrane; 2. progressive inflammation and beginning of cartilage destruction; 3. complete loss of synovial membrane; 4. complete joint loss.

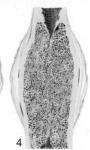
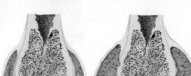
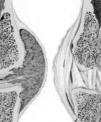
(b) 1   2   3   4

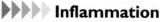

DID YOU KNOW ?

▶▶▶▶ **Inflammation**

The Latin word *inflammatio* is the origin of this term, which literally means "to ignite or set ablaze." Because the symptoms of inflammation are heat, swelling, redness, and pain, this term is aptly named!

arthrochondritis
AHR throh kon DRY tiss

6.19 In the joint disease **arthrochondritis**, the articular cartilage within synovial joints undergoes inflammation, resulting in joint pain during movements. Unlike arthritis, _____ is usually a temporary condition caused by a localized infection. As a constructed term, it can be written arthr/o/chondr/itis by putting together the combining form *arthr/o* ("joint") with the word root *chondr* ("gristle, cartilage") and the suffix *-itis* ("inflammation").

bunion
BUN yun

6.20 A **bunion** is an abnormal enlargement of the joint at the base of the big toe. A _____ is caused by an inflammation of a bursa near the big toe.

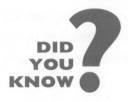

▶▶▶▶▶ **Bunion**

The term *bunion* is derived from the Old French word *buigne,* which means "a swelling caused by a blow to the head." However, the modern meaning is limited to a swelling of the big toe.

bursitis ber SIGH tiss	**6.21** Remember that the suffix *-itis* means "inflammation," and the word root *burs* means "purse or sac" and refers to a saclike bursa that cushions certain joints. So the inflammation of a bursa is known as _____. The constructed form of this term is written as burs/itis.
bursolith BER soh lith	**6.22** A calcium deposit within a bursa of the foot is known as a **bursolith**. The diagnosis of a _____ is confirmed with an X-ray and is typically surgically removed. The word root *lith* is derived from the Greek word, *lithos,* which means "a stone." The constructed form of this term is written as burs/o/lith. (Note that no suffix is used in this term.)
carpal tunnel syndrome KAR pahl * TUN ul * SIN drohm	**6.23** People working at computer stations for extended periods of time increase their risk of a repetitive stress injury of the wrist. Commonly known as _____ _____ _____, or **CTS**, it is characterized by inflammation of the wrist (tenosynovitis, see Frame 6.57) that causes pressure against the median nerve, resulting in local pain and restricted movement.
carpoptosis KAR pop TOH siss	**6.24** Also known as "wrist drop," the condition **carpoptosis** is a weakness of the wrist resulting in difficulty supporting the hand. _____ is a constructed term, which can be written as carp/o/ptosis. It literally means "drooping of the wrist" (*-ptosis* is the suffix that means "drooping" and the combining form *carp/o* means "wrist").
cramps	**6.25** Prolonged, involuntary muscular contractions cause pain wherever they occur, often striking the stomach wall or thigh muscles after strenuous exercise. The painful contractions are called _____.
DJD	**6.26** A general term describing a disease of joints in which the cartilage undergoes degeneration is called **degenerative joint disease**, abbreviated _____. This type of disease is progressive, becoming worse in time. During the process of joint degeneration, the articular cartilage degrades and is often replaced with bone. Arthritis (Frame 6.18) is the most common form of DJD.

Duchenne muscular dystrophy doo SHEN * MUS kyoo lar * DIS troh fee	**6.27** Children are occasionally born with a disease causing skeletal muscle degeneration, resulting in progressive muscle weakness and deterioration. Abbreviated **DMD**, it is called **Duchenne muscular dystrophy**. Unfortunately, _____ _____ _____ has no known cure.
epicondylitis ep ih kon dih LYE tiss	**6.28** When the suffix that means "inflammation" is combined with the word root *condyl* ("knuckle of a joint") and the prefix *epi-* ("upon, over, above, on top"), it forms the term _____. The epicondyles are small bony elevations on the humerus near the elbow joint. In epicondylitis this area of the elbow becomes inflamed, usually due to an injury. The constructed form of this term is written as epi/condyl/itis.
fibromyalgia FIE broh my AHL jee ah	**6.29** A disease of unknown origin that produces widespread pain of musculoskeletal structures of the limbs, face, and trunk is known as **fibromyalgia**. This term is constructed of the combining form *fibr/o*, the word root *my*, and the suffix *-algia*, which together mean "condition of pain of the fibers and muscles." _____ can be written as fibr/o/my/algia. Also known as **fibromyalgia syndrome**, there is some evidence that it may be, at least in part, caused by sleep deprivation.
fracture FRAK sher	**6.30** The clinical term for a break in a bone is _____. There are numerous types of fractures, many of which are described further in Table 6.1■ and illustrated in Figure 6.6■.

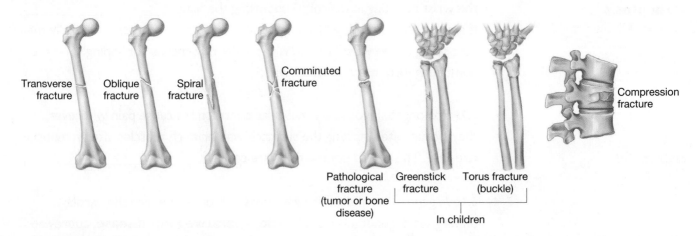

Transverse fracture   Oblique fracture   Spiral fracture   Comminuted fracture   Pathological fracture (tumor or bone disease)   Greenstick fracture   Torus fracture (buckle)   In children   Compression fracture

Figure 6.6 ■
Common bone fractures.

Table 6.1 ■ Categories of Fractures

Category	Definition
Colles' (KOH leez)	a break in the distal part of the radius
comminuted (KOM ih noo ted)	a break resulting in fragmentation of the bone
compression (kom PREH shun)	a crushed break, often due to weight or pressure applied to a bone during a fall
displaced	a break causing an abnormal alignment of bone pieces
epiphyseal (eh PIFF ih see al)	a break at the location of the growth plate, which can affect growth of the bone
greenstick	a slight break in a bone that appears as a slight fissure in an X-ray
nondisplaced	a break in which the broken bones retain their alignment
Pott's	a break at the ankle that affects both bones of the leg
spiral	a spiral-shaped break often caused by twisting stresses along a long bone

gout
  GOWT

6.31 In **gout**, a person experiences sharp pain in the joints of the toes, especially the big toe. See Figure 6.7■. The pain of _____ is often exacerbated by a diet high in protein because the disorder is caused by an abnormal accumulation of uric acid crystals in the joints, which are waste products of protein metabolism. Roughly 3 million people are currently diagnosed with gout in the United States, most of whom are males.

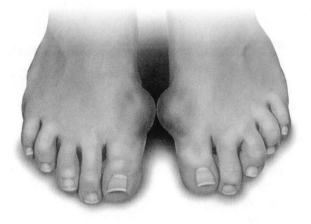

Figure 6.7 ■
Gout. Also known as gouty arthritis, it often strikes the big toe, as seen in this illustration.

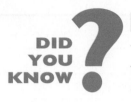

▶▶▶▶▶ **Gout**

The term *gout* is derived from the Latin word *gutta,* which means "a drop." The foot pain that characterizes gout was thought to be caused by a body fluid dripping internally onto the joint. It was a malady common to European aristocracy prior to the 20th century, made worse by poor dietary habits that included diets high in protein and low in fresh vegetables and fruits.

herniated disk
HER nee ay ted * disk

6.32 The rupture of an intervertebral disk is called **herniated disk**. It causes pressure against spinal nerves or the spinal cord to produce back pain and is regarded as the most common musculoskeletal disease. A _____ _____ is a back injury often caused by a sudden movement or an attempt to lift a heavy object. See Figure 6.8■.

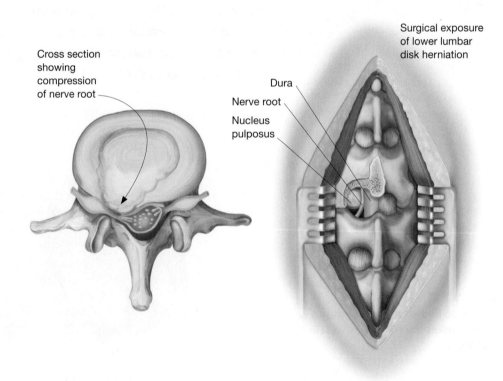

Cross section showing compression of nerve root

Surgical exposure of lower lumbar disk herniation

Dura

Nerve root

Nucleus pulposus

Figure 6.8 ■
Herniated disk. A herniated disk is a protrusion of the disk's gelatinous center, called the nucleus pulposus, which often pushes into the spinal cord or spinal nerves to cause pain and loss of movement (left illustration). The illustration on the right shows the back surgery necessary to access the injury.

kyphosis
kih FOH siss

lordosis
lor DOH siss

scoliosis
SKOH lee OH siss

6.33 Spinal curvatures are normal and help us to stand erect. However, some individuals suffer from a deformity of the spine that alters the normal curves. The three primary spinal deformities are **kyphosis**, **lordosis**, and **scoliosis**. A _____ occurs when the upper thoracic curve bends posteriorly, causing an abnormal hump at the upper back (*kyph* means "hump") that often accompanies osteoporosis (see Frame 6.46). A _____ is an exaggerated anterior spinal curve in the lumbar area (*lord* means "bent forward"). A _____ is a lateral curvature of the spine with a congenital origin, usually in the thoracic or lumbar regions (*scoli* means "curved"). See Figure 6.9■. All three terms for abnormal spinal curvatures are constructed terms. For example, scoliosis can be written as scoli/osis.

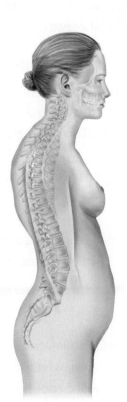 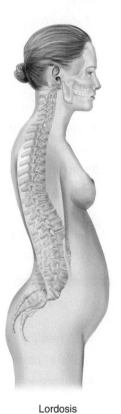 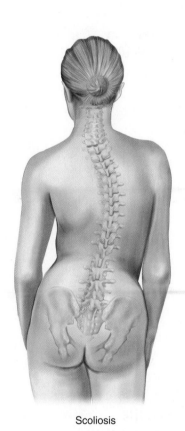

Kyphosis   Lordosis   Scoliosis

Figure 6.9 ■
Spinal disfigurements. Kyphosis, or humpback, in which the upper thoracic curve bends posteriorly; lordosis, an exaggerated anterior curve in the lumbar region; and scoliosis, a lateral curvature.

Marfan's syndrome
mahr FAHNZ * SIN drohm

6.34 The congenital disease called **Marfan's syndrome** results in excessive cartilage formation at the epiphyseal plates (growth plates), forming abnormally long limbs and a tall, thin body form. The heart valves of those suffering from _____ _____ are also deformed, resulting in valvular heart disease. Some forensic scientists have postulated that Abraham Lincoln suffered from this syndrome.

meniscitis MEN ih SIGH tiss	**6.35** A meniscus is a crescent-shaped band of cartilage that supports certain joints, such as the knee and shoulder. Inflammation of a meniscus results in joint pain and is called _____. As a constructed term, it is written as menisc/itis.
myasthenia gravis my ass THEE nee ah * GRAHV iss	**6.36 Myasthenia gravis** is characterized by a progressive failure of muscles to respond to nerve stimulation. The term _____ _____ means "serious muscle weakness." The word _gravis_ means "serious," and you may recognize _myasthenia_ as a constructed term that can be written as my/asthenia.
myeloma my ah LOH mah	**6.37** The red bone marrow is the site of blood cell formation. A malignant tumor arising from this tissue is known as **myeloma**. The term literally means "tumor of red bone marrow," in which _myel_ means "bone marrow" and _-oma_ means "tumor." The constructed form of _____ is written as myel/oma.
myocele MY oh seel	**6.38** A muscle is surrounded by a layer of tough connective tissue, known as fascia. An injury to a muscle may cause the muscle to tear through the fascia, causing a protrusion. This condition is known as a **myocele**. The constructed form of the term _____ is written as my/o/cele, which is composed of the combining form for muscle, _my/o_, and the suffix _-cele_, which means "protrusion."
myositis my oh SYE tiss	**6.39** A common result of muscle injury is a local inflammation known as **myositis**. Combining _myos_ (which means "muscle") and _-itis_ ("inflammation"), the constructed form of _____ is written as myos/itis.
osteitis OSS tee EYE tiss	**6.40** When injured or exposed to infection, bone tissue often responds with inflammation. This condition, which combines the suffix that means "inflammation" and _oste,_ the word root meaning "bone," is known as _____, which literally means "inflammation of bone." The constructed form is written as oste/itis.

osteitis deformans

OSS tee EYE tiss * day FOR manz

6.41 Also called **Paget's disease**, **osteitis deformans** results in bone deformities due to a failure of bone remodeling, which is a balance between bone loss and bone deposition. Common symptoms of _____ _____ include severe bone pain and frequent fractures. Recent evidence suggests this disease is inherited but requires a trigger by a virus. It strikes roughly 1% of the adult population in the United States.

osteosarcoma

OSS tee oh sar KOH mah

6.42 An **osteosarcoma** is bone cancer arising from connective tissue, usually within the bone itself. It is an aggressive form of cancer, striking mostly in the young and middle teens. The constructed form of bone cancer arising from connective tissue, or _____, is oste/o/sarc/oma. A second form of malignant bone cancer arises from the cells of the red bone marrow and is called **leukemia** (loo KEE mee ah). This term literally means "condition of white blood," named because of the high levels of deformed white blood cells in a blood sample that are a diagnostic of the disease.

osteogenesis imperfecta

OSS tee oh jen eh siss * im per FEK tah

6.43 An inherited disease resulting in impaired bone growth and fragile bones is known as **osteogenesis imperfecta**. The term means "imperfect bone development." Tragically, _____ _____ is progressive, leading to severe bone pain, skeletal deformities, and frequent fractures.

osteomalacia

OSS tee oh mah LAY she ah

6.44 The suffix -malacia means "softening," and the combining form oste/o means "bone." A disease resulting in the softening of bones is generally known as _____. It is a constructed term that is written as oste/o/malacia. The cause is usually a hormonal imbalance, resulting in the gradual loss of calcium to bone tissue.

osteomyelitis

OSS tee oh my eh LYE tiss

6.45 The word root myel means "bone marrow." Inflammation of the red bone marrow is a painful disease known as _____, which literally means "inflammation of red bone marrow and bone." The usual cause is a bacterial infection. Osteomyelitis is a constructed term that can be written as oste/o/myel/itis.

osteoporosis

OSS tee oh por ROH siss

6.46 The abnormal loss of bone density is a common result of aging, especially among postmenopausal women. The condition is called **osteoporosis** and results in a loss of posture and flexibility. See Figure 6.10■. The term _____ literally means "condition of holes in bone." The constructed term includes four word parts and is written as oste/o/por/osis. (The word root por means "hole.")

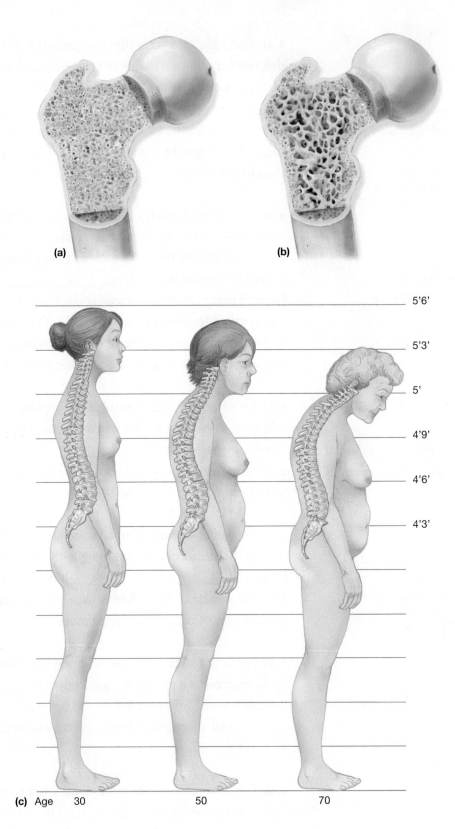

(a)

(b)

5'6'

5'3'

5'

4'9'

4'6'

4'3'

(c) Age   30   50   70

Figure 6.10 ■

Osteoporosis. (a) A section through normal spongy bone. (b) A section through a bone with osteoporosis reveals a reduction of bone spicules and additional space. (c) Spinal curvatures resulting from osteoporosis of the vertebral column with advancing age.

paraplegia
PAIR ah PLEE jee ah

quadriplegia
KWAHD rih PLEE jee ah

6.47 The suffix -*plegia* means "paralysis." One form of paralysis is _____, in which there is a loss of sensation or voluntary movement of the area of the body below the hips, including both legs. In another form of paralysis, all four limbs are without sensation or voluntary movement. It utilizes a prefix that means "four" and is called _____.

polymyositis
PALL ee my oh SYE tiss

6.48 The term _____ means "inflammation of many muscles." It is a condition caused by bacterial infection in which a group of muscles become infected and react with inflammation. The constructed form of this term is written as poly/myos/itis, in which the prefix *poly-* means "many," *myos* means "muscle," and the suffix -*itis* means "inflammation."

rickets
RIHK ehts

6.49 In the disease **rickets**, the bones become softened due to the excessive removal of calcium for other body functions. _____ is caused by a lack of calcium and/or vitamin D in the diet. Rickets is a disease of childhood, resulting in bowing of the legs and growth retardation.

rotator cuff injury

6.50 The rotator cuff is a combination of four muscles and their tendons that surround and stabilize the shoulder joint: teres minor, supraspinatus, infraspinatus, and subscapularis. A trauma to the shoulder can tear one or more tendons and muscles, resulting in a _____ _____ _____ that can cause local inflammation, pain, and joint dislocation.

spinal cord injury

6.51 A trauma to the vertebral column may result in _____ _____ _____, which is abbreviated **SCI**. If severe, the injury can cause paralysis of areas of the body below the vertebral level of the injury.

spondylarthritis
SPON dill ahr THRYE tiss

6.52 The clinical term that is formed by combining the suffix meaning "inflammation," the word root *arthr,* meaning "joint," and the word root spondyl, meaning "vertebra" is _____, which means "inflammation of joints of vertebrae." It is a relatively uncommon condition of intervertebral joints that leads to a gradual inability to flex and bend the back. The constructed form of this term is written spondyl/arthr/itis.

sprain

6.53 A _____ is a tear of collagen fibers within a ligament. See Figure 6.11 ■. It usually is caused by stretching the ligament beyond its normal range without warming or slow stretching.

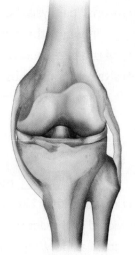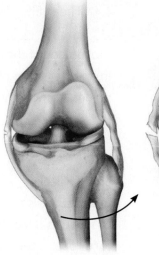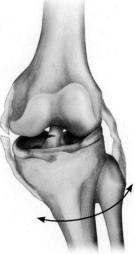

1st-degree sprain
Localized joint pain and
tenderness, but no joint laxity.

2nd-degree sprain
Detectable joint laxity, plus
localized pain and tenderness.

3rd-degree sprain
Complete disruption of
ligaments and gross joint
instability.

Figure 6.11 ■
Sprain. A sprain involves damage to one or more ligaments, and is categorized into three degrees of injury as shown.

strain	**6.54** Similar to a sprain but involving a muscle, a _____ usually is caused by stretching a muscle beyond its normal range. It often causes a bruise due to the tearing of muscle tissue and capillary damage.
temporomandibular joint disease TEMP or oh man DIH byoo lahr * JOYNT * DIS eez	**6.55** The temporomandibular joint is the junction of the mandible and the temporal bone, which allows the lower jaw to move when speaking and chewing. A disease of this joint is known as _____ _____ _____, or **TMJ**, and results in frequent dislocations that make it difficult and painful to move the jaw during speaking and chewing.
tendonitis TEN dunn EYE tiss	**6.56** Inflammation of a tendon is a common sports injury and is known as _____. An example occurs when damage is caused by throwing a ball without warming up, which is known as **rotator cuff tendonitis**. *Tendonitis* is a constructed term, written as tendon/itis.
tenosynovitis TEN oh sin oh VYE tiss	**6.57** A form of tendonitis that also involves inflammation of the synovial membrane surrounding the joint is known as _____. This term has four word parts and is written as ten/o/synov/itis, in which *ten/o* means "stretch, tendon," *synov* means "synovial," and *-itis* means "inflammation."

PRACTICE: Diseases and Disorders of the Skeletal and Muscular Systems

The Right Match

Match the term on the left with the correct definition on the right.

_____ 1. Pott's

_____ 2. gout

_____ 3. bunion

_____ 4. Duchenne muscular dystrophy

_____ 5. cramps

_____ 6. sprain

_____ 7. fracture

_____ 8. strain

_____ 9. comminuted

_____ 10. rotator cuff injury

a. an abnormal enlargement of the joint at the base of the big toe

b. a condition that causes skeletal muscle degeneration, which results in progressive muscle weakness and deterioration; abbreviated DMD

c. prolonged, involuntary muscular contractions

d. a trauma that causes tearing of tendons and/or muscles of the shoulder

e. caused by an abnormal accumulation of uric acid crystals in the joints; usually affects the big toe joints

f. an injury that results from stretching a muscle beyond its normal range

g. a type of fracture that involves a break resulting in fragmentation of the bone

h. a tear of collagen fibers within a ligament

i. a type of fracture that involves a break at the ankle that affects both bones of the leg

j. clinical term for a break in the bone

Linkup

Link the word parts in the list to create the terms that match the definitions. You may use word parts more than once. Remember to add combining vowels when needed—and that some terms do not use any combining vowel. The first one is completed as an example.

Prefix	Combining Form	Suffix
epi-	arthr/o	-asthenia
poly-	burs/o	-itis
	condyl/o	-malacia
	lith/o	-osis
	lord/o	
	menisc/o	
	my/o, myos/o	
	oste/o	
	synov/o	
	ten/o	

Definition

Term

1. weakness in the muscles — *myasthenia*

2. inflammation of many muscles simultaneously — _____

3. a spine deformity with an anterior curve of the spine — _____

4. inflammation of bony elevations (epicondyles) near the elbow joint — _____

5. inflammation and degeneration of a joint — _____

6. a gradual and painful softening of bones — _____

7. inflammation of a bursa — _____

8. inflammation of bone tissue — _____

9. a calcium deposit or stone within a bursa — _____

10. inflammation of a meniscus — _____

11. form of tendonitis that also involves inflammation of the synovial membrane — _____

Treatments, Procedures, and Devices of the Skeletal and Muscular Systems

Here are the word parts that specifically apply to the treatments, procedures, and devices associated with the skeletal and muscular systems that are covered in the following section. Note that the word parts are color-coded to help you identify them: combining forms are red, and suffixes are blue.

Combining Form	Definition
arthr/o	joint
burs/o	purse or sac, bursa
chondr/o	gristle, cartilage
cost/o	rib
crani/o	skull, cranium
electr/o	electricity
fasci/o	fascia
lamin/o	thin, lamina
my/o	muscle
orth/o	straight
ost/o, oste/o	bone
spondyl/o	vertebra
syn/o	connect
ten/o	stretch, tendon
vertebr/o	vertebra

Suffix	Definition
-centesis	surgical puncture
-clasia, -clasis	break apart
-desis	surgical fixation, fusion
-ectomy	surgical excision, removal
-gram	a record or image
-graphy	recording process
-iatry	treatment, specialty
-ist	one who specializes
-lysis	loosen, dissolve
-pathy	disease
-plasty	surgical repair
-rrhaphy	suturing
-scope	instrument used for viewing
-scopy	process of viewing
-tic	pertaining to
-tomy	incision, to cut

KEY TERMS A–Z

arthrocentesis
AHR throh sen TEE siss

6.58 The suffix *-centesis* means "surgical puncture," and the combining form *arthr/o* means "joint." Many joint injuries result in the condition of inflammation, which may slow healing and lead to additional complications. In the procedure known as _____, excess fluids are **aspirated**, or withdrawn by suction, through a surgical puncture into the synovial cavity of the joint. See Figure 6.12■. This constructed term is written as arthr/o/centesis.

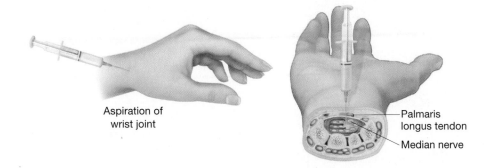

Figure 6.12 ■
Arthrocentesis. The aspiration of fluid is a common treatment for joint injuries resulting in inflammation, such as carpal tunnel syndrome (CTS) in this illustration.

Aspiration of wrist joint

Palmaris longus tendon

Median nerve

arthroclasia ahr throh KLAY see ah	**6.59** Occasionally, an abnormally stiff joint must be broken during surgery to increase the **range of motion**, or **ROM**. This procedure is called _____, in which the suffix -*clasia* means "break apart." After surgery, it is common to undergo ROM exercises to increase muscle strength and joint mobility. *Arthroclasia* is a constructed term with three word parts that is written as arthr/o/clasia.
arthrodesis ahr throh DEE siss	**6.60** The suffix -*desis* means "surgical fixation, fusion." Thus, the term _____ means "surgical fixation of a joint." The constructed form of this term is written as arthr/o/desis.
arthrogram AHR throh gram	**6.61** Prior to joint surgery, it is common to obtain an X-ray of the joint after injection of contrast media, air, or both to highlight the synovial joint. The image is printed on a film and is called an _____ because the suffix -*gram* means "a record or image." The constructed form of this term is arthr/o/gram.
arthrolysis ahr THROH loh siss	**6.62** The suffix -*lysis* means "loosen, dissolve." During an _____, a joint is loosened of abnormal restrictions, such as calcium deposits and bursoliths (see Frame 6.22). The constructed form of this term is arthr/o/lysis.
arthroplasty AHR throh PLASS tee	**6.63** The suffix -*plasty* means "surgical repair." The goal of an _____ procedure is to repair a joint. A complete arthroplasty refers to a joint replacement, the most common of which is a hip replacement. The constructed form of this term is arthr/o/plasty.

arthroscopy
ahr THROSS koh pee

6.64 An endoscopic visual examination of a joint cavity uses an instrument that integrates fiber optics, live-action photography, and computer enhancement, known as an **arthroscope**. The viewing process is called _____. When arthroscopy is part of a surgery, the procedure is called **arthroscopic surgery**. See Figure 6.13■.

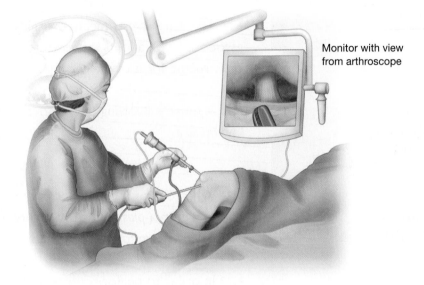

Monitor with view from arthroscope

Figure 6.13 ■
Arthroscopic surgery. In this illustration, the knee joint is undergoing surgery with a specialized endoscope called an arthroscope in the procedure known as arthroscopic surgery.

arthrotomy
ahr THROTT oh mee

6.65 The suffix -*tomy* means "incision, to cut." A surgical incision into the synovial cavity of a joint is known as _____. The constructed form of the term is arthr/o/tomy.

bursectomy
ber SEK toh mee

6.66 A surgery involving the removal of a bursa from a joint is known as a _____. The constructed form of the term is burs/ectomy, in which *burs* means "purse or sac" and -*ectomy* means "surgical excision or removal."

chiropractic
KIGH roh PRAK tik

6.67 The field of therapy that is centered on manipulation of bones and joints, most commonly the vertebral column, is known as _____. A practitioner of this therapy is called a **chiropractor** (KIGH roh prak tor).

chondrectomy
kon DREK toh mee

6.68 Surgical excision, or removal, of the cartilage associated with a joint is a common procedure known as _____. The surgery commonly uses arthroscopy to reduce the size of the incision and improve the surgeon's view. It is a constructed term that can be written as chondr/ectomy to reveal its two word parts: *chondr*, which means "gristle, cartilage," and -*ectomy*, which means "surgical excision or removal."

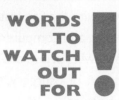

▶▶▶▶▶ *-ectomy* or *-tomy*?

These two suffixes look very similar, but how do you tell them apart? One easy way is to remember that *-ectomy* means "**e**xcision" (see how they both start with an e?). The suffix *-tomy* means "incision" or "to cut," and this meaning does not start with an e.

---

chondroplasty
KON droh plass tee

6.69 The suffix *-plasty* means "surgical repair." Surgical repair of cartilage associated with a joint is known as _____. The constructed form of the term is chondr/o/plasty.

---

costectomy
koss TEK toh mee

6.70 A surgery involving the removal of a rib (the combining form is *cost/o*) is known as a _____.

---

cranioplasty
KRAY nee oh plass tee

6.71 When one or more bones of the cranium (*crani/o*) undergo repair during surgery (*-plasty*), the procedure is called _____. The constructed term for this procedure is crani/o/plasty.

---

craniotomy
KRAY nee OTT oh mee

6.72 In order to perform surgery of the brain, a **craniotomy** is required, during which the surgeon enters the cranial cavity. The constructed form of _____ is written as crani/o/tomy, in which the combining form *crani/o* means "skull, cranium," and the suffix *-tomy* means "incision, to cut."

---

diskectomy
disk EK toh mee

6.73 A surgical procedure that is used frequently to reduce the pain of a herniated disk by surgically removing the intervertebral disk is a _____. It may also be called a **spinal fusion** when the adjacent vertebrae are fused together following the removal of the disk. An alternate term for spinal fusion is **spondylosyndesis** (SPON dih loh sin DEE siss), which literally means "surgical fixation to connect vertebrae." This constructed term is written as spondyl/o/syn/desis, in which the combining form *spondyl/o* means "vertebra," *syn* means "connect," and the suffix *-desis* means "surgical fixation, fusion." Also performed to treat a herniated disk is a **laminectomy** (lahm ih NEK toh mee), during which the part of a vertebra known as the lamina is surgically removed to relieve pressure on the spinal cord.

electromyography
ee LEK troh my OG rah fee

6.74 The strength of a muscle contraction can be measured and recorded by a procedure called **electromyography**. It utilizes an instrument that electrically stimulates a muscle, and the resulting contraction is recorded and analyzed on a computer. In this term, *electr/o* means "electricity," *my/o* means "muscle," and *-graphy* means "recording process." _____ includes five word parts and is written as electr/o/my/o/graphy.

fasciotomy
FASH ee OTT oh mee

6.75 A surgical incision into the connective tissue sheath surrounding a muscle, called fascia, is known as a _____. The constructed form of this term is fasci/o/tomy.

fracture reduction

6.76 Orthopedic surgeons, or orthopedists, treat fractures by aligning the broken bones to their normal positions in a procedure known as **reduction**. Manipulating the bone without surgery during reduction is known as **closed** _____ _____. If surgical intervention is needed to align the broken area, the procedure is called **open fracture reduction**. During this procedure, pins, screws, rods, or plates may be used to stabilize the alignment, known as **internal fixation**. In **external fixation**, metal rods and pins are attached from outside the skin surface. External fixation carries the advantage of avoiding the use of a plaster cast for immobilization. If the normal healing process is impeded, **bone grafting** or **electrical bone stimulation** may be applied to stimulate the healing process.

myoplasty
MY oh plass tee

myorrhaphy
my OR ah fee

6.77 The combining form *my/o* means "muscle." A muscle may become torn during a serious injury and require surgical intervention to promote healing. During a _____, a muscle undergoes surgical repair (*-plasty*). The constructed form of the term is written my/o/plasty. The repair often includes suturing the torn ends together in the procedure known as _____. The constructed form of the term is my/o/rrhaphy, in which the suffix *-rrhaphy* means "suturing."

NSAIDs

6.78 The most common pharmacological treatment for any condition, including inflammation or pain of muscle or bone tissue, is the use of **nonsteroidal anti-inflammatory** drugs, commonly abbreviated _____. Examples of NSAIDs are aspirin and ibuprofen.

orthotics or THOTT iks	**6.79** The field of medical support involving the construction and fitting of orthopedic appliances to assist a patient, such as lifts, artificial limbs, and retraction devices, is known as **orthotics**. Formed from the combining form *orth/o*, which means "straight," and the suffix *-tic*, which means "pertaining to," this constructed term is written as orth/o/tics. A specialist in _____ is called an **orthotist** (or THOTT ist). The medical term for an artificial limb is **prosthesis** (pross THEE siss).
ostectomy oss TEK toh mee	**6.80** An _____ is the surgical removal, or excision, of bone tissue. It is performed to remove unwanted bony formations. The constructed form of this term is ost/ectomy, in which the suffix meaning "surgical excision or removal" is added to the word root for bone (*ost*).
osteoclasis OSS tee oh KLAY siss	**6.81** In some cases, it becomes necessary to break a bone purposely to correct a defect or an improperly healed fracture. Formed by adding the suffix *-clasis*, meaning "break apart," to the combining form that means "bone," the name of the procedure is _____. It is a constructed term that is written oste/o/clasis.
osteopathy OSS tee OPP ah thee	**6.82** A medical field that emphasizes the relationship between the musculoskeletal system and overall health with an emphasis on body alignment and nutrition is called **osteopathy**. The constructed form is oste/o/pathy. A physician trained in _____ is known as an **osteopath** or **osteopathic surgeon**, and is symbolized by the abbreviation **DO**.
osteoplasty OSS tee oh plass tee	**6.83** The surgical repair of bone is a general procedure known as _____. This term is formed by adding the suffix *-plasty* ("surgical repair") to the combining form *oste/o* ("bone"). The constructed form is oste/o/plasty.

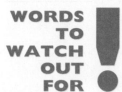

WORDS TO WATCH OUT FOR

▶▶▶▶▶ *-pathy* or *-plasty*?

These two suffixes look very similar, but how do you tell them apart? The suffix *-pathy* means "disease," whereas the meaning of the suffix *-plasty* is "surgical repair." One easy way to tell them apart is to think of the sound of *-plasty*: it sounds like "plaster," which is a home product that is used to repair walls.

podiatry poh DYE ah tree	**6.84** The Greek word for foot is *podos*. This word root, combined with the suffix *-iatry*, which means "treatment or specialty," is used to construct the term _____, which is the specialty that focuses on foot health. A healthcare professional trained in this field is called a **podiatrist** (poh DYE ah trist).
tenomyoplasty TEN oh MY oh plass tee	**6.85** Some injuries involve damage to both the muscle and its associated tendon. The surgical procedure involving the repair of both muscle and tendon is called a _____. This constructed term may be written as ten/o/my/o/plasty to reveal its word parts: the combining forms *ten/o*, meaning "stretch, tendon," and *my/o*, meaning "muscle"; and the suffix *-plasty*, meaning "surgical repair."
tenorrhaphy ten OR ah fee	**6.86** Stepping into a hole and falling can cause a serious injury to the calcaneal tendon of the ankle. This tendon, also known as the Achilles tendon, attaches the powerful calf muscles to the large heel bone (calcaneus). If it tears, mobility of the affected leg becomes impossible until surgical intervention corrects the injury. The surgery is called a _____ and involves the suturing of a tendon to close a tear. This constructed term is written as ten/o/rrhaphy to reveal its word parts. In this term, the suffix *-rrhaphy*, which means "suturing," is added to the combining form that means "stretch, tendon."
tenotomy ten OTT oh mee	**6.87** A tenorrhaphy often includes the _____ procedure, during which one or more incisions are made into a tendon. Also a constructed term, it is written as ten/o/tomy, using the combining form that means "stretch, tendon" and the suffix that means "incision, to cut."
vertebroplasty VERT eh broh plass tee	**6.88** A surgical procedure that repairs damaged or diseased vertebrae is called a _____. Adding the combining form that means "vertebra" with the suffix that means "surgical repair" creates this constructed term, which is written vertebr/o/plasty.

PRACTICE: Treatments, Procedures, and Devices of the Skeletal and Muscular Systems

The Right Match

Match the term on the left with the correct definition on the right.

_____ 1. reduction

_____ 2. aspiration

_____ 3. arthrocentesis

_____ 4. nonsteroidal anti-inflammatory drugs

_____ 5. spinal fusion

_____ 6. arthroscopy

_____ 7. chondroplasty

_____ 8. tenorrhaphy

_____ 9. podiatry

_____ 10. arthrogram

a. the most common pharmacological treatment for inflammation or pain of muscle or bone tissue

b. a procedure in which adjacent vertebrae are fused together following a diskectomy

c. withdrawing by suction

d. a procedure in which excess fluids are aspirated through a surgical puncture in the joint

e. a procedure that aligns broken bones to their normal positions

f. an X-ray image of a joint that is printed on a film

g. healthcare specialty that focuses on foot health

h. an endoscopic visual examination of a joint cavity

i. surgical repair of cartilage

j. a surgery that sutures a tear in a tendon

Break the Chain

Analyze these medical terms:

a) Separate each term into its word parts; each word part is labeled for you (**p** = prefix, **r** = root, **cf** = combining form, and **s** = suffix).

b) For the Bonus Question, write the requested word part or definition in the blank that follows.

1. a) arthrodesis   _____ / ___ / _____
                                      cf   s

   b) *Bonus Question:* What is the definition of the suffix?_____

2. a) chondrectomy   _____ / _____
                                   r   s

   b) *Bonus Question:* What is the definition of the word root?_____

3. a) craniotomy   _____ / ___ / _____
                                      cf   s

   b) *Bonus Question:* Does this term contain a prefix?_____

4. a) laminectomy   _____ / _____
                                   r   s

   b) *Bonus Question:* What is the definition of the suffix?_____

5. a) electromyography   _____ / ___ / _____ / ___ / _____
                                      cf   cf   s

   b) *Bonus Question:* What is the definition of the second combining form?_____

6. a) orthotics   _____ / ___ / _____
                                      cf   s

   b) *Bonus Question:* What is the definition of the combining form?_____

7. a) osteoclasis   _____ / ___ / _____
                                      cf   s

   b) *Bonus Question:* What is the definition of the suffix?_____

8. a) tenomyoplasty   _____ / ___ / _____ / ___ / _____
                                      cf   cf   s

   b) *Bonus Question:* What is the definition of the suffix?_____

9. a) osteoplasty   _____ / ___ / _____
                                      cf   s

   b) *Bonus Question:* What is the definition of the combining form?_____

Abbreviations of the Skeletal and Muscular Systems

The abbreviations that are associated with the skeletal and muscular systems are summarized here. Study these abbreviations, and review them in the exercise that follows.

Abbreviation	Definition
ACL	anterior cruciate ligament, a ligament that stabilizes the knee joint
CTS	carpal tunnel syndrome
DJD	degenerative joint disease
DMD	Duchenne muscular dystrophy
DO	physician specializing in osteopathy
EMG	electromyography
HNP	herniated nucleus pulposus, a herniated intervertebral disk
MG	myasthenia gravis
NSAIDs	nonsteroidal anti-inflammatory drugs

Abbreviation	Definition
OA	osteoarthritis
ortho	orthopedics
RA	rheumatoid arthritis
ROM	range of motion
SCI	spinal cord injury
THR	total hip replacement
TKA	total knee arthroplasty
TKR	total knee replacement
TMJ	temporomandibular joint
Vertebrae	
C1 through C7	the seven cervical vertebrae
T1 through T12	the twelve thoracic vertebrae
L1 through L5	the five lumbar vertebrae

PRACTICE: Abbreviations

Fill in the blanks with the abbreviation or the complete medical term.

Abbreviation	Medical Term
1. _____	spinal cord injury
2. TKA	_____
3. _____	rheumatoid arthritis
4. DMD	_____
5. _____	herniated nucleus pulposus
6. EMG	_____
7. _____	anterior cruciate ligament
8. THR	_____
9. _____	the five lumbar vertebrae
10. CTS	_____
11. _____	range of motion
12. OA	_____
13. _____	total knee replacement
14. T1–T12	_____
15. _____	degenerative joint disease
16. TMJ	_____
17. _____	myasthenia gravis

Chapter Review

Word Building

Construct medical terms from the following meanings. The first question has been completed for you as an example.

1. a gradual and painful softening of bone   osteo_malacia_____

2. abnormal loss of bone density   osteo_____

3. paralysis of lower body, including both legs   _____plegia

4. abnormal lateral curve of the spine   scoli_____

5. inflammation of a tendon and synovial membrane   teno_____

6. X-ray film of a joint   arthro_____

7. inflammation of a meniscus   _____itis

8. surgical incision into a joint   arthro_____

9. muscular weakness   my_____

10. protrusion of muscle through its fascia   myo_____

11. a repetitive stress injury of the wrist   _____tunnel syndrome

12. a therapy in which a joint is loosened of its restrictions   arthro_____

13. a viral infection of bone that accelerates bone loss   _____'s disease

14. a rupture of an intervertebral disk   _____ disk

15. surgical repair of a joint   arthro_____

16. pain in a tendon   teno_____

17. a calcium deposit within a bursa   burso_____

18. abnormal condition of joint stiffness   _____osis

19. abnormally slow movements   _____kinesia

20. an abnormal reduction of calcium in bone   _____ (do this one on your own!)

21. surgical stabilization of a joint   arthro_____

22. a progressive disease of the joints in which the cartilage degenerates; abbreviated DJD   degenerative _____

23. an orthopedic procedure in which metal rods and pins are attached from outside the skin surface to align a bone fracture   external _____

24. a disease of unknown origin that produces widespread pain of musculoskeletal structures of the limbs, face, and trunk (but not joints)   _____myalgia

25. a tumor that forms in the red bone marrow   myel_____

26. lacking development, or wasting   _____trophy

▶▶▶▶ **Medical Report Exercises**

Jorge Johnson _____

Read the following medical report, then answer the questions that follow.

PEARSON GENERAL HOSPITAL

PGH

5500 University Avenue, Metropolis, TX
Phone: (211) 594-4000 • Fax: (211) 594-4001

Medical Consultation: Orthopedics

Date: 6/15/2011

Patient: Jorge Johnson

Patient Complaint: Severe pain of the right ankle with any movement of the lower limb, which began during an injury while playing touch football 10 hours prior to check-in. The patient has also reported bleeding of the right ankle.

History: 35-year-old male African-American with no prior histories of musculoskeletal challenges. Social History: The patient is physically active, and reports the injury occurred during a weekend touch football game.

Family History: Father deceased at 82 years of age, Type 2 diabetic with COPD. Mother Type 2 diabetic with right amputation of lower limb at knee.

Allergies: None

Physical Examination: All vital signs are normal, with slightly elevated blood pressure of 127/84. Broken skin at right ankle at distal end of the tibia and fibula. Erythema and edema surrounding the right ankle and into the foot. Edema at the Achilles tendon. X-rays taken shortly after check-in indicate compound Pott's fracture of right ankle.

Diagnosis: Compound Pott's fracture of the distal end of the right tibia and fibula with tendinitis of Achilles tendon.

Treatment: Apply ice to wound and Achilles tendon immediately and elevate right leg. Prep for surgery. Ortho surgery to remove bone fragments and realign fracture. Close with sutures and cast right ankle and leg below the knee in plaster. Schedule follow-up in two weeks.

Jonathan McIntyre, M.D.
Jonathan McIntyre, M.D.

Photo Source: Monkey Business Images/Shutterstock

Comprehension Questions

1. What is the evidence supporting a diagnosis of a compound fracture? _____

_____

_____

2. Why are X-rays required before treatment can begin? _____

_____

_____

3. In what area of the body might a Pott's fracture occur? _____

_____

_____

Case Study Questions

The following case study provides further discussion regarding the patient in the medical report. Fill in the blanks with the correct terms. Choose your answers from the list of terms that precedes the case study. (Note that some terms may be used more than once.)

compound	myalgia	myositis
polymyositis	Pott's	tendonitis

A 35-year-old patient named Jorge Johnson received injuries during a weekend touch football game in the park. Upon his arrival at emergency, he presented an open, or (a) _____ fracture of the distal end of the right tibia and fibula, pain, and discoloration of the ankle that suggested damage to a tendon, or (b) _____, and muscle tenderness or (c) _____ that suggested damaged muscle fibers or (d) _____, and inflammation of all muscles of the right lower extremity, or (e) _____. An X-ray examination revealed a fracture at the right ankle, called a (f) _____ fracture, with associated inflammation of the Achilles tendon, or generalized (g) _____.

Debra Simpson _____

For a greater challenge, read the following medical report and answer the critical thinking questions that follow.

PEARSON GENERAL HOSPITAL

PGH

5500 University Avenue, Metropolis, ID
Phone: (211) 594-4000 • Fax: (211) 594-4001

Medical Consultation: Orthopedics

Date: 10/22/2011

Patient: Debra Simpson

Patient Complaint: Difficulty moving, loss of ability to stand erect. Pain in both hands with a loss of dexterity.

History: 85-year-old widowed female with 3 adult children; complete hysterectomy at age 65.

Family History: Father and mother deceased in automobile accident 35 years ago; no histories on file.

Allergies: None

Physical Examination: All vital signs are normal. Kyphosis with dyskinesia observed. Hardened swelling and erythema in the joints of the fingers. X-rays indicate a reduced bone density.

Diagnosis: Osteoporosis, osteoarthritis.

Treatment: Hormone therapy with calcium supplements and mild exercise for osteoporosis. Recommend NSAIDs to help manage the OA.

Paula S. Medina, M.D.

Paula S. Medina, M.D.

Photo Source: absolut/Shutterstock

Comprehension Questions

1. What is the diagnosis? _____

_____

_____

2. What term is abbreviated OA? _____

_____

_____

3. What is the meaning of the term *osteoporosis*? _____

_____

_____

Case Study Questions

The following case study provides further discussion regarding the patient in the medical report. Recall the terms from this chapter to fill in the blanks with the correct terms.

Debra Simpson, an 85-year-old female, was initially seen by her personal general practitioner when she complained of

difficulty in movement, or (h) _____, and joint pain, or (i) _____, of both wrists. The

GP referred her to (j) _____ due to an abnormal bent-over posture, called a

(k) _____, the presence of a minor back hump, or (l) _____, and X-ray exams

that indicated a loss of bone density. Based on these findings, the initial diagnosis was (m) _____. The

orthopedist also reported advanced joint degeneration in her carpometacarpal and metacarpophalangeal joints that was

diagnosed as (n) _____ due to her advanced age. Treatments were prescribed to include hormone

therapy with calcium supplements and mild exercise for the bone loss, and NSAIDs for OA management.

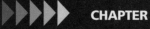

CHAPTER 7

Blood and the Lymphatic System

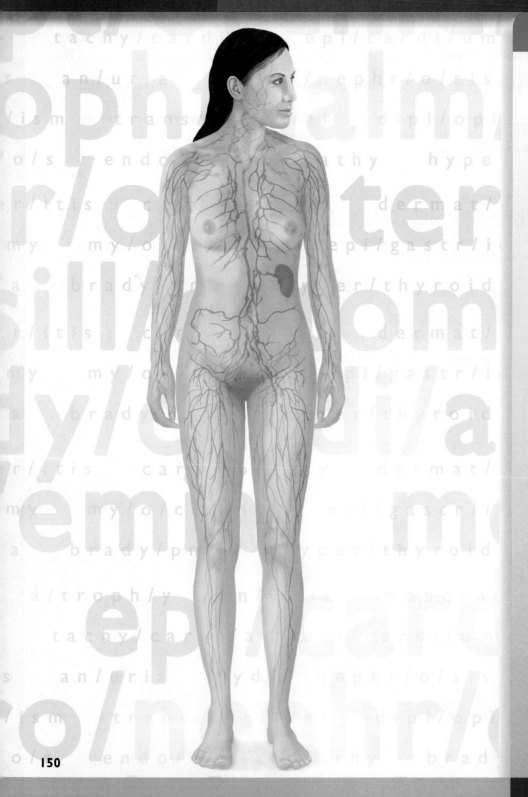

LEARNING OBJECTIVES

After completing this chapter, you will be able to:

1 Define and spell the word parts used to create terms for the blood and the lymphatic system.

2 Break down and define common medical terms used for symptoms, diseases, disorders, procedures, and treatments associated with the blood and the lymphatic system.

3 Build medical terms from the word parts associated with the blood and the lymphatic system.

4 Pronounce and spell common medical terms associated with the blood and the lymphatic system.

Anatomy and Physiology Terms ▶▶▶▶▶

The following table provides the combining forms that specifically apply to the anatomy and physiology of the blood and the lymphatic system. Note that the combining forms are colored red to help you identify them when you see them later in the chapter.

Combining Form	Definition	Combining Form	Definition
aden/o	gland	lymph/o	clear water or fluid
bacteri/o	bacteria	path/o	disease
blast/o	germ, bud, developing cell	splen/o	spleen
erythr/o	red	thromb/o	clot
hem/o, hemat/o	blood	thym/o	wartlike, thymus gland
immun/o	exempt, immunity	tox/o	poison
leuk/o	white		

blood

lymph

7.1 Although the blood is a tissue that is part of the cardiovascular system, the blood is also closely associated with another system, the lymphatic system. Therefore, the blood and lymphatic system are combined in this chapter. In the human body, blood is normally found only within the heart and blood vessels of the cardiovascular system. As _____ courses through these organs, it performs its primary function of transport. Its components include red blood cells, white blood cells, platelets, and plasma. Another type of body fluid, known as lymph, also transports substances throughout the body, but this fluid is found only within lymphatic vessels. Lymphatic vessels and _____ are important parts of the lymphatic system, along with the lymph nodes, spleen, and thymus gland. Lymph carries the components of immunity, such as white blood cells and the products they use to fight infection. Amazingly, blood and lymph are intertwined because lymph is formed from blood during capillary exchange and rejoins the bloodstream later. And, because both blood and lymph carry white blood cells, both fluids are involved in the fight against infection.

transport

protection

7.2 The primary function of blood is the _____ of substances throughout the body. Vital substances carried by the blood include oxygen, carbon dioxide, hormones, enzymes, nutrients, and waste materials. The blood also protects against infectious disease and helps regulate body temperature. The primary function of the lymphatic system is _____ from infectious disease. It also recycles fluids from the extracellular environment to the bloodstream.

1. **neutrophil**
2. **platelets**
3. **red blood cells**

7.3 Use the anatomy terms that appear in the left column to fill in the corresponding blanks in Figures 7.1■ and 7.2■.

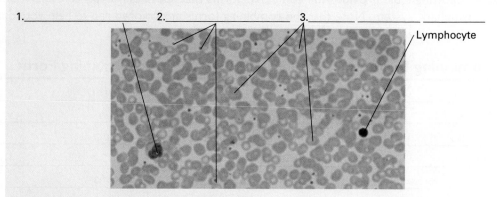

1._____ 2._____ 3._____ _____ _____

Lymphocyte

Figure 7.1 ■
A blood smear. The smear reveals representative cells from each formed element group: red blood cells, platelets, and two white blood cells (shown is a lymphocyte and a neutrophil).

4. **lymphatic vessel**
5. **thymus gland**
6. **spleen**
7. **lymph nodes**

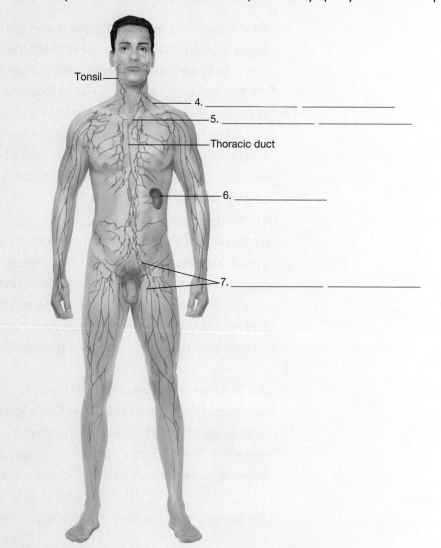

Tonsil

4. _____ _____

5. _____ _____

Thoracic duct

6. _____

7. _____ _____

Figure 7.2 ■
The lymphatic system. Lymphatic vessels, major lymph nodes, and lymphatic organs. The direction of lymph flow is toward the heart.

Medical Terms of the Blood and the Lymphatic System ▶▶▶▶▶

transport

diagnostic

7.4 Because blood is a vital fluid, making sure it is healthy is an important part of healthcare management. Like any other tissue, blood can become diseased from any one of several sources, including inherited abnormalities, infection, or tumor development. The loss of blood itself can become a life-threatening situation if intervention is not provided in time, due to its important function as a _____ medium for gases, enzymes, nutrients, hormones, blood cells, and other substances. Fortunately, blood serves as an important diagnostic tool. Because blood can be conveniently removed from a blood vessel and analyzed, it is an important avenue for testing body chemistry as well as blood cells during a _____ evaluation.

hemat/o/logy

hematologist

7.5 The general field of medicine focusing on blood-related disease is known as **hematology** (HEE mah TALL oh jee). You should recognize this term as being constructed of three word parts and shown as _____/_____/_____. It includes the combining form _hemat/o_, which is derived from the Greek word for blood, _haima_, and the suffix _-logy_ that means "study or science of." A physician specializing in the treatment of disease associated with blood is called a _____ (HEE mah TALL oh jist), or alternatively a **hematopathologist** (hee MAH toh path ALL oh jist).

infection

lymph

7.6 The lymphatic system has dual functions: the filtering and recycling of fluid to the bloodstream and the battle against _____. A disease of the lymphatic system can affect either function, or perhaps both. Also, because the lymphatic system components are distributed throughout the body, a lymphatic disease can spread quickly to distant areas of the body. In fact, metastasizing cancer cells often use the low-pressure current of the _____ to travel from one area of the body to another. In addition to tumors, lymphatic disease also includes infections that may overwhelm the immune response and inherited conditions that result in deficiencies in immune protection.

immun/o/logy

bacteriology

7.7 Our understanding of infectious disease has grown rapidly during the past 50 years, due mainly to new information coming from research labs. The field of medicine that treats this form of disease is generally called **immunology** (IM yoo NALL oh jee) or, at some hospitals, **infectious disease**. The term *immunology* refers to the body's ability to defend against infection and includes a variety of mechanisms. This is a constructed term, written as _____/_____/_____, where *immun/o* is a combining form derived from the Latin word *immunis,* which means "exempt or immunity," and *-logy* is the often-used suffix that means "study or science of." Subspecialties in the field of infectious disease include **virology** (vih RALL oh jee; study of viruses), and _____ (bak TEER ee ALL oh jee; study of bacteria).

lymphatic
lim FAT ik

7.8 In the following sections, we will review the prefixes, combining forms, and suffixes that combine to build the medical terms of the blood and the _____ system.

Signs and Symptoms of the Blood and the Lymphatic System

Here are the word parts that specifically apply to the signs and symptoms of the blood and the lymphatic system that are covered in the following section. Note that the word parts are color-coded to help you identify them: prefixes are green, combining forms are red, and suffixes are blue.

Prefix	Definition
an-	without, absence of
iso-	equal
macro-	large
poly-	excessive, over, many

Combining Form	Definition
bacteri/o	bacteria
cyt/o	cell
erythr/o	red
hem/o	blood
leuk/o	white
poikil/o	irregular
splen/o	spleen
thromb/o	clot
tox/o	poison

Suffix	Definition
-emia	condition of blood
-ia	condition of
-lysis	loosen, dissolve
-megaly	abnormally large
-osis	condition of
-penia	abnormal reduction in number, deficiency
-rrhage	abnormal discharge

KEY TERMS A–Z

anisocytosis
an EYE soh sigh TOH siss

7.9 The presence of red blood cells of unequal size in a sample of blood is an abnormal finding. It is a sign known as **anisocytosis**. The constructed form of this term is an/iso/cyt/osis, in which *an-* is a prefix that means "without or absence of," *iso-* is a prefix that means "equal," *cyt/o* is the combining form for "cell," and *-osis* means "condition of." Thus, _____ literally means "condition of without equal cells."

bacteremia
bak ter EE mee ah

7.10 The presence of bacteria in a sample of blood is a sign of an infection and is called **bacteremia**. The constructed form of this term reveals two word parts, bacter/emia. Because the suffix -emia means "condition of blood," _____ literally means "condition of bacteria in the blood."

erythropenia
ee RITH roh PEE nee ah

erythr/o/cyt/o/penia

7.11 The suffix -penia means "abnormal reduction in number, deficiency." It is used in the term _____ to describe an abnormally reduced number of red blood cells in a sample of blood. This constructed term is written erythr/o/penia. It is also called **erythrocytopenia**, which is also a constructed term and is written _____/___/_____/___/_____.

hemolysis
hee MALL ih siss

7.12 The rupture of red blood cells may occur if a blood transfusion is not compatible with the recipient's blood. The rupture of the red blood cell membrane is called **hemolysis**. The constructed form of _____ is written hem/o/lysis, which literally means "dissolve blood."

hemorrhage
HEM eh rihj

7.13 The abnormal loss of blood from the circulation is a sign of trauma or illness. It is called _____, which is a constructed term written hem/o/rrhage.

leukopenia
loo koh PEE nee ah

leuk/o/cyt/o/penia

7.14 An abnormally reduced number of white blood cells in a sample of blood is a sign of disease called _____. The constructed form of this term is leuk/o/penia. It is also called **leukocytopenia** (LOO koh SIGH toh PEE nee ah), which is also a constructed term and is written _____/___/_____/___/_____.

macrocytosis
MAK roh sigh TOH siss

7.15 The presence of abnormally large red blood cells in a sample of blood is a sign of disease and is called **macrocytosis**. The constructed form of _____ is written macro/cyt/osis, which literally means "condition of large cell."

poikilocytosis
POY kih loh sigh TOH siss

7.16 The combining form poikil/o means "irregular." The presence of tear-shaped red blood cells in a sample of blood is called _____. The constructed form of this term is poikil/o/cyt/osis, which literally means "condition of irregular cell."

polycythemia
pall ee sigh THEE mee ah

7.17 The prefix *poly-* means "excessive, over, many." When combined with the word roots that mean cell (*cyt*) and blood (*hem*) and the suffix that means "condition of" (*-ia*), the term _____ is formed. This constructed term is written poly/cyt/hem/ia. Polycythemia, which is an abnormal increase in the number of red blood cells in the blood, may also be called **erythrocytosis** (eh RITH roh sigh TOH siss). This is also a constructed term, written erythr/o/cyt/osis, that literally means "condition of red cell."

splenomegaly
splee noh MEG ah lee

7.18 The suffix *-megaly* means "abnormally large." Abnormal enlargement of the spleen is a symptom of injury or infection and is called _____. The constructed form is written splen/o/megaly, which literally means "abnormally large spleen."

thrombopenia
throm boh PEE nee ah

thromb/o/cyt/o/penia

7.19 An abnormally reduced number of platelets in a sample of blood is a symptom of disease called **thrombopenia**. The constructed form of _____ is thromb/o/penia. It is also called **thrombocytopenia** (THROM boh SIGH toh PEE nee ah), which is also a constructed term and is written _____/___/_____/___/_____.

toxemia
tahk SEE mee ah

7.20 The presence of toxins in the bloodstream is a symptom known as _____. The constructed form is tox/emia, which literally means "condition of blood poison."

PRACTICE: Signs and Symptoms of the Blood and the Lymphatic System

The Right Match

Match the term on the left with the correct definition on the right.

_____ 1. anisocytosis

_____ 2. bacteremia

_____ 3. splenomegaly

_____ 4. toxemia

_____ 5. erythropenia

_____ 6. macrocytosis

_____ 7. poikilocytosis

_____ 8. polycythemia

_____ 9. hemorrhage

a. presence of bacteria in the blood

b. abnormally reduced number of red blood cells

c. abnormally large red blood cells

d. presence of red blood cells of unequal size

e. abnormal increase in number of red blood cells

f. irregularly shaped red blood cells

g. presence of toxins in the bloodstream

h. abnormal loss of blood from the circulation

i. abnormal enlargement of the spleen

Break the Chain

Analyze these medical terms:

a) Separate each term into its word parts; each word part is labeled for you (**p** = prefix, **r** = root, **cf** = combining form, and **s** = suffix).

b) For the Bonus Question, write the requested definition in the blank that follows.

The first set has been completed as an example.

1. a) polycythemia
    <u>poly/cyt/hem/ia</u>
       p   r   r   s

    b) *Bonus Question:* What is the definition of the suffix? *condition of*

2. a) thrombopenia
    _____/___/_____
         cf   s

    b) *Bonus Question:* What is the definition of the combining form? _____

3. a) leukopenia
    _____/___/_____
         cf   s

    b) *Bonus Question:* What is the definition of the suffix? _____

4. a) hemolysis
    _____/___/_____
         cf   s

    b) *Bonus Question:* What is the definition of the suffix? _____

5. a) leukocytopenia
    _____/___/_____/___/_____
         cf   cf   s

    b) *Bonus Question:* What is the definition of the first combining form? _____

Diseases and Disorders of the Blood and the Lymphatic System

Here are the word parts that specifically apply to the diseases and disorders of the blood and the lymphatic system that are covered in the following section. Note that the word parts are color-coded to help you identify them: prefixes are green, combining forms are red, and suffixes are blue.

Prefix	Definition	Combining Form	Definition	Suffix	Definition
an-	without, absence of	aden/o	gland	-emia	condition of blood
ana-	up, toward	aut/o	self	-genic	pertaining to producing
mono-	one	botul/o	sausage		
		fung/o	fungus	-ial	pertaining to
		globin/o	protein	-ic	pertaining to
		hem/o, hemat/o	blood	-ism	condition or disease
		hydr/o	water	-itis	inflammation
		iatr/o	physician	-oma	tumor
		idi/o	individual	-osis	condition of
		immun/o	exempt, or immunity	-pathy	disease
		leuk/o	white	-philia	loving, affinity for

(continued)

Combining Form	Definition
lymph/o	clear water or fluid
necr/o	death
nosocom/o	hospital
nucle/o	kernel, nucleus
path/o	disease
sept/o	putrefying; wall or partition
staphylococc/o	Staphylococcus (bacterium)
streptococc/o	Streptococcus (bacterium)
thym/o	wartlike, thymus gland

Suffix	Definition
-phobia	fear
-phylaxis	protection
-rrhagic	pertaining to abnormal discharge

KEY TERMS A–Z

AIDS

7.21 The acronym for **acquired immunodeficiency syndrome** is _____. This devastating disease is caused by the human immunodeficiency virus (**HIV**), which disables the immune response by destroying important white blood cells known as helper T cells. The loss of immune function allows opportunistic diseases to proliferate, such as pneumonia caused by *Pneumocystis jiroveci,* dementia, Kaposi's sarcoma, and many others, which eventually cause death.

allergy
AL er jee

7.22 An **allergy** is the body's immune response to allergens, which are foreign substances that produce a reaction including immediate inflammation. An _____ may strike in different forms, the most common of which are **allergic rhinitis** (hay fever), which affects the mucous membranes of the nasal cavity and throat, and **allergic dermatitis**, which affects the skin where it has been in physical contact with the allergen (Figure 7.3■).

Figure 7.3 ■
The patient is undergoing an allergy skin test by receiving subdermal inoculations of allergens. Inflammation (redness, swelling, heat, and pain) of the inoculated area is evidence of an allergic reaction.
Source: kiep/Shutterstock

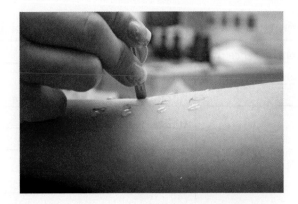

anaphylaxis
AN ah fih LAK siss

7.23 An immediate reaction to a foreign substance that includes rapid inflammation, vasodilation, bronchospasms, and spasms of the GI tract is called **anaphylaxis**. In severe cases it can become life threatening if medical intervention is not available. This term is constructed from the prefix *ana-* that means "up, toward" and the suffix *-phylaxis* that means "protection." Thus, the constructed form of _____ is written ana/phylaxis.

anemia
ah NEE mee ah

7.24 The prefix *an-* means "without, absence of," and the suffix *-emia* means "condition of blood." Combining these two word parts forms the term **anemia**, which literally means "without blood." The constructed form of this term is written an/emia. _____ is the reduced ability of red blood cells to deliver oxygen to tissues. It may be the result of a reduced number of normal circulating red blood cells or a reduction in the amount of the oxygen-binding protein in red blood cells called hemoglobin. Some common forms of anemia include **aplastic anemia**, in which the red bone marrow fails to produce sufficient numbers of normal blood cells; **iron deficiency anemia**, caused by a lack of available iron, resulting in the body's inability to make adequate amounts of hemoglobin; **sickle cell anemia**, in which the hemoglobin is defective within cells, resulting in misshaped red blood cells that cause obstructions in blood vessels; and **pernicious** (per NISH us) **anemia**, caused by a failure to acquire vitamin B12 into the bloodstream for its delivery to red bone marrow, which requires it in order to produce new red blood cells.

anthrax
AN thraks

7.25 A bacterial disease that has been threatened to be used in **bioterrorism**, which is the application of disease-causing microorganisms (pathogens) to cause harm to a population, is **anthrax**. The spores of the bacteria can survive within a powder that can be distributed through the air, making it very dangerous. If inhaled, _____ can become fatal. The term is derived from the Greek word *anthrakos,* which means "coal," referring to the blackening effect the infection has on the skin and lungs.

autoimmune disease
au toe im YOON * dis EEZ

7.26 A disease that is caused by a person's own immune response attacking otherwise healthy tissues is called **autoimmune disease**. The term *autoimmune* is a constructed term, written aut/o/immune, and literally means "self-exempt" or "self-immunity." Examples of _____ _____ include rheumatoid arthritis, systemic lupus erythematosus, and multiple sclerosis. The triggering mechanism that results in autoimmune disease is not yet known.

botulism
BAHT yoo lizm

7.27 One lethal form of food-borne illness is called **botulism**. It is caused by the ingestion of food contaminated with the neurotoxin produced by the bacterium *Clostridium botulinum*. _____ usually occurs when canned food is not prepared properly and is often fatal due to the extreme toxic nature of the botulism neurotoxin.

communicable disease
co MYOON ik ah bul * dis EEZ

7.28 A disease that is capable of transmission from one person to another is called a _____ _____. Also known as a **contagious disease**, it may be transmitted by direct contact with an infected person, indirectly by way of contact with infected body fluids or other materials, or by way of vectors, usually biting arthropods such as mosquitoes, ticks, and fleas.

diphtheria
diff THEER ee ah

7.29 Diphtheria is an infectious disease resulting in acute inflammation of the mucous membranes, primarily in the mouth and throat. Derived from the Greek word for "leather," _____ is characterized by the formation of an obstructive, leatherlike membrane in the throat. It is illustrated in Figure 7.4■.

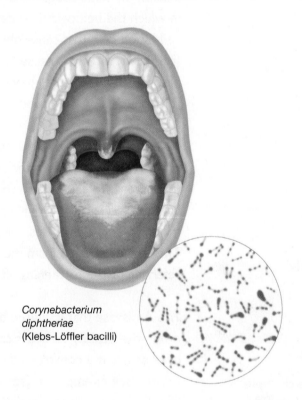

Corynebacterium diphtheriae (Klebs-Löffler bacilli)

Figure 7.4 ■
Diphtheria. The bacteria that cause this disease, called *Corynebacterium diphtheriae*, proliferate in the mucous membranes of the throat to establish a leathery, white covering.

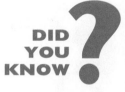

▶▶▶▶▶ **Diphtheria**

Before the availability of antibiotics, diphtheria was a life-threatening scourge among children, killing thousands each year within the United States. It is caused by the toxins produced by the bacterium *Corynebacterium diphtheriae,* which produces inflammation of the throat and the formation of a thick secretion. Because the infected throat becomes covered with a leathery membrane, it was named after the Greek word for leather, *diphthera.*

dyscrasia diss KRAY zee ah	**7.30** Derived from the Greek word *dyskrasia,* which means "difficult temperament," the clinical term _____ is any abnormal condition of the blood. Apparently, the ones who named this condition observed a correlation between a difficult temperament and blood disease.
edema eh DEE mah	**7.31** The leakage of fluid from the bloodstream into the interstitial space between body cells causes swelling and is one aspect of inflammation. The swelling is called _____. The term is derived from the Greek word, *oidema,* which means "swelling."
fungemia fun JEE mee ah	**7.32** The combining form for fungus is *fung/o,* and the suffix *-emia* means "condition of blood." Putting these word parts together forms the term **fungemia**, which is a fungal infection that spreads throughout the body by way of the bloodstream. As a constructed term, _____ is written fung/emia and literally means "condition of blood fungus." Another common term for this infection is **fungal septicemia**.
gas gangrene gas * GANG green	**7.33** Infection of a wound may be caused by various anaerobic bacteria, which cause additional damage to local tissues when blood flow is reduced due to some reason, including frostbite or diabetes. The condition is called **gas gangrene**, which can become life threatening if it is allowed to spread. If antibiotics fail to control the _____ _____ infection, amputation may become a lifesaving option. The term *gangrene* is derived from the Greek word *gangraina,* which means "eating sore." The term *gas* is included in the term because of the fermentation gas that is a diagnostic of the disease.
hematoma HEE mah TOH mah	**7.34** When a word root for blood, *hemat/o,* is combined with the suffix that means "tumor" (*-oma*), the term _____ is formed. It is a mass of blood outside blood vessels and confined within an organ or space within the body, usually in a clotted form (Figure 7.5■). Commonly known as a bruise or a contusion when it is visible through the skin, a hematoma is usually the result of injury or disease. The constructed form of this term is written hemat/oma.

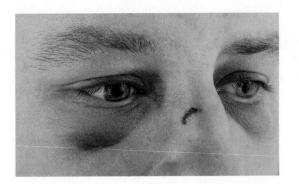

Figure 7.5 ■
Hematoma. A hematoma around the right eye caused by an injury. A hematoma is the result of bleeding below the surface of the skin and is also known as a contusion or bruise when it is visible through the skin. *Source: Molodec/Shutterstock.*

hemoglobinopathy
HEE moh gloh bin AH path ee

7.35 A general term for a disease that affects hemoglobin within red blood cells is **hemoglobinopathy**. This constructed term contains five word parts, as shown when it is written as hem/o/globin/o/pathy. It literally means "disease of blood protein." Because sickle cell anemia is a disease that affects hemoglobin (Frame 7.24), it is a form of _____.

hemophilia
HEE moh FILL ee ah

7.36 An inherited bleeding disorder that results from defective or missing blood-clotting proteins that are necessary components in the coagulation process is known as **hemophilia**. Because the clotting proteins normally stop the loss of blood after minor injuries, a patient suffering from _____ experiences an abnormal loss of blood. The term is a constructed term, written hem/o/philia, which literally means "love for blood."

hemorrhagic fever
HEM or AJ ik

7.37 An infectious disease that causes internal bleeding, or internal hemorrhage (Frame 7.13), and high fevers is generally known as _____ _____. The disease is often caused by viruses, such as Ebola, and some forms exhibit a high rate of mortality.

Hodgkin's disease

7.38 In 1832, the British physician Thomas Hodgkin first described a malignant form of cancer of lymphatic tissue that is characterized by the progressive enlargement of lymph nodes, fatigue, and deficiency of the immune response. Known as _____ _____ or **Hodgkin's lymphoma**, about 1,300 Americans die of the disease each year, usually from opportunistic infections. It is less common than **non-Hodgkin's lymphoma**, which had approximately 66,360 estimated new cases in 2011 compared to the 8,830 estimated new cases of Hodgkin's disease.

iatrogenic disease EYE a troh JEN ik * dis EEZ	**7.39** A condition that is caused by a medical treatment is called an **iatrogenic disease**. This constructed term combines the combining form that means "physician," *iatr/o*, with the suffix that means "pertaining to producing, forming," *-genic*. The resulting constructed form of _____ _____ is written iatr/o/genic.
idiopathic disease id ee oh PATH ik * dis EEZ	**7.40** A disease that develops without a known or apparent cause is called an _____ _____. The constructed form of this term is idi/o/path/ic, which literally means "pertaining to individual disease."
immunodeficiency IM yoo noh dee FISH ehn see	**7.41** A condition resulting from a defective immune response is called an **immunodeficiency**. It occurs when there are insufficient numbers of functional white blood cells, especially lymphocytes, available to defend the body from sources of infection. A closely related term is **immunocompromised**, which is used to describe a patient suffering from an _____.
immunosuppression IM yoo noh suh PREH shun	**7.42** A reduction of an immune response may be caused by disease or by the use of chemical, pharmacological, or immunologic agents. The suppressed status of the immune response that results is called _____.
incompatibility IN com PAT ih BILL ih tee	**7.43** The combination of two blood types that result in the destruction of red blood cells is called _____. It may occur during a blood transfusion causing severe consequences, including the possibility of death if the donor blood antibodies attack the recipient's red blood cells.
infection in FEK shun	**7.44** A multiplication of disease-causing microorganisms, or pathogens, in the body is called an **infection**. The term is derived from the Latin word *infectus,* which means "to color, stain, or dye," referring to the discoloration of skin during an infection. A disease caused by _____ is called an **infectious disease**. The reaction of the body against an infection is illustrated in Figure 7.6■.

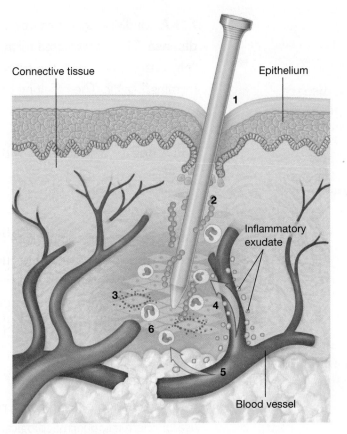

Connective tissue

Epithelium

Inflammatory exudate

Blood vessel

Figure 7.6 ■
Reaction against infection. Pathogens may invade the body by a pierce through the skin. The result of invasion is the proliferation of pathogens within body tissues, or infection. The body responds to the infection by mounting an attack that begins with inflammation, which promotes the movement of phagocytes to the site of the infection. Phagocytes localize the pathogens and destroy them by phagocytosis. Pus is released, which is composed of dead bacteria and phagocytes.

1. Dirty nail punctures skin.
2. Bacteria enter and multiply.
3. Injured cells release histamine.
4. Blood vessels dilate and become permeable, releasing inflammatory exudate.
5. Blood flow to the damaged site increases.
6. Neutrophils (polymorphs) move toward bacteria (chemotaxis) and destroy them (phagocytosis).

inflammation
in flah MAY shun

7.45 The physiological process that serves as the body's initial response to injury and many forms of illness involves the swelling of body tissue. Known as **inflammation**, the swelling results from the movement of plasma from capillaries into the extracellular space to produce edema (Frame 7.31), or fluid accumulation in tissue (Figure 7.7■). The common symptoms of _____ include swelling, redness, heat, and pain. The term *inflammation* is derived from the Latin word *inflammatio,* which means "to ignite" or "to set ablaze."

Figure 7.7 ■

Inflammation. Inflammation is characterized by the presence of swelling, redness, heat, and pain. Swelling is caused by the accumulation of fluid in tissue spaces and is also known as edema. In this photograph, the patient exhibits severe edema of both legs caused by infection of a parasitic worm.

Source: Courtesy of CDC Public Health Image Library.

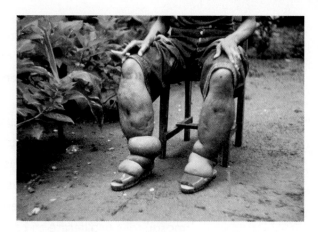

influenza

in floo EHN zah

7.46 A viral disease characterized by fever and an acute inflammation of respiratory mucous membranes is called **influenza**. Commonly called "the flu," _____ is highly contagious, and the virus is capable of mutating to escape detection by white blood cells.

leukemia

loo KEE mee ah

7.47 A form of cancer that literally means "condition of white blood cells" is _____. Leukemia originates from cells within the blood-forming tissue of the red marrow. The constructed form of the term is written leuk/emia. The primary tumor of leukemia spreads throughout the red marrow, transforming the blood-forming tissue into a dysfunctional mass that produces abnormal white blood cells (Figure 7.8■). As a result, common symptoms of leukemia include immunodeficiency and the development of opportunistic infections.

Figure 7.8 ■

Leukemia. A blood smear from a patient suffering from leukemia demonstrates the abundance of enlarged, nonfunctional leukocytes that serve as a diagnostic characteristic of this disease.

Source: Courtesy of CDC Public Health Image Library/Stacy Howard.

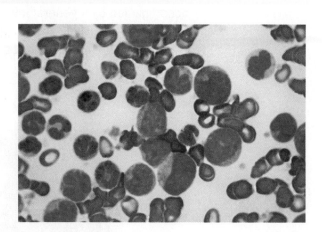

lymphadenitis

limm fad eh NYE tiss

7.48 Inflammation of the lymph nodes is a condition called **lymphadenitis**. The constructed form of this term is lymph/aden/itis. The acute form of _____ is common during infections. The chronic form indicates a more serious disorder may be the cause, such as lymphoma (Frame 7.49).

lymphoma
limm FOH mah

7.49 A malignant tumor originating in lymphatic tissue is called _____. The constructed form uses the suffix *-oma*, which means "tumor," and is written lymph/oma.

malaria
mah LAIR ee ah

7.50 A disease caused by a parasitic protozoan that infects red blood cells and the liver during different parts of its life cycle is called **malaria**. The vector, or carrier, of the protozoan is the *Anopheles* mosquito, and the symptoms of malaria include periodic flares of high fever. The term _____ literally means "bad air," referring to the swampy marshlands where the mosquitoes proliferate to cause higher incidences of the disease.

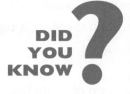

▶▶▶▶ Malaria

The term *malaria* is derived from combining the Italian word for bad, *mal,* with that of air, *aria.* It was first used during the Middle Ages, when malaria was believed to have been caused by breathing bad air near swamplands. We now know that this dreaded disease is caused by the bite of an *Anopheles* mosquito carrying the protozoan known as *Plasmodium.* According to the U.S. Centers for Disease Control (CDC), malaria caused 708,000 to 1,003,000 deaths in the last year it was counted, 2008.

measles

7.51 Measles is an acute viral disease that often begins as a fever, followed by the development of a skin rash containing numerous vesicles and often accompanied by a general inflammation of the respiratory tract (Figure 7.9■). Prior to the availability of a widely distributed vaccine, _____ killed thousands of children and adults each year in the United States. A clinical synonym is **rubeola**.

Figure 7.9 ■
Measles. A photograph of a child stricken with measles, showing the tell-tale sign of the skin rash.
Source: Courtesy of CDC Public Health Image Library.

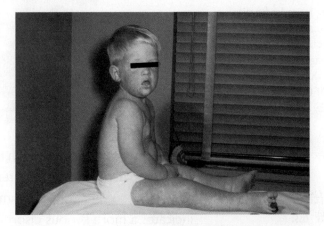

mononucleosis
MAHN oh nook lee OH siss

7.52 A viral disease characterized by enlarged lymph nodes and spleen, atypical lymphocytes, throat pain, pharyngitis, fever, and fatigue is called **mononucleosis**. Also called **infectious mononucleosis**, it is caused by the Epstein-Barr virus and is a communicable disease (Figure 7.10■). The term _____ is a constructed term made up of the prefix *mono-*, meaning "one," the word root *nucle*, meaning "kernel, nucleus," and the very common suffix *-osis*, meaning "condition of." It is written as mono/nucle/osis.

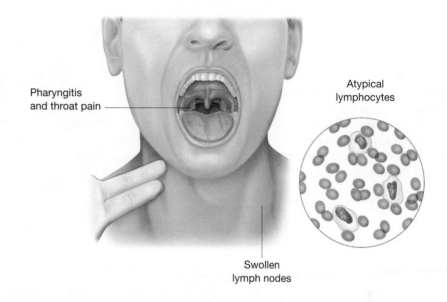

Figure 7.10 ■
Mononucleosis. Infectious mononucleosis is caused by the Epstein-Barr virus and produces the symptoms of swollen palatine tonsils (pharyngitis), swollen cervical lymph nodes (lymphadenopathy), high fever, and a blood sample that reveals atypical lymphocytes.

Pharyngitis and throat pain

Atypical lymphocytes

Swollen lymph nodes

necrosis
neh KROH siss

7.53 The death of one or more cells or a portion of a tissue or organ is called **necrosis**. The term _____ is derived from the Greek word *nekrosis*, which means "death." A cell or cells, tissue, or organ that is dead is often called **necrotic**.

nosocomial infection
noh soh KOH mee al * in FEK shun

7.54 An infectious disease that is contracted during a hospital stay is called a **nosocomial infection**. The term *nosocomial* is derived from the Greek word *nosokomeion*, which means "hospital." The most common cause of _____ _____ in recent years has been a lack of hand washing, made worse by the development of antibiotic-resistant strains of *Staphylococcus* (Frame 7. 59).

plague
playg

7.55 Any infectious disease that is widespread and causes extensive mortality is called a **plague**. The term is derived from the Latin word *plago,* which means "to strike or beat." The term originated from the first recorded outbreak of bubonic plague in 542 AD. Today, the term also applies to the bubonic _____, which is caused by the bacterium *Yersinia pestis* and is characterized by high fever, skin eruptions (called buboes) and discoloration, internal hemorrhage, and pneumonia. The bacteria are transmitted by the bite of a flea that may jump from small mammals, such as rats, to humans, shown in Figure 7.11■.

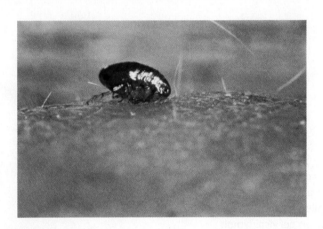

Figure 7.11 ■
Photograph of the flea that transmits *Yersinia pestis* to cause bubonic plague, called the oriental rat flea, *X. cheopsis*. The flea hops from rats and other small mammals to humans, transmitting the disease by taking a human blood meal.
Source: Courtesy of CDC Public Health Image Library.

rabies
RAY beez

7.56 A viral infection that is spread from the saliva of an infected animal, usually by way of a bite, is known as **rabies**. In Latin, *rabies* means "savage, fierce," which refers to the ferocity of infected animals. The virus acts on the central nervous system to cause paranoia and paralysis and is usually fatal. _____ has also been called **hydrophobia** (HIGH droh FOH bee ah), which literally means "fear of water" and refers to the symptom of a fear of water appearing during the stage of mental deterioration. *Hydrophobia* is a constructed term, written as hydr/o/phobia.

septicemia
sep tih SEE mee ah

7.57 A systemwide disease caused by the presence of bacteria and their toxins in the circulating blood is called **septicemia**. This is a constructed term written sept/ic/emia and literally means "condition of putrefying blood." The word root, *sept*, is derived from the Greek word *sepsis*, which means "putrefying." Thus, _____ may also be called by its Greek origin, **sepsis**. A person suffering from this condition is referred to as **septic**.

smallpox

7.58 A viral disease caused by the *variola* virus that was the scourge of the human population prior to its eradication in 1975 is known as **smallpox**. The term was first used around 1400 AD to distinguish the disease from syphilis, the "great pox," which at the time was characterized by the formation of large pustules on the skin that exceeded the pustules of smallpox in size and number. The eradication of _____ was the crowning achievement of the World Health Organization, which battled the disease with an aggressive vaccination (Frame 7.90) campaign for about 8 years. Although it is eradicated from the population, reserves of *variola* remain in storage for research purposes.

staphylococcemia
STAFF ih loh kok SEE mee ah

7.59 The presence of the bacterium *Staphylococcus* in the blood is a condition known as **staphylococcemia**. Only two word parts, the word root *staphylococc* and the suffix meaning "condition of blood," *-emia*, are used to construct _____, which is written staphylococc/emia. *Staphylococcus* is a frequent cause of infections in wounds, a complication of normal healing. An infection caused by *Staphylococcus* is commonly called a **staph infection**. It is also the most common cause of food-borne illness, skin inflammation, osteomyelitis (infection of bone), and nosocomial infections (Frame 7.54). Varieties of *Staphylococcus* that are resistant to antibiotics are one of the greatest challenges to antiseptic medical procedures. These resistant strains are abbreviated **MRSA**, for methicillin-resistant *Staphylococcus aureus,* and are often referred to as "**mersa**."

streptococcemia
STREP toh kok SEE mee ah

7.60 The presence of the bacterium *Streptococcus* in the blood is known as **streptococcemia**. The constructed term _____ is written streptococc/emia. An infection caused by *Streptococcus* (a bacterium) is commonly called a **strep infection**. It frequently begins in the throat as a form of pharyngitis called **strep throat** or in the mouth following a dental procedure and, if not managed, may spread to the bloodstream, which distributes the infection to vital organs. The heart valves in particular are a potential target of *Streptococcus* and are subject to permanent damage if infected.

tetanus
TETT ah nuss

7.61 A disease caused by a powerful neurotoxin released by the common bacterium *Clostridium tetani* is called **tetanus**. The toxin acts on the central nervous system to cause convulsions and spastic paralysis (in which muscles are unable to relax). The term _____ is derived from the Latin word *tetanos,* which means "convulsive tension." Infection can be obtained from a puncture wound that is not properly cleaned, but is easily prevented with periodic vaccination (Frame 7. 89). (See Figure 7.6.)

thymoma

thigh MOH mah

7.62 A tumor originating in the thymus gland is called a **thymoma**. The constructed form of _____ uses the word root _thym_ and the suffix _-oma_ and is written _thym/oma_.

PRACTICE: Diseases and Disorders of the Blood and the Lymphatic System

The Right Match

Match the term on the left with the correct definition on the right.

_____ 1. sickle cell anemia

_____ 2. rabies

_____ 3. botulism

_____ 4. Hodgkin's disease

_____ 5. tetanus

_____ 6. immunodeficiency

_____ 7. fungemia

_____ 8. plague

_____ 9. diphtheria

_____ 10. malaria

a. disease caused by a neurotoxin released by _Clostridium tetani_

b. anemia resulting from defective hemoglobin within cells, resulting in misshaped red blood cells

c. viral infection that is spread from the saliva of an infected animal

d. condition resulting from a defective immune response

e. any infectious disease that is widespread and causes extensive mortality

f. fungal infection that spreads throughout the body by way of the bloodstream

g. a cancer of lymph nodes

h. caused by a neurotoxin produced by _Clostridium botulinum_

i. disease caused by a parasitic protozoan that infects red blood cells and the liver

j. infectious disease resulting in acute inflammation with formation of a leathery membrane in the throat

Linkup

Link the word parts in the list to create the terms that match the definitions. You may use word parts more than once. Remember to add in combining vowels when needed—and that some terms do not use any combining vowel. The first one is completed for you as an example.

Prefix	Combining Form	Suffix
mono-	aden/o	-emia
	botul/o	-genic
	globin/o	-ia
	hemat/o	-ic
	hem/o	-ism
	hydr/o	-itis
	iatr/o	-oma
	leuk/o	-osis
	lymph/o	-pathy
	nucle/o	-philia
	sept/o	-phobia
	thym/o	

Definition

Term

1. systemwide disease caused by the presence of bacteria and their toxins in the circulating blood
   septicemia

2. tumor originating in the thymus gland
   _____

3. reduced ability of red blood cells to deliver oxygen to tissues
   _____

4. poisoning caused by the ingestion of food contaminated with the toxin produced by the bacterium *Clostridium botulinum*
   _____

5. blood outside the blood vessels and confined within an organ or space within the body, usually in a clotted form
   _____

6. a condition that is caused by a medical treatment
   _____

7. an inherited bleeding disorder that results from missing or deficient blood-clotting proteins
   _____

8. general term for a disease that affects hemoglobin within red blood cells
   _____

9. inflammation of the lymph nodes
   _____

10. a viral disease characterized by enlarged lymph nodes, atypical lymphocytes, throat pain, pharyngitis, fever, and fatigue
    _____

11. another term for rabies that refers to infected animals' inability to drink water due to progressive paralysis
    _____

Treatments and Procedures of the Blood and the Lymphatic System

Here are the word parts that specifically apply to the treatments and procedures of the blood and the lymphatic system that are covered in the following section. Note that the word parts are color-coded to help you identify them: prefixes are green, combining forms are red, and suffixes are blue.

Prefix	Definition	Combining Form	Definition	Suffix	Definition
anti-	against, opposite of	aden/o	gland	-crit	to separate
pro-	before	aut/o	self	-ectomy	surgical excision, removal
		bi/o	life	-ic	pertaining to
		globin/o	protein	-logous	pertaining to study
		hem/o, hemat/o	blood	-logy	study or science of
		hom/o	same	-lysis	loosen, dissolve
		immun/o	exempt, immunity	-phylaxis	protection
		lymph/o	clear water or fluid	-stasis	standing still
		splen/o	spleen	-therapy	treatment
		thromb/o	clot	-tic	pertaining to

KEY TERMS A–Z

antibiotic therapy
AN tih bye AHT ik * THAIR ah pee

7.63 A therapeutic treatment involving the use of a substance with known toxicity to bacteria is called **antibiotic therapy**. The constructed form of the term *antibiotic* is written anti/bi/o/tic, which literally means "pertaining to against life." The antibiotic may be obtained from a fungus, usually a mold, or other bacteria. _____ _____ is effective only against bacteria, many types of which are capable of developing resistance, especially when antibiotics are not administered properly.

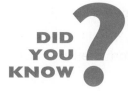

 Discovery of Antibiotics

The first antibiotic was discovered in 1928 by Sir Alexander Fleming, who found that a common bread mold (a fungus) could produce toxins capable of killing bacterial colonies (Figure 7.12 ■). The *Penicillium* mold produces an antibacterial toxin that is now known as penicillin. In time, the fungal toxins were proven to be effective against many strains of bacteria, and their use as antibiotics has been hailed as the single most important treatment against bacterial infections ever.

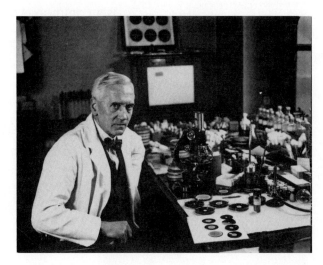

Figure 7.12 ■
Alexander Fleming photographed in his lab where he observed the natural competition between a fungus and bacteria in 1928, which gave rise to the discovery of antibiotics.
Source: © Daily Herald Archive/NMeM/Science & Society Picture Library—All rights reserved.

anticoagulant
AN tye koh AG yoo lant

7.64 A chemical agent that delays or prevents the clotting process in blood is called an anticoagulant. It is often administered to reduce the likelihood of clot formation after surgery. The constructed form of anticoagulant is written anti/coagulant. The most common _____ agent is **warfarin** (Coumadin).

antiretroviral therapy
AN tye REH troh VYE ral *
THAIR ah pee

7.65 A pharmacological therapy that is useful in battling a class of viruses that tend to mutate quickly, called retroviruses, is often called _____ _____. It is used against the virus that causes AIDS (Frame 7. 21), HIV. The drugs form a cocktail that includes nucleotide analog reverse transcriptase inhibitors and protease inhibitors, which block HIV replication by a variety of means.

attenuation
ah TEN yoo AY shun

7.66 The process in which pathogens are rendered less virulent, or infectious, prior to their incorporation into a vaccine preparation is called _____. The term is derived from the Latin word *attenuatus,* which means "to make thin."

autologous transfusion
aw TALL oh guss * trans FYOO zhun

7.67 A transfusion of blood donated by a patient for their personal use is called an **autologous transfusion.** The term includes a constructed term that is written aut/o/logous and means "pertaining to study of self." _____ _____ is a common procedure before a surgery to avoid potential incompatibility or contamination of blood. (See Figure 7.13■.)

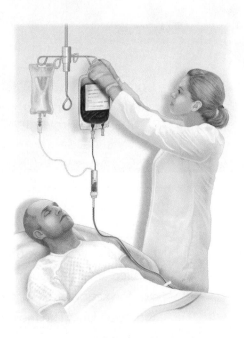

Figure 7.13 ■
Blood transfusion. A transfusion of one's own blood is called an autologous transfusion (see Frame 7.67). A transfusion of donated blood from another person is called a homologous transfusion (see Frame 7.79).

blood chemistry

7.68 A test or series of tests on a sample of plasma to measure the levels of its composition, including glucose, albumin, triglycerides, pH, cholesterol, and electrolytes is called _____ _____.

blood culture

7.69 A clinical test to determine infection in the blood is called a _____ _____. It is performed by placing a sample of blood in a nutrient-rich liquid medium in an effort to grow populations of bacteria for analysis.

blood transfusions

7.70 The introduction of blood, blood products, or a blood substitute into a patient's circulation to restore blood volume to normal levels is called **blood transfusion.** The two main types of _____ _____ are **autologous transfusion** (Frame 7.67) and **homologous transfusion** (Frame 7.79). (See Figure 7.13.)

bone marrow transplant

7.71 A common procedure to treat leukemia (Frame 7.47), or injury resulting from radiation therapy or chemotherapy, is a _____ _____ _____. It involves the removal of a sample from a compatible donor, usually from red marrow in the pelvis, and its inoculation into the donor's red marrow (Figure 7.14■).

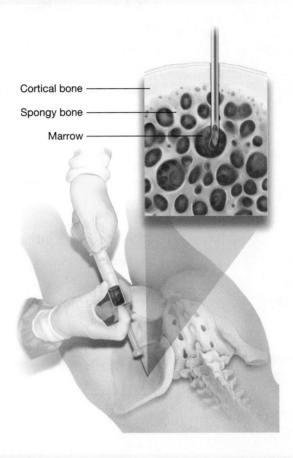

Cortical bone

Spongy bone

Marrow

Figure 7.14 ■
Bone marrow transplant. A bone marrow transplant is usually extracted from red bone marrow within a donor's pelvis with a syringe due to its fluid state, then inoculated into the recipient's red bone marrow.

coagulation time
koh ahg yoo LAY shun

7.72 A timed blood test to determine the time required for a blood clot to form is called **coagulation time**. One form of this _____ _____ test, called **prothrombin time (PT)**, measures the time required for prothrombin, a precursor protein, to form thrombin. Thrombin then acts on the blood protein fibrinogen to form fibrin, a threadlike protein that coagulates blood. This procedure is often used to monitor the effects of anticoagulants (Frame 7.64). Another type of test is used to evaluate clotting ability and is called **partial thromboplastin time (PTT)**.

complete blood count

7.73 A common laboratory test that evaluates a sample of blood to provide diagnostic information about a patient's general health is abbreviated CBC, which means **complete blood count**. A _____ _____ _____ includes several more specific tests, including hematocrit (Frame 7.75), hemoglobin (Frame 7.77), red blood count (Frame 7.86), and white blood count. Sometimes a platelet count (PLT) is also included (Frame 7.84).

differential count	**7.74** A microscopic count of the number of each type of white blood cell in a sample of blood is called _____ _____. The procedure uses staining techniques to highlight the features of white blood cells, allowing the hematologist to distinguish between the types.
hematocrit hee MAT oh krit	**7.75** A procedure included in a complete blood count that measures the percentage of red blood cells in a volume of blood is called **hematocrit**. This constructed term includes the suffix -*crit*, which means "to separate," and is written hemat/o/crit. Abbreviated **HCT** or **Hct**, a _____ is obtained by centrifuging a sample of blood to separate the cells from plasma in the centrifuge tube.
hematology HEE mah TALL oh jee	**7.76** The general field of medicine focusing on blood-related disease is called _____. The constructed form of this term is hemat/o/logy.
hemoglobin HEE moh gloh binn	**7.77** A procedure included in a complete blood count that measures the level of hemoglobin in red blood cells (in grams) is simply called _____ and is abbreviated **HGB** or **Hgb**. Any level below normal is diagnosed as a form of anemia (Frame 7.24).
hemostasis HEE moh STAY siss	**7.78** The stoppage of bleeding is a physiological process known as **hemostasis**. It literally means "standing still blood." The constructed form of _____ is written hem/o/stasis.
homologous transfusion hoh MALL oh gus * trans FYOO zhun	**7.79** Transfusion of blood that is voluntarily donated by another person is called a _____ _____. The term *homologous* is a constructed term written hom/o/logous and means "pertaining to study of the same." It requires blood-type work called **crossmatching** to prevent incompatibility (Frame 7.43). See Figure 7.13.

immunization

IM yoo nih ZAY shun

7.80 A treatment that establishes immunity against a particular foreign substance that may otherwise cause disease is called _____. The treatment includes inoculation of antigen components that stimulate the patient's immune response to produce memory lymphocytes and antibodies, which will be available in the blood to provide immune protection when a future exposure occurs (Figure 7.15■).

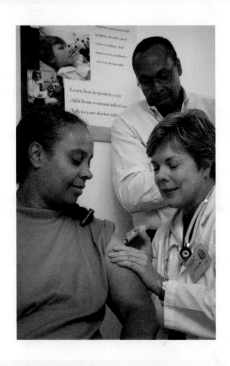

Figure 7.15 ■
Immunization with a vaccine. A healthcare professional is injecting a vaccine into the patient's arm to provide her with acquired immunity against the influenza virus.
Source: James Gathany/CDC Public Health Image Library/Judy Schmidt.

immunology

IM yoo NALL oh jee

7.81 The science concerned with immunity and allergy is called _____. The constructed form of this term is immun/o/logy.

immunotherapy

IM yoo noh THAIR ah pee

7.82 The treatment of infectious disease by the administration of pharmacological agents, such as serum, gamma globulin, treated antibodies, and suppressive drugs is called _____. This constructed term is written immun/o/therapy.

lymphadenectomy

limm fad eh NEK toh mee

7.83 The suffix -*ectomy* means "surgical excision, removal." Placing this suffix at the end of a word root for an organ describes the procedure that surgically removes the organ. For example, the surgical removal of one or more lymph nodes is called _____. The constructed form of this term reveals three word parts, lymph/aden/ectomy.

platelet count

7.84 A laboratory procedure that calculates the number of platelets in a known volume of blood is called a **platelet count**, or **PLT**. A reduced _____ _____ suggests a potential failure of hemostasis (Frame 7.78) because platelets play a major role in blood clot formation and coagulation.

prophylaxis proh fih LAK siss	**7.85** Any treatment that tends to prevent the onset of an infection or other type of disease is called **prophylaxis**. The constructed form of _____ is written as pro/phylaxis, which literally means "protection before."
red blood count	**7.86** A lab test included in a complete blood count that measures the number of red blood cells within a given volume of blood is called a _____ _____ _____, or **RBC**.
splenectomy splee NEK toh mee	**7.87** The surgical removal of the spleen is often necessary if it has ruptured, which may occur during a physical injury to the left side of the trunk. The procedure is called _____. The constructed form of this term is written splen/ectomy.
thrombolysis throm BALL ih siss	**7.88** A treatment that is performed to dissolve an unwanted blood clot, or **thrombus**, is called _____. The constructed form of this term is thromb/o/lysis, which literally means "dissolve clot."
vaccination VAK sih NAY shun	**7.89** The inoculation of a foreign substance that has reduced virulence, or a reduced ability to cause infection, as a means of providing a cure or prophylaxis (Frame 7.85), is called a _____.
vaccine vak SEEN	**7.90** A preparation that is used to activate an immune response to provide acquired immunity against an infectious agent is called a _____.

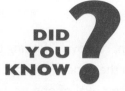

DID YOU KNOW?

▶▶▶▶▶ **Vaccines**

Vaccines have been in use since the Middle Ages or possibly earlier, when scrapings from smallpox sores were given to people as prophylaxis against this deadly disease. The use of the term *vaccine* (derived from the Latin word *vaccinus*, which means "relating to a cow") began in 1796, when Edward Jenner published his findings that scrapings of skin pustules from people infected with a similar virus that produced a different disease contracted from milking cows, known as cowpox, provided immunity against the *variola* virus that causes smallpox.

PRACTICE: Treatments and Procedures of the Blood and the Lymphatic System

The Right Match

Match the term on the left with the correct definition on the right.

_____ 1. attenuation

_____ 2. hematocrit

_____ 3. vaccine

_____ 4. immunization

_____ 5. red blood count

_____ 6. prothrombin time

_____ 7. blood chemistry

_____ 8. antiretroviral therapy

_____ 9. prophylaxis

_____ 10. antibiotic therapy

a. measures the number of red blood cells

b. procedure that establishes immunity against a particular antigen

c. process in which pathogens are rendered less virulent, or infectious, prior to their incorporation into a vaccine

d. tests on a sample of plasma to measure the levels of certain chemicals

e. a timed test for coagulation rate

f. measures the percentage of red blood cells in a volume of blood by centrifuging a sample

g. drugs used to battle retroviruses

h. a preventive treatment

i. a therapy against bacterial infections

j. a preparation used to activate an immune response

Break the Chain

Analyze these medical terms:

    a.   Separate each term into its word parts; each word part is labeled for you (**p** = prefix, **r** = root, **cf** = combining form, and **s** = suffix).

    b.   For the Bonus Question, write the requested definition in the blank that follows.

1. a. immunotherapy   _____/___/_____
                                          cf   s

    b. *Bonus Question:* What is the definition of the suffix? _____

2. a. splenectomy   _____/_____
                                  r   s

    b. *Bonus Question:* What is the definition of the word root? _____

3. a. lymphadenectomy   _____/_____/_____
                                  r   r   s

    b. *Bonus Question:* What is the definition of the second word root? _____

4. a. immunology   _____/___/_____
                                   cf   s

    b. *Bonus Question:* What is the definition of the combining form? _____

5. a. homologous   _____/___/_____
                                   cf   s

    b. *Bonus Question:* What is the definition of the combining form? _____

6. a. hematology   _____/___/_____
                                   cf   s

    b. *Bonus Question:* What is the definition of the suffix? _____

7. a. autologous   _____/___/_____
                                   cf   s

    b. *Bonus Question:* What is the definition of the combining form? _____

8. a. antibiotic   _____/_____/___/_____
                                p   cf   s

    b. *Bonus Question:* What is the definition of the prefix? _____

9. a. hemostasis   _____/___/_____
                                   cf   s

    b. *Bonus Question:* What is the definition of the suffix? _____

10. a. thrombolysis   _____/___/_____
                                   cf   s

    b. *Bonus Question:* What is the definition of the suffix? _____

Abbreviations of the Blood and the Lymphatic System

The abbreviations that are associated with the blood and the lymphatic system are summarized here. Study these abbreviations, and review them in the exercise that follows.

Abbreviation	Definition
AIDS	acquired immunodeficiency syndrome
CBC	complete blood count
HCT, Hct	hematocrit
HGB, Hgb	hemoglobin
HIV	human immunodeficiency virus
MRSA	methicillin-resistant *Staphylococcus aureus*

Abbreviation	Definition
PLT	platelet count
PT	prothrombin time
PTT	partial thromboplastin time
RBC	red blood cell or red blood count
WBC	white blood cell or white blood count

PRACTICE: Abbreviations

Fill in the blanks with the abbreviation or the complete medical term.

Abbreviation

1. _____
2. CBC
3. _____
4. RBC
5. _____
6. PT
7. _____
8. WBC
9. _____
10. HIV

Medical Term

acquired immunodeficiency syndrome

_____

platelet count

_____

hemoglobin

_____

partial thromboplastin time

_____

hematocrit

_____

▶▶▶▶ # Chapter Review

Word Building _____

Construct medical terms from the following meanings. (Some are built from word parts, some are not.) The first question has been completed as an example.

1. reduced ability of blood to deliver oxygen   an*emia*_____

2. presence of red blood cells of unequal size   _____cytosis

3. any abnormal condition of the blood   dys_____

4. a serious protozoan infection of red blood cells   _____ia

5. abnormal reduction of red blood cells   erythro_____

6. inherited defect in blood coagulation   _____philia

7. cancer originating in red bone marrow, producing abnormal white blood cells   _____emia

8. abnormally large red blood cells   macro_____

9. a condition of staphylococci (bacteria) in the blood   staphylococc_____

10. disease caused by immune reaction against own tissues   _____disease

11. abnormal increase in number of red blood cells   _____emia

12. red blood cells that are tear-shaped   _____cytosis

13. presence of bacteria and toxins in the blood   septic_____

14. a drug that reduces blood clotting   anti_____

15. transfusion of blood donated by another person   _____logous transfusion

16. measures percentage of red blood cells in a sample   hemato_____

17. stoppage of bleeding   _____stasis

18. calculation of the number of platelets in blood   _____count

19. cancer of lymphatic tissue   _____disease

20. inflammation of the lymph nodes   _____itis

21. bacterial disease that causes a membrane in the throat to form   _____ia

▶▶▶▶ **Medical Report Exercises**

Millie Nyugen _____

Read the following medical report, then answer the questions that follow.

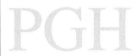

PEARSON GENERAL HOSPITAL

5500 University Avenue, Phone: (211) 594-4000
Metropolis, TX • Fax: (211) 594-4001

Medical Consultation: Hematology

Date: 10/02/2011

Patient: Millie Nyugen

Patient Complaint: Mild fever for two weeks with general body aches; tenderness of the armpit and groin regions to pressure that was first noticed more than one month previous.

History: 55-year-old female of Asian-American descent with no prior hospitalization or serious complaints.

Family History: Father deceased at 62 years with primary hepatic cancer. Mother, 77 years, with complete hysterectomy following diagnosis of stage 1 cervical cancer; no reported conditions otherwise.

Allergies: Dietary restrictions to sesame seeds and milk products.

Physical Examination: Vital signs include mild fever of 99.98°F, blood pressure elevated at 130/90, pulse 75/min. Possible swollen lymph nodes in cervical, axillary, and inguinal regions. Differential count: neutrophils, monocytes, lymphocytes elevated 25%. Blood culture positive for *Staphylococcus*.

Diagnosis: Staphylococcemia

Treatment: Antibiotic treatment with two IV antibiotics with daily reevaluation until cleared. Follow-up in two weeks after discharge.

Sylvia S. Hernandez, M.D.

Sylvia S. Hernandez, M.D.

Photo Source: Monkey Business Images/Shutterstock

Comprehension Questions

1. What complaints support the diagnosis?_____

_____

_____

2. Why do you think antibiotics might fail as a treatment? _____

_____

_____

3. What does the term *staphylococcemia* mean? _____

_____

_____

Case Study Questions

The following Case Study provides further discussion regarding the patient in the medical report. Fill in the blanks with the correct terms. Choose your answers from the list of terms that precedes the case study. (Note that some terms may be used more than once.)

antibiotic	Hodgkin's disease	lymphadenitis	septicemia
blood culture	immunodeficiency	immunotherapy	splenomegaly
differential count	infection	lymphoma	staphylococcemia

A 55-year-old female, Millie Nyugen, was admitted to the infectious disease wing of the clinic after having been

referred by her personal physician, due to a prolonged fever and mild inflammation of the lymph nodes, called

(a) _____, in the neck, armpit, and groin regions. The doctor's initial diagnosis was an unspecified

disease of the lymph nodes, or lymphadenopathy, and she was concerned about a possible tumor originating in the lymph

nodes, or (b) _____, which might include cancer of the nodes, or (c) _____. Upon

more thorough examinations, no evidence of a tumor was found. However, an abnormal enlargement of the spleen, or

(d) _____, was observed. Blood tests including a(n) (e) _____ were ordered to

look for multiplication of pathogens, or a(n) (f) _____. The tests were positive for bacteria, indicating

the patient suffered from (g) _____, or bacterial infection of the blood. Further tests identified the

common bacterium *Staphylococcus* as the causative pathogen, providing the diagnosis of (h) _____.

The patient was administered (i) _____ therapy. However, after two weeks, the symptoms failed

to lessen. The patient had developed a deficient immune response, or (j) _____. To combat this,

(k) _____ was begun immediately that included antibody treatments in combination with antibiotic

therapy. A complete recovery resulted after three months of treatment.

Shane Alexander _____

For a greater challenge, read the medical report provided and answer the critical thinking questions that follow.

PGH **PEARSON GENERAL HOSPITAL**

5500 University Avenue, Phone: (211) 594-4000
Metropolis, MN • Fax: (211) 594-4001

Medical Consultation: Infectious Disease

Date: 11/08/2011

Patient: Shane Alexander

Patient Complaint: Lethargy, frequent acute infections

History: 17-year-old African-American male with no prior history of disease; childhood vaccinations complete.

Family History: Mother and father negative for immunological and hematological disease.

Allergies: None

Physical Examination: Hct and HGB with low RBCs and correspondingly low hemoglobin levels; dietary supplements with folic acid did not resolve. Microscopic evaluation of red blood cells revealed poikilocytosis and anisocytosis. Bone marrow bx positive for myelodysplastic cells.

Diagnosis: Aplastic anemia

Treatment: Stabilize with whole blood homologous transfusion. If patient fails to resolve in two weeks, prepare for bone marrow transplant.

T. R. McBain, M.D.

T. R. McBain, M.D.

Photo Source: Tracy Whiteside/Shutterstock

Comprehension Questions

1. Why were dietary supplements administered to the patient?_____

_____

_____

2. What is aplastic anemia?_____

_____

_____

3. How would you describe the symptoms of poikilocytosis and anisocytosis?_____

_____

_____

Case Study Questions

The following case study provides further discussion regarding the patient in the medical report. Recall the terms from this chapter to fill in the blanks with the correct terms.

A 17-year-old male named Shane Alexander was seen by his personal physician after complaining of low energy and

susceptibility to infections. Prior to seeing the patient, the physician suspected that a nonspecific blood disorder,

or (l) _____, was the cause of the symptoms and ordered tests to measure the levels of blood

components, known as a (m) _____, including a test for the percentage of red blood cells, called a

(n) _____, and a test for the levels of hemoglobin in the blood, called a (o) _____.

The tests showed low hemoglobin and low numbers of red blood cells, but low numbers of red blood cells, suggesting a

general condition of (p) _____. Dietary supplements of iron and folic acid were administered. About

two weeks later, the dietary supplements failed to correct the symptoms, thereby ruling out (q) _____

_____ anemia. A microscopic evaluation of cells was then ordered. This test revealed that red blood

cells were of unequal size, a condition known as (r) _____, and were irregularly shaped, a condition

called (s) _____. Samples from red bone marrow were then examined, which showed that abnormal

stem cells were producing the defective red blood cells, a condition known as (t) _____ anemia.

Because this condition was identified early, before the cells became cancerous (which would have resulted in the cancer

known as (u) _____), treatment by irradiation was successful in restoring the patient's health.

MEDICAL TERMINOLOGY INTERACTIVE

Medical Terminology Interactive is a premium online homework management system that includes a host of features to help you study. Registered users will find:

- Fun games and activities built within a virtual hospital
- Powerful tools that track and analyze your results—allowing you to create a personalized learning experience
- Videos, flashcards, and audio pronunciations to help enrich your progress
- Streaming video lesson presentations and self-paced learning modules

www.pearsonhighered.com/mti

The Cardiovascular System

8

LEARNING OBJECTIVES

After completing this chapter, you will be able to:

1 Define and spell the word parts used to create terms for the cardiovascular system.

2 Break down and define common medical terms used for symptoms, diseases, disorders, procedures, treatments, and devices associated with the cardiovascular system.

3 Build medical terms from the word parts associated with the cardiovascular system.

4 Pronounce and spell common medical terms associated with the cardiovascular system.

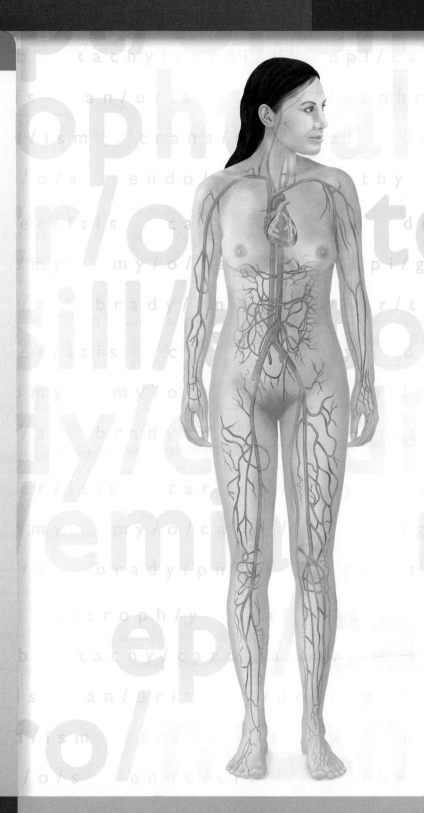

Anatomy and Physiology Terms ▶▶▶▶▶

The following table provides the combining forms that specifically apply to the anatomy and physiology of the cardiovascular system. Note that the combining forms are colored red to help you identify them when you see them again later in the chapter.

Combining Form	Definition	Combining Form	Definition
angi/o	blood vessel	pector/o	chest
aort/o	aorta	valvul/o	little valve
arter/o, arteri/o	artery	vas/o	vessel
atri/o	atrium	vascul/o	little vessel
cardi/o	heart	ven/o	vein
coron/o	crown or circle, heart	ventricul/o	little belly, ventricle
my/o, myos/o	muscle		

cardiovascular
  kar dee oh VAS kyoo lar

blood

8.1 Every one of the 30 trillion or so cells in your body requires a continuous supply of oxygen and nutrients and an unending removal of waste materials. To meet these demands, the blood carries these materials in the body's circulation within a series of closed tubes, called blood vessels, pushed along mainly by the movements of the heart. The movement and transport of blood is thereby achieved by the _____ system, which consists of the heart and blood vessels, as the word parts that form the term *cardiovascular* suggest. The constructed form is written cardi/o/vascul/ar, in which *cardi/o* is a combining form that means "heart," and *vascul* is a word root that means "little vessel." The continuous flow of _____ to all tissues is vital to maintain normal body functions. If the supply of oxygen or nutrients or the removal of carbon dioxide is reduced or cut off, even for a few minutes, the affected cells will die. Thus, a disease of the cardiovascular system can pose life-threatening risks to health and survival.

heart

blood vessels

8.2 The functions of the cardiovascular system may be summarized as:

- Propulsion of blood by the _____

- Transport of blood to all body tissues by the _____
  _____

- Exchange of materials between the blood and body tissues

1. capillaries
2. heart
3. artery
4. vein

8.3 Use the anatomy terms that appear in the left column to fill in the corresponding blanks in Figures 8.1■ and 8.2■.

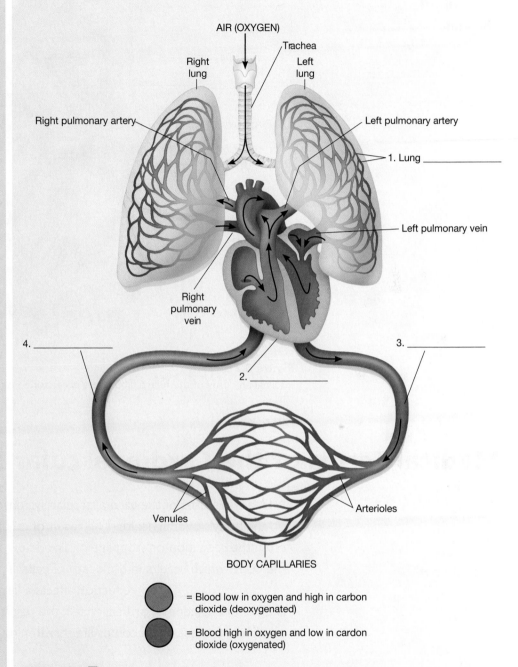

Figure 8.1 ■
The cardiovascular system. A schematic view of the closed circulation of blood. The heart is sectioned, and the capillaries are enlarged to enable you to see them.

5. aorta
6. right
7. mitral
8. left

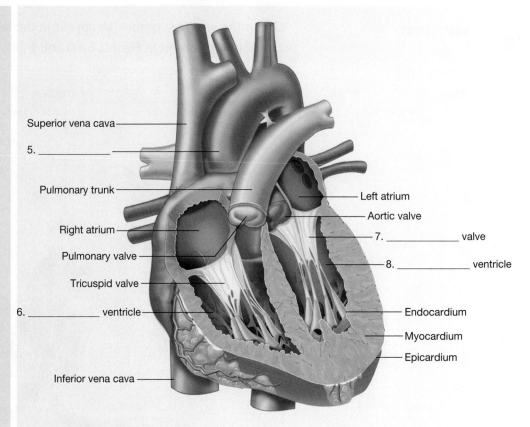

Superior vena cava

5. _____

Pulmonary trunk

Left atrium

Aortic valve

Right atrium

7. _____ valve

Pulmonary valve

8. _____ ventricle

Tricuspid valve

6. _____ ventricle

Endocardium

Myocardium

Epicardium

Inferior vena cava

Figure 8.2 ■
Internal anatomy of the heart. The heart is sectioned to reveal its internal features.

Medical Terms of the Cardiovascular System ▶▶▶▶

blood flow

8.4 Many diseases of the cardiovascular system have a profound effect on the body's overall health. The result of cardiovascular disease is often the reduction or stoppage of blood flow to one or more parts of the body, which results in the death of cells. If _____ _____ reduction affects a large area or a critical organ like the brain, kidneys, or heart itself, the resulting cell death can produce a condition that quickly becomes life threatening.

cardi/o/logy

cardiologist
  kar dee ALL oh jist

8.5 The division of medicine known as **cardiology** (kar dee ALL oh jee) provides clinical treatment for heart disease. *Cardiology* is a constructed term, _____/_____/_____, where the combining form *cardi/o* means "heart" and the suffix *-logy* means "study or science of." A physician specializing in this field is called a **cardiologist.** Generally, a _____ also treats conditions associated with blood vessels, due to the close functional relationship between blood vessels and the heart.

cardiovascular

8.6 In the following sections, we will review the prefixes, combining forms, and suffixes that combine to build the medical terms of the _____ system.

Signs and Symptoms of the Cardiovascular System

Here are the word parts that specifically apply to the signs and symptoms of the cardiovascular system that are covered in the following section. Note that the word parts are color-coded to help you identify them: prefixes are green, combining forms are red, and suffixes are blue.

Prefix	Definition
a-	without, absence of
brady-	slow
dys-	bad, abnormal, painful, difficult
tachy-	rapid, fast

Combining Form	Definition
angi/o	blood vessel
cardi/o	heart
cyan/o	blue
pect/o, pector/o	chest
rhythm/o, rrhythm/o	rhythm
sten/o	narrow

Suffix	Definition
-a	singular
-algia	condition of pain
-dynia	condition of pain
-genic	pertaining to producing, forming
-ia	condition of
-osis	condition of
-plegia	paralysis
-sis	state of
-spasm	sudden involuntary muscle contraction

KEY TERMS A–Z

angina pectoris
an JYE nah * pek TOR iss

8.7 The primary symptom of an insufficient supply of oxygen to the heart is chest pain called _____ _____. This Latin term literally means "chest choke." The level of chest pain varies with the patient, varying from a very slight pressure to an overbearing pain that radiates to the shoulders, upper left arm, and back.

angiospasm
AN jee oh spazm

8.8 The common combining form of "blood vessel" is *angi/o*. Blood vessel disorders may include abnormal muscular contractions, or spasms, of the smooth muscles forming the vessel walls. This sign is called _____. The constructed form of this term is angi/o/spasm.

angiostenosis
AN jee oh sten OH siss

8.9 Narrowing of a blood vessel is a sign of cardiovascular disease, causing a reduction of blood flow to the part of the body at the receiving end of the narrowed vessel. This sign is called **angiostenosis.** The constructed form of this term is written angi/o/sten/osis and includes one combining form: *angi/o*, which means "blood vessel"; and the word root *sten*, which means "narrow." Thus, the literal meaning of _____ is "condition of a narrow blood vessel."

arrhythmia
ah RITH mee ah

8.10 The prefix *a-* means "without, absence of," and the prefix *dys-* means "bad, abnormal, painful, difficult." In some cases, they may be used interchangeably. For example, a loss of the normal rhythm of the heart is called _____, which means "condition of without rhythm" and is written a/rrhythm/ia. An alternate term for an abnormal heart rhythm is **dysrhythmia.** The constructed form of this term is written dys/rhythm/ia.

WORDS TO WATCH OUT FOR ▶▶▶▶ **Arrhythmia and Dysrhythmia**

These two medical terms relating to the abnormal rhythm of the heart appear to function similarly. As you have learned, the prefix *a-* means "without, absence of," and the prefix *dys-* means "bad, abnormal, painful, difficult." Now look closer at the word roots. They are not identical. Both *rrhythm* and *rhythm* mean "rhythm." The term arrhythmia ("condition of without rhythm") has an extra **r.** To remember which term is spelled with two *r*s, it might help to think of the expression "without rhyme or reason." A condition of arrhythmia is a heartbeat "***without** rhyme or reason,*" whereas a condition of dysrhythmia is a heartbeat with an abnormal rhythm.

---

bradycardia
brad ee KAR dee ah

8.11 The common word root for heart is *cardi.* You will find it used in many terms in this chapter. In the term **bradycardia,** the prefix that means "slow" is used to form the meaning "slow heart." _____ is an abnormally slow heart rate, usually under 60 beats per minute. The normal resting heart rate ranges from 60 to 90 beats per minute.

cardiodynia
kar dee oh DIN ee ah

8.12 The most common term for chest pain is, simply, **chest pain,** abbreviated **CP.** An alternate term may also be used for this symptom. This term, **cardiodynia,** uses the suffix *-dynia,* which means "condition of pain." The constructed form of _____ is written cardi/o/dynia.

cardiogenic
kar dee oh JENN ik

8.13 The suffix *-genic* means "pertaining to producing, forming." When combined with the word part for heart, the term _____ is formed. The constructed form of the term is written cardi/o/genic. It refers to a symptom or sign that originates from a condition of the heart. For example, the pain sensation of angina pectoris (Frame 8.7) is a cardiogenic symptom because it is caused by insufficient blood flow to the heart.

cardioplegia
kar dee oh PLEE jee ah

8.14 The suffix *-plegia* means "paralysis." Therefore, a sign in which the heart has become paralyzed is called _____. The constructed form of this term is cardi/o/plegia.

cyanosis sigh ah NOH siss	**8.15** A symptom in which a blue tinge is seen in the skin and mucous membranes is called **cyanosis,** which literally means "condition of blue." It is written cyan/osis. _____ is caused by oxygen deficiency in tissues and is a common sign of respiratory failure often caused by cardiovascular disease.
palpitation pal pih TAY shun	**8.16** A symptom of pounding, racing, or skipping of the heartbeat is called _____. The term is derived from the Latin word *palpitatus,* which means "a throbbing."
tachycardia tack ee KAR dee ah	**8.17** The opposite of the prefix *brady-* is the prefix *tachy-,* which means "rapid, fast." A rapid heart rate is called _____. It may be a symptom of heart disease if the heart exceeds 100 beats per minute at rest.

PRACTICE: Signs and Symptoms of the Cardiovascular System

Break the Chain

Analyze these medical terms:

   a) Separate each term into its word parts; each word part is labeled for you (**p** = prefix, **r** = root, **cf** = combining form, and **s** = suffix).

   b) For the Bonus Question, write the requested definition in the blank that follows.

The first set has been completed for you as an example.

1. a. angiostenosis
    <u>angi/o/sten/osis</u>
       cf   r   s

    b. *Bonus Question:* What is the definition of the suffix? <u>*condition of*</u>

2. a. bradycardia
    _____/_____/_____
         p   r   s

    b. *Bonus Question:* What is the definition of the word root? _____

3. a. cardiodynia
    _____/___/_____
         cf   s

    b. *Bonus Question:* What is the definition of the suffix? _____

4. a. cardiogenic
    _____/___/_____
         cf   s

    b. *Bonus Question:* What is the definition of the suffix? _____

5. a. cyanosis
    _____/_____
        r   s

    b. *Bonus Question:* What is the definition of the word root? _____

6. a. angiospasm
    _____/___/_____
         cf   s

    b. *Bonus Question:* What is the definition of the suffix? _____

The Right Match

Match the term on the left with the correct definition on the right.

_____ 1. cyanosis

_____ 2. angina pectoris

_____ 3. cardioplegia

_____ 4. cardiogenic

_____ 5. cardiodynia

_____ 6. arrhythmia

_____ 7. tachycardia

_____ 8. palpitation

a. sign or symptom that originates from a condition of the heart

b. pounding, racing, or skipping of the heartbeat

c. opposite of bradycardia; fast heartbeat

d. pain associated with the heart

e. chest pain or pressure

f. blue tinge in the skin and mucous membranes

g. paralyzed heart

h. term that literally means "condition of without rhythm"

Diseases and Disorders of the Cardiovascular System

Here are the word parts that specifically apply to the diseases and disorders of the cardiovascular system that are covered in the following section. Note that the word parts are color-coded to help you identify them: prefixes are green, combining forms are red, and suffixes are blue.

Prefix	Definition
endo-	within
epi-	upon, over, above, on top
hyper-	excessive, abnormally high, above
hypo-	deficient, abnormally low, below
peri-	around
poly-	excessive, over, many

Combining Form	Definition
angi/o	blood vessel
aort/o	aorta
arter/o, arteri/o	artery
ather/o	fatty
atri/o	atrium
cardi/o	heart
coron/o	crown or circle, heart
hem/o	blood
isch/o	hold back
my/o	muscle
phleb/o	vein
scler/o	hard
sept/o	putrefying; wall, partition
sten/o	narrow
tampon/o	plug
tens/o	pressure
thromb/o	clot
valvul/o	little valve
varic/o	dilated vein
ventricul/o	little belly, ventricle

Suffix	Definition
-ac	pertaining to
-ade	process
-al	pertaining to
-ar	pertaining to
-emia	condition of blood
-ic	pertaining to
-ion	process
-itis	inflammation
-megaly	abnormally large
-oma	tumor
-osis	condition of
-pathy	disease

KEY TERMS A-Z

aneurysm
AN yoo rism

8.18 An abnormal bulging of an arterial wall is called an **aneurysm** and is shown in Figure 8.3■. The term is derived from the Greek word *aneurysma*, which means "a widening." An _____ is usually caused by a congenital defect or an acquired weakness of the arterial wall, which worsens in time as blood is pushed against it. The bursting of a large aneurysm is usually life threatening, resulting in massive hemorrhage.

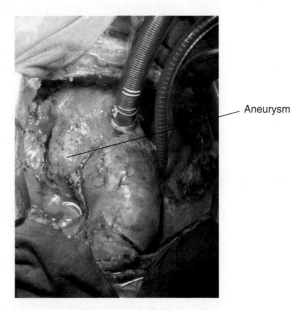

Aneurysm

Figure 8.3 ■
Aneurysm. Photograph of the aorta, the large blood vessel arising from the heart, with a large bulge, or aneurysm, in its wall (just to the left of the tubing). An aneurysm is a weakened blood vessel wall that is in danger of bursting, which often results in a life-threatening hemorrhage.
Source: kalewa/Shutterstock

angiocarditis
AN jee oh kar DYE tiss

8.19 Inflammation of the heart and blood vessels is a disease called **angiocarditis.** It is usually caused by a widespread bacterial infection of the blood, or septicemia (Frame 8.55). The four word parts of _____ are shown when it is written angi/o/card/itis.

angioma
an jee OH mah

8.20 A term describing a tumor arising from a blood vessel combines the word root for blood vessel, *angi*, with the suffix for tumor, *-oma*, to form _____. This constructed term is written angi/oma. Also known as **hemangioma** (heh MAN gee OH mah), it is a benign clump of endothelium forming a mass. In some cases the mass can obstruct the flow of blood through the vessel, although the term carries a second meaning of a red or purple birthmark on the skin that does not obstruct blood flow.

aortic insufficiency
a OR tik * in suf FISH un see

8.21 The aortic valve is the semilunar valve located at the base of the aorta, which normally prevents blood from returning to the left ventricle. If it fails to close completely during ventricular diastole, blood may return to the left ventricle, causing the left ventricle to work harder. This condition is called **aortic insufficiency.** The long-term result of _____ _____, abbreviated **AI,** is a chronic condition of the heart known as congestive heart failure, which is described in Frame 8.36. An alternate term for AI is **aortic regurgitation.**

aortic stenosis
a OR tik * sten OH siss

8.22 The word root *sten* means "narrow." An **aortic stenosis** is a narrowing of the aorta that reduces the flow of blood through this large vessel, which causes the left ventricle to work harder than normal. It is usually a more serious condition than aortic insufficiency, although the long-term effect is similar by leading to congestive heart failure (Frame 8.36). The constructed form of _____ _____ is written aort/ic sten/osis.

aortitis
ay or TYE tiss

8.23 Inflammation of the aorta is called _____. The constructed form of this term is aort/itis. Often caused by a bacterial infection, it can lead to acute aortic insufficiency (Frame 8.21).

arteriopathy
ahr tee ree AH path ee

8.24 A general term for a disease of an artery is _____. This constructed term uses the suffix -*pathy* (meaning "disease") and is written arteri/o/pathy.

arteriosclerosis
ahr TEE ree oh skleh ROH siss

8.25 One common form of arteriopathy occurs when an artery wall becomes thickened and loses its elasticity, resulting in a reduced flow of blood to tissues. The risk of developing this disease, known as **arteriosclerosis,** increases with advanced age. The constructed form of _____ is written arteri/o/scler/osis, which literally means "condition of hard artery." If coronary arteries supplying the heart are damaged by this disease, the condition is called **arteriosclerotic heart disease (ASHD).**

atherosclerosis

ATH er oh skleh ROH siss

8.26 A term describing a specific form of arteriosclerosis (Frame 8.25), in which one or more fatty plaques form along the inner walls of arteries, uses the combining form that means "fatty" to form the term **atherosclerosis.** The plaques thicken with time, which reduces the flow of blood through the affected vessel (Figure 8.4■). The constructed form of this term is written ather/o/scler/osis, which literally means "condition of hard fat." A major cause of coronary artery disease (Frame 8.38), _____ poses an immediate threat to life if a plaque disrupts blood flow and releases blood clots, which may trigger an acute myocardial infarction (Frame 8.49).

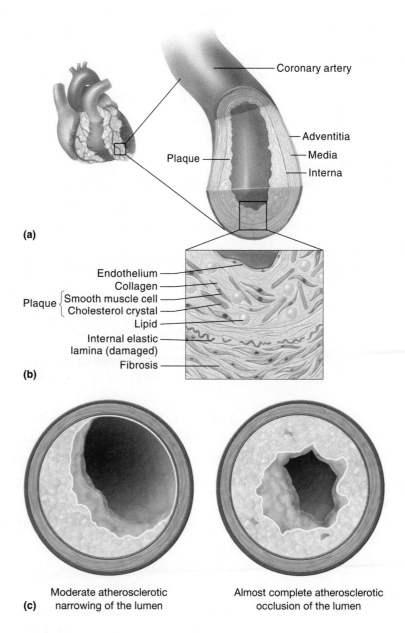

Figure 8.4 ■

Atherosclerosis. (a) A sectioned coronary artery that exhibits an accumulation of fatty plaque, which reduces the internal diameter of the vessel. (b) In this close-up, you can see that the plaque consists of cholesterol, triglycerides, phospholipids, collagen, and smooth muscle cells. (c) Two types and degrees of atherosclerotic narrowing, or stenosis.

atrial septal defect
AY tree al * SEP tal * DEE fekt

8.27 A congenital condition characterized by a failure of the foramen ovale to close at birth, producing an opening in the septum (*sept/o*) that separates the right and left atria, is called _____ _____ _____. It allows blood to pass between the two atria, which bypasses the pulmonary circulation. *Atrial* and *septal* are constructed terms, as you can see when they are written as atri/al and sept/al.

atriomegaly
AY tree oh MEG ah lee
atri/o/megaly

8.28 The suffix *-megaly* means "abnormally large." In the condition **atriomegaly,** the atria have become abnormally enlarged or dilated, reducing their ability to push blood into the ventricles. The constructed form of _____ reveals three word parts when written ____/____/____. It is a form of cardiomegaly (Frame 8.32).

atrioventricular block
AY tree oh ven TRIK yoo lar

8.29 An injury to the atrioventricular node (AV node), which normally receives impulses from the sinoatrial node (SA node) and transmits them to the ventricles to stimulate ventricular contraction, is called an _____ _____, or **AV block.** The injury is usually caused by a myocardial infarction (Frame 8.49), during which the cells of the AV node die due to a loss of blood flow. The term *atrioventricular* is a constructed term, written atri/o/ventricul/ar.

cardiac arrest
KAR dee ak * ah REST

8.30 The cessation of heart activity is called _____ _____. As you should know, *cardiac* is a constructed term written cardi/ac. *Arrest* means "stop." In **sudden cardiac arrest,** abbreviated **SCA,** the patient often has little or no warning signs, and it is a major killer: roughly 325,000 die each year in the United States. Most deaths occur within minutes, primarily due to a sudden loss of blood flow to the heart.

cardiac tamponade
KAR dee ak * tamp oh NAHD

8.31 Acute compression of the heart due to the accumulation of fluid within the pericardial cavity is known as **cardiac tamponade.** The term is constructed from word parts and is shown as cardi/ac tampon/ade. It literally means "pertaining to heart plug process." _____ _____ is a complication of an inflammatory disease of the pericardium known as pericarditis (Frame 8.52).

cardiomegaly
KAR dee oh MEG ah lee

8.32 Recall that the suffix *-megaly* means "abnormally large." The abnormal enlargement of the heart is called _____, which occurs when the heart must work harder than normal to meet the oxygen demands of body cells. The constructed form of this term is cardi/o/megaly.

cardiomyopathy
KAR dee oh my OPP ah thee

8.33 A general term for a disease of the myocardium of the heart is **cardiomyopathy.** The constructed form of _____ reveals five word parts and is written cardi/o/my/o/pathy. The most common causes of cardiomyopathy include hypertension (Frame 8.46), chronic alcoholism, bacterial infection, and congenital defects of the myocardial cells.

cardiovalvulitis
KAR dee oh val vyoo LYE tiss

8.34 An inflammation of the valves of the heart is called **cardiovalvulitis.** The constructed form of this term is cardi/o/valvul/itis. As you know, *cardi/o* means "heart," and the suffix *-itis* means "inflammation." The word root *valvul* means "little valve." The most common causes of this disease are bacterial infection, which leads to the deposition of calcium deposits on heart valves, and congenital defects, which results in abnormally shaped valves. _____ is usually diagnosed from the presence of a heart murmur (Frame 8.44), which is a gurgling sound detected during auscultation (Frame 8.68).

coarctation
ko ark TAY shun

8.35 A congenital defect that is present at birth is known as **coarctation of the aorta.** The term *coarctation* is derived from the Latin word *coarcto,* which means "to press together." _____ of the aorta causes reduced systemic circulation of blood and accumulation of fluid in the lungs and requires surgical repair.

congestive heart failure

8.36 A chronic form of heart disease characterized by the failure of the left ventricle to pump enough blood to supply systemic tissues is called **congestive heart failure (CHF).** Also known as **left ventricular failure,** the reduced function of the left ventricle characteristic of

_____ _____ _____

makes the heart work harder, resulting in cardiomegaly (Frame 8.32), pulmonary congestion, and reduced stroke volume that eventually leads to cardiac arrest (Frame 8.30).

cor pulmonale
kor * pull moh NAY lee

8.37 A chronic enlargement of the right ventricle resulting from congestion of the pulmonary circulation is called **cor pulmonale.** A French word that literally means "heart lung," _____ _____ is also known as **right ventricular failure.**

coronary artery disease

8.38 A general term for a disease that afflicts the coronary arteries supplying the heart is _____ _____ _____ **(CAD).** The most common form of CAD is atherosclerosis (Frame 8.26).

coronary occlusion

8.39 *Occlusion* is a general term that means "blockage." A **coronary occlusion** is a blockage within a coronary artery, resulting in a reduced blood flow to an area of the heart muscle. The most common single cause of a _____ _____ is atherosclerosis (Frame 8.26). Atherosclerosis or other diseases may also lead to emboli (drifting blood clots), and a congenital stenosis may also contribute to coronary occlusion.

embolism

EM boh lizm

8.40 A blockage or occlusion that forms when a blood clot or other foreign particle (including air or fat) moves through the circulation is called an **embolism.** The term is derived from the Greek word *embolisma,* which means "piece or patch." An _____ can produce a severe circulatory restriction when the blood clot or particle, called an **embolus** (plural form is **emboli**), lodges in an artery.

endocarditis

EHN doh kar DYE tiss

8.41 Inflammation of the endocardium, the thin membrane lining the inside walls of the heart chambers, is an acute disease called _____ (Figure 8.5■). The constructed form of this term is endo/card/itis. Because the endocardium also covers the heart valves, endocarditis often results in cardiovalvulitis (Frame 8.34). It is usually caused by a bacterial infection.

Figure 8.5 ■

Endocarditis. The human heart has been sectioned to reveal the left ventricle and origin of the aorta, with the aortic valve between them. The yellow growths, called vegetations, on the aortic valve have been caused by a *Streptococcus* infection, rendering the aortic valve nonfunctional. Because the heart valve is affected, the condition is also called cardiovalvulitis. *Source: Courtesy of the Public Health Image Library, Centers for Disease Control, Atlanta, Georgia/ Dr. Edwin P. Ewing, Jr.*

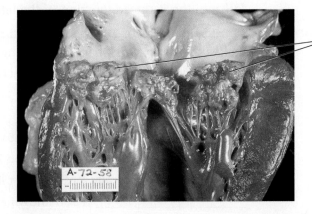

Mitral valve vegetations

fibrillation fih bril AY shun	**8.42** A condition of uncoordinated, rapid contractions of the muscle forming the ventricles or atria is called _____. It is a severe form of arrhythmia (Frame 8.10). **Atrial fibrillation** leads to a reduction of blood expelled from the atria and is usually not fatal. However, **ventricular fibrillation** results in circulatory collapse due to the failure of the ventricles to expel blood.
heart block	**8.43** A block or delay of the normal electrical conduction of the heart is called _____ _____. It is often the result of a myocardial infarction (Frame 8.49) that damages the SA node or AV node.
heart murmur	**8.44** An abnormal soft, gurgling or blowing sound heard during auscultation (Frame 8.68) of the heart is called **heart murmur.** It often indicates the regurgitation of blood through one or more heart valves. The most common source of _____ _____ occurs when the mitral valve leaks during ventricular contraction, called **mitral valve prolapse (MVP).**
hemorrhoids HEM oh roydz	**8.45** The presence of dilated, or varicose, veins in the anal region is called _____. It produces symptoms of local pain and itching.
hypertension HIGH per TEN shun	**8.46** Persistently high blood pressure is an abnormal condition called _____. This constructed term is written hyper/tens/ion and means "process of abnormally high pressure." It includes **essential hypertension,** in which the condition is not traceable to a single cause, and **secondary hypertension,** in which the high blood pressure is caused by the effects of another disease, such as atherosclerosis.
hypotension HIGH poh TEN shun	**8.47** A condition of abnormally low blood pressure is called _____, which includes the prefix hypo- that means "deficient, abnormally low, below." It is an acute reaction to hemorrhage or septicemia (Frame 8.55).
ischemia iss KEE mee ah	**8.48** An abnormally low flow of blood to tissues is the condition known as **ischemia.** The term is a constructed term, isch/emia, which literally means "condition of holding back blood." Coronary _____ is a temporary deficiency caused by an occlusion, such as atherosclerotic plaque (Frame 8.26), emboli (Frame 8.40), or congenital stenosis.

myocardial infarction
my oh KAR dee al * in FARK shun

8.49 Death of a portion of the myocardium is called **myocardial infarction.** The term *infarction* is derived from the Latin word *infarctus,* which means "stuff into." In medicine it is used to describe a death of cells resulting from a sudden loss of blood flow (Figure 8.6■). The term *myocardial* is constructed from word parts, as shown when it is written as my/o/cardi/al, which means "pertaining to heart muscle." If the _____ _____, or **MI,** affects a large or functionally critical part of the heart, arrhythmia (Frame 8.10), cardiac arrest (Frame 8.30), or both may follow. The common name for an MI is a **heart attack.**

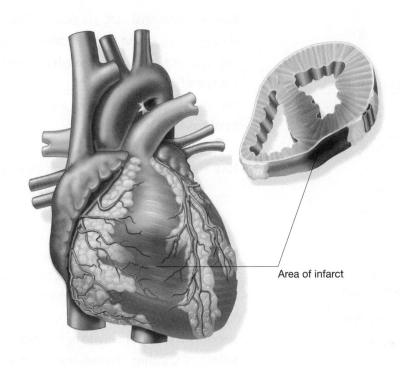

Area of infarct

Figure 8.6 ■
Myocardial infarction. A heart with a myocardial infarction of the left ventricle wall, in which cardiac cells have died and surrounding tissues have become damaged. The right image is a section through the heart.

myocarditis
my oh kar DYE tiss

8.50 Inflammation of the myocardium of the heart is an acute condition called _____. The constructed form of this term is my/o/card/itis. Often caused by bacterial infection, it is a form of cardiomyopathy (Frame 8.33).

patent ductus arteriosus
PAY tent * DUCK tuss *
ahr tee ree OH siss

8.51 A congenital condition characterized by an opening between the pulmonary artery and the aorta at birth due to a failure of the fetal vessel, called the ductus arteriosus, to close is called **patent ductus arteriosus.** The term *patent* means "open." The condition _____ _____ _____ permits the flow of blood from the pulmonary artery to the aorta, which bypasses the pulmonary circulation.

pericarditis pair ih kar DYE tiss	**8.52** Inflammation of the membrane surrounding the heart, the pericardium, is called _____. The constructed form of the term is written peri/card/itis. It is usually caused by bacterial infection and affects both layers of the pericardium (the pericardial sac and the epicardium).
phlebitis fleh BYE tiss	**8.53** A word root for vein is _phleb_, and it is used in the construction of the term that means "inflammation of a vein." The term is _____, and its constructed form is written phleb/itis. In the related condition **thrombophlebitis** (THROM boh fleh BYE tiss), the inflammation of the vein includes an obstruction by a blood clot.
polyarteritis PALL ee ahr ter EYE tiss	**8.54** Simultaneous inflammation of many arteries is a condition known as _____. The constructed form of this term reveals three word parts and is written poly/arter/itis.
septicemia SEP tih SEE mee ah	**8.55** A bacterial infection of the bloodstream is called **septicemia.** Because the bacteria are carried throughout the body by way of the infected blood, it becomes widespread and life threatening quickly. The constructed form of _____ is written sept/ic/emia, which literally means "condition of putrefying blood." Recall that **sepsis** is a Greek word that means "putrefying."
tetralogy of Fallot teh TRALL oh jee * of * fah LOH	**8.56** A severe congenital disease in which four defects associated with the heart are present at birth is called **tetralogy of Fallot.** The four defects are pulmonary stenosis (narrowing of the pulmonary valve), ventricular septal defect (Frame 8.59), incorrect position of the aorta, and right ventricular hypertrophy. As a result of _____ _____, the pulmonary circulation is partially bypassed.
thrombosis throm BOH siss	**8.57** The presence of stationary blood clots within one or more blood vessels is called **thrombosis.** The term is the Greek word for clotting, _thrombosis_. A coronary _____ is often caused by atherosclerosis (Frame 8.26), and its rupture can result in sudden death due to an acute myocardial infarction (Frame 8.49).

varicosis

vair ih KOH siss

8.58 An abnormally dilated vein is called _____, or varicose vein. *Varicosis* is a constructed term, written varic/osis, which literally means "condition of dilated vein." It results when valves within a superficial vein of the leg or elsewhere fail, allowing blood to pool in response to gravitational forces (Figure 8.7■).

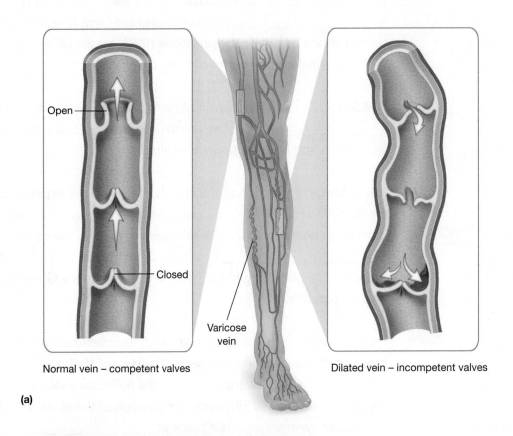

Open

Closed

Varicose vein

Normal vein – competent valves

Dilated vein – incompetent valves

(a)

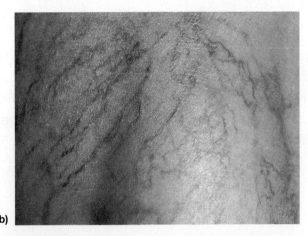

(b)

Figure 8.7 ■

Varicosis. (a) Varicose veins develop due to the failure of valves in the superficial veins of the leg, which leads to blood accumulation in response to gravity and vein dilation. (b) Photograph of spider veins (small varicose veins) of the leg.

Source: Courtesy of Jason L. Smith, MD.

ventricular septal defect
vehn TRIK yoo lar * SEPP tal *
DEE fekt

8.59 A congenital disease in which an opening in the septum (*sept/o* in this case means "wall, partition") separating the right and left ventricles is present at birth is called _____ _____ _____, abbreviated **VSD.** The opening allows some blood to flow from the left ventricle to the right ventricle, reducing blood flow to body organs while dangerously increasing blood flow to the lungs.

PRACTICE: Diseases and Disorders of the Cardiovascular System

Linkup

Link the word parts in the list to create the terms that match the definitions. You may use word parts more than once. Remember to add in combining vowels when needed—and that some terms do not use any combining vowel. The first one is completed as an example.

Prefix	Combining Form	Suffix
hyper-	angi/o	-ion
peri-	ather/o	-ism
	cardi/o	-itis
	embol/o	-oma
	my/o	-osis
	scler/o	-pathy
	tens/o	
	thromb/o	
	varic/o	

Definition

1. An occlusion of blood flow

2. A general term for a disease of the myocardium of the heart

3. A specific form of arteriosclerosis in which one or more fatty plaques form along the inner walls of arteries

4. A tumor arising from a blood vessel

5. Inflammation of the membrane surrounding the heart

6. Inflammation of the heart and blood vessels

7. An abnormally dilated vein

8. The presence of a stationary blood clot within a blood vessel

9. Persistently high blood pressure

Term

embolism

_____

_____

_____

_____

_____

_____

_____

_____

The Right Match

Match the term on the left with the correct definition on the right.

_____ 1. aneurysm

_____ 2. cardiac tamponade

_____ 3. cor pulmonale

_____ 4. heart murmur

_____ 5. cardiac arrest

_____ 6. coronary artery disease

_____ 7. coronary occlusion

_____ 8. atrial septal defect

_____ 9. congestive heart failure

_____ 10. heart block

_____ 11. fibrillation

a. a disease of the coronary vessels

b. a congenital heart defect

c. a block of the heart conduction system

d. a blockage in a coronary vessel

e. abnormal bulging of an arterial wall

f. soft, gurgling, or blowing sound heard through auscultation

g. cessation of heartbeat

h. uncoordinated, rapid heartbeat

i. literally, "heart lung"

j. left ventricular failure

k. caused by fluid within pericardial cavity

Treatments, Procedures, and Devices of the Cardiovascular System

Here are the word parts that specifically apply to the treatments, procedures, and devices associated with the cardiovascular system that are covered in the following section. Note that the word parts are color-coded to help you identify them: prefixes are green, combining forms are red, and suffixes are blue.

Prefix	Definition
endo-	within

Combining Form	Definition
angi/o	blood vessel
aort/o	aorta
arter/o, arteri/o	artery
cardi/o	heart
coron/o	crown or circle, heart
ech/o	sound
electr/o	electricity
embol/o	plug
man/o	thin, scanty
phleb/o	vein
pulmon/o	lung
son/o	sound
sphygm/o	pulse
thromb/o	clot
valvul/o	little valve

Suffix	Definition
-ac	pertaining to
-ary	pertaining to
-ectomy	surgical excision, removal
-gram	a record or image
-graphy	recording process
-lytic	pertaining to loosen, dissolve
-meter	measure, measuring instrument
-metry	measurement, process of measuring
-plasty	surgical repair
-rrhaphy	suturing
-scopy	process of viewing
-stomy	surgical creation of an opening
-tomy	incision, to cut

KEY TERMS A-Z

angiography
an jee OG rah fee

8.60 A diagnostic procedure that includes X-ray photography, MRI, or CT scan images of a blood vessel after injection of a contrast medium is called **angiography.** This constructed term is written angi/o/graphy. The image resulting from _____ is called an **angiogram** (AN jee oh gram), which is written angi/o/gram. When the procedure is focused on the heart, it is called **cardiac** or **coronary angiography.**

angioplasty
AN jee oh plass tee

8.61 The surgical repair of a blood vessel is generally known as _____. The constructed form of this term is angi/o/plasty. It includes procedures to reopen blocked vessels, such as **balloon angioplasty,** in which an inflatable balloon is inserted into a blocked vessel and inflated (Figure 8.8■), and **laser angioplasty,** which uses a laser beam to open a blocked artery.

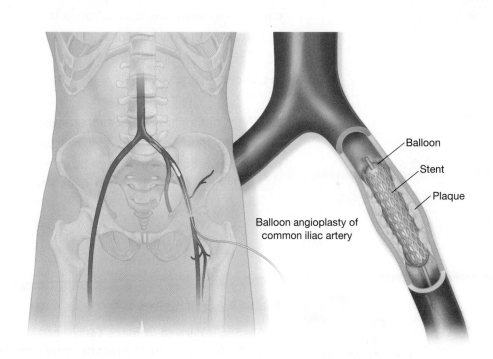

Figure 8.8 ■
Angioplasty. One form is called balloon angioplasty, shown here. A balloon catheter is threaded into the blocked coronary artery and positioned into the obstructed area. The balloon is then inflated, which presses the plaque against the vessel wall. After the balloon catheter is withdrawn, the plaque remains flattened, improving the flow of blood through the vessel.

Balloon
Stent
Plaque
Balloon angioplasty of common iliac artery

angioscopy
AN jee OS koh pee

8.62 The use of a flexible fiber-optic instrument, or endoscope, to observe a diseased blood vessel and to assess any lesions is a procedure called _____. This constructed term is written angi/o/scopy. The endoscope is often a modified instrument, called an **angioscope,** which includes a camera at one end and video monitor at the opposite end.

angiostomy
an jee OS toh mee

8.63 The suffix -*stomy* means "surgical creation of an opening." The surgical procedure that involves the creation of an opening into a blood vessel, usually for the insertion of a catheter, is called _____. The constructed form of this term is angi/o/stomy.

angiotomy an jee OT oh mee	**8.64** The surgical incision into a blood vessel is called _____, which uses the suffix *-tomy* that means "incision, to cut." The constructed form of this term reveals three word parts, as shown in angi/o/tomy.
aortography AY or TOG rah fee	**8.65** A procedure that obtains an X-ray image, MRI, or CT scan image of the aorta is called _____. The constructed form of this term is aort/o/graphy. The image is called an **aortogram.**
arteriography ahr tee ree OG rah fee	**8.66** A procedure that obtains an image of an artery is known as _____. The constructed form of this term is arteri/o/graphy, which literally means "process of recording an artery." The image is called an **arteriogram.**
arteriotomy ahr tee ree OT oh mee	**8.67** An incision into an artery is called an _____. This constructed term is written arteri/o/tomy. It is usually performed to repair an injured artery during a procedure known as an **arterioplasty.** The conclusion of the procedure is achieved by suturing the opening, called **arteriorrhaphy.**
auscultation oss kull TAY shun	**8.68** A part of a physical examination that involves listening to internal sounds using a **stethoscope** (STETH oh skope) is called _____. Certain sounds suggest abnormalities of heart function, especially arrhythmias and valve disorders.

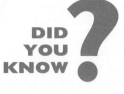

DID YOU KNOW ?

▶▶▶▶▶ **Auscultation**

Auscultation is derived from the Latin word *ausculto,* which means "to listen." During the ancient times of Aristotle, early physicians practiced this form of evaluation by pressing an ear against the patient's chest. The stethoscope, which literally means "to view the chest," is a device that made this procedure much more efficient after its first use around 1725.

cardiac catheterization
KAR dee ak *
kath eh ter ih ZAY shun

8.69 Insertion of a narrow flexible tube, called a **catheter,** through a blood vessel leading into the heart is called _____ _____ (Figure 8.9■). The procedure is performed to withdraw blood samples from heart chambers, measure pressures, and inject contrast medium for imaging purposes. The term *catheter* is derived from the Greek word *katheter,* which means "to send down."

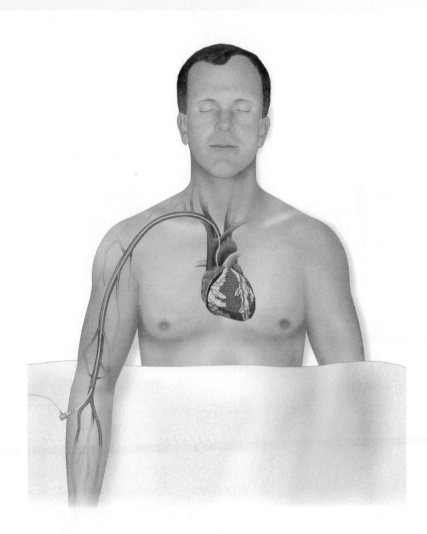

Figure 8.9 ■
Cardiac catheterization. Insertion of a tube called a catheter through a blood vessel. In this example, the catheter is inserted into the brachial artery of the arm and extends to the heart.

cardiac pacemaker
KAR dee ak * PAYS maker

8.70 A **cardiac pacemaker** is a battery-powered device that is implanted under the skin and wired to the wall of the heart (Figure 8.10■). It produces timed electric pulses that replace the function of the SA node as a treatment for a heart block and certain other arrhythmias. Recently, the _____ _____ has been improved to adjust to the patient's physical activity and SA node function. This is called an "on-demand" pacemaker.

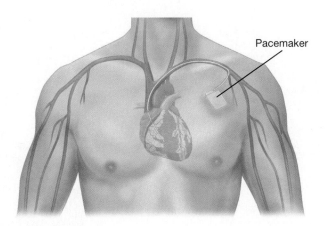

Pacemaker

Figure 8.10 ■
Cardiac pacemaker. The pacemaker device is implanted beneath the skin near the heart, and the electrode is surgically connected to the heart wall.

cardiopulmonary resuscitation
KAR dee oh PULL mon air ee *
ree SUSS ih TAY shun

8.71 An emergency procedure that is used to restore breathing by applying a combination of chest compression and artificial ventilation at intervals is commonly abbreviated **CPR,** which means _____ _____. The constructed form of this term is written cardi/o/pulmon/ary resuscitation. The term *resuscitation* is derived from the Latin word *resuscitatio,* which means "to revive."

coronary artery bypass graft

8.72 A surgical procedure that involves removing a blood vessel from another part of the body and inserting it into the coronary circulation is called _____-_____ _____ _____, or **CABG.** The grafted vessel restores blood flow to an oxygen-deprived area of the heart by carrying blood around an occluded (blocked) coronary artery (Figure 8.11■).

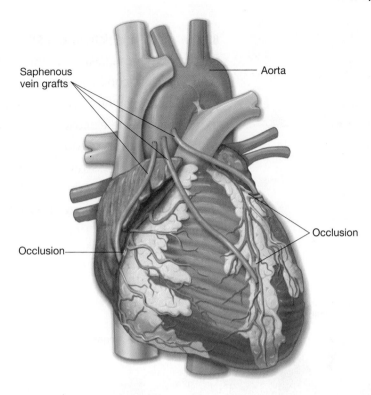

Saphenous vein grafts

Aorta

Occlusion

Occlusion

Figure 8.11 ■
Coronary artery bypass graft (CABG). The grafts are often obtained from the patient's saphenous veins in the legs and are inserted to carry blood around the blockage (occlusion).

coronary stent

8.73 An artificial, metallic scaffold that is used to anchor a surgical implant, or graft, is called a **stent** (Figure 8.12■). In coronary circulation, a **coronary stent** may be implanted into a coronary artery that is occluded to restore blood flow to an oxygen-deprived part of the heart. A _____ _____ may also be used to prevent closure of a coronary artery after angioplasty (Frame 8.61).

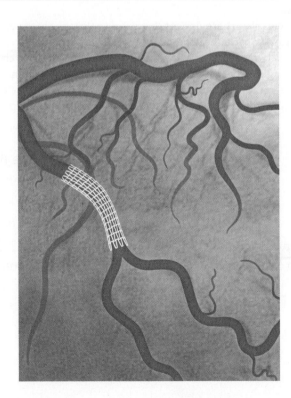

Figure 8.12 ■
Coronary stent. Illustration of an angiogram revealing a coronary stent, which helps prevent closure of the coronary vessel supplying the heart.

defibrillation

dee fib rih LAY shun

8.74 In cases in which an arrhythmia progresses to the state of ventricular fibrillation (Frame 8.42), an electric charge may be applied to the chest wall to stop the heart conduction system momentarily, then restart it with a more normal heart rhythm. This procedure is called _____.
In most cases, the electric charge is applied to the skin of the chest with paddles using an **automated external defibrillator.** Abbreviated **AED,** a portable unit is illustrated in Figure 8.13a■. It may also be performed with electrodes directly on the heart if the defibrillation is needed during surgery, using an **implantable cardioverter defibrillator (ICD),** illustrated in Figure 8.13b■.

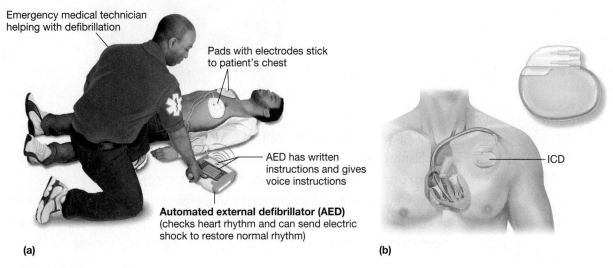

Emergency medical technician helping with defibrillation

Pads with electrodes stick to patient's chest

AED has written instructions and gives voice instructions

Automated external defibrillator (AED) (checks heart rhythm and can send electric shock to restore normal rhythm)

ICD

(a)

(b)

Figure 8.13 ■
Defibrillator. Defibrillators are devices that supply a voltage charge to the heart in the hope of restarting the cardiac cycle (heartbeat). (a) A portable automated external defibrillator (AED). The unit includes two paddles that are pressed against the external chest wall, which deliver a brief voltage charge from a generator to the patient. AEDs are given credit for saving thousands of lives every year, mainly from sudden cardiac arrest (SCA). (b) An implantable cardioverter defibrillator. ICDs are used during surgery and may be inserted for postsurgical maintenance.

Doppler sonography

DOP ler * son OG rah fee

8.75 An ultrasound procedure that evaluates blood flow through a blood vessel is called **Doppler sonography.** It is often performed on the heart to evaluate coronary circulation in a noninvasive manner and may also be used to monitor pulse rate from peripheral arteries. In the term _____ _____, *sonography* is a constructed term, written son/o/graphy, which literally means "recording process of sound."

8.76 An ultrasound procedure that directs sound waves through the heart to observe heart structures in an effort to evaluate heart function is called _____. This is a constructed term with five word parts that is written ech/o/cardi/o/graphy. The procedure may also be called **cardiac ultrasonography** (KAR dee ak * ul trah son OG rah fee). The record or image of the data is typically called an **echocardiogram** (ek oh KAR dee oh gram). If a heart condition is suspected, it is often performed during and after exercise to reproduce the dysfunction for closer evaluation, in the procedure known as a **stress ECHO.**

echocardiography
ek oh kar dee OG rah fee

8.77 In the procedure known as **electrocardiography,** electrodes are pasted to the skin of the chest to detect and record the electrical events of the heart conduction system (Figure 8.14■). The constructed form of _____ is written electr/o/cardi/o/graphy. The record or image of the data is called an **electrocardiogram** and abbreviated **ECG** or **EKG** (the K is from the Greek word for heart, *kardia*). Electrocardiography is used extensively to evaluate heart function. It is particularly useful in diagnosing cardiac arrhythmias (Frame 8.10). When measured during physical activity using a treadmill or stationary bicycle, it is called a **stress ECG.**

electrocardiography
ee LEK troh KAR dee AWG rah fee

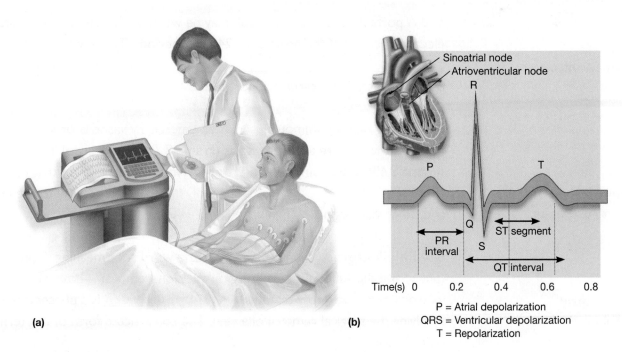

(a)

(b)

P = Atrial depolarization
QRS = Ventricular depolarization
T = Repolarization

Figure 8.14 ■
Electrocardiography. (a) Electrodes are placed on the patient's chest to record the electrical events within the heart. (b) A normal electrocardiogram includes three peaks or waves, called the P wave, QRS wave, and T wave.

WORDS TO WATCH OUT FOR ▶▶▶▶▶ Echocardiography and Electrocardiography

Echocardiography and electrocardiography are both methods of measuring heart function. The two medical terms are similar enough in construction and in meaning to be confusing. Let the word parts provide the clue. Remember that one *hears* an echo, and thus, *echocardiography* is the procedure that uses ultra*sound* technology to make measurements of heart function. Also remember a synonym for *ultrasound* is *sonography,* which means "recording process of sound."

embolectomy EM boh LEK toh mee	**8.78** The suffix *-ectomy* means "surgical excision, removal." The surgical removal of a floating blood clot, or embolus (Frame 8.40), is called _____. The constructed form of this term is embol/ectomy.
endarterectomy END ahr teh REK toh mee	**8.79** The removal of the inner lining of an artery to remove a fatty plaque is a surgical procedure called **endarterectomy.** The constructed form of _____ is end/arter/ectomy, which literally means "surgical excision or removal of within artery." The most common surgical site for this procedure is the carotid artery in the neck, which is subject to developing atherosclerotic plaques (Frame 8.26). Note that the *o* ending in the prefix *endo-* is deleted from this constructed term for ease of pronunciation.
Holter monitor	**8.80** A portable electrocardiograph may be worn by the patient to monitor electrical activity of the heart over 24-hour periods. The device is called a _____ _____ and is useful in detecting periodic or transient cardiac abnormalities.
nitroglycerin NIGH troh GLIH ser ihn	**8.81** A drug that is commonly used as an emergency vasodilator as a treatment for severe angina pectoris (Frame 8.7) or myocardial infarction (Frame 8.49) is the compound **nitroglycerin.** The vasodilation that results from _____ temporarily improves blood flow to the heart and other vital organs.
phlebectomy fleh BEK toh mee	**8.82 Phlebectomy** is constructed from the word root meaning "vein" (*phleb*) and the suffix meaning "surgical excision, removal" (*-ectomy*). From its word parts, we know that a _____ is a procedure involving the surgical removal of a vein. The constructed form of this term is phleb/ectomy.

phlebotomy
fleh BOT oh mee

8.83 A puncture into a vein to remove blood for sampling or donation is called **phlebotomy** (Figure 8.15■). This constructed term combines the word root for vein, the combining vowel *o*, and the suffix meaning "incision or to cut" to create the term _____, which is written phleb/o/tomy. Although the word part for incision is included, a small puncture is made rather than an incision when withdrawing blood (called a **venipuncture**). A healthcare professional who performs this procedure is called a **phlebotomist** (fleh BOT oh mist).

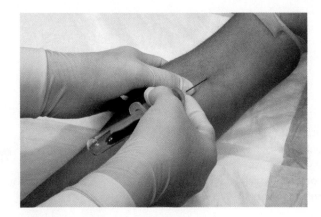

Figure 8.15 ■
Phlebotomy. In this common procedure, a syringe needle punctures a vein, usually in the arm, and withdraws blood for sampling or donation.
Source: Courtesy of the Public Health Image Library, Centers for Disease Control, Atlanta, Georgia/Jim Gathany

positron emission tomography scan
PAHZ ih tron * ee MISH uhn * toh MOG rah fee

8.84 A noninvasive procedure that provides blood flow images using positron emission tomography (**PET**) techniques combined with radioactive isotope labeling may be used to produce images of the heart to reveal functional defects. The procedure is called _____ _____ _____ _____,

or **PET scan.**

sphygmomanometry
SFIG moh mah NOM eh tree

8.85 A common procedure that measures arterial blood pressure is called _____. This constructed term is written sphygm/o/man/o/metry, which literally means "the process of measuring pulse gas." It utilizes a device called a **sphygmomanometer** (sfig moh mah NOM eh ter), which consists of an arm cuff and air pressure pump with a pressure gauge (Figure 8.16■). In recent years, the mercury pressure gauge has been replaced by aneroid dials and digital technology.

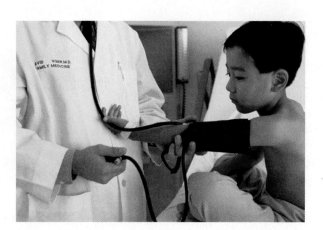

Figure 8.16 ■
Sphygmomanometry. Photograph of a physician taking blood pressure readings with the use of a sphygmomanometer, which includes an arm cuff and pressure gauge.
Source: Keith Brofsky/Photodisc/Thinkstock.

thrombolytic therapy
throm boh LITT ik * THAIR ah pee

8.86 Treatments to dissolve unwanted blood clots are often necessary after surgery to prevent the development of emboli (Frame 8.40). It is also performed soon after a myocardial infarction (Frame 8.49) to minimize damage to the heart and is credited with saving many lives. Known as _____ _____, it includes the use of drugs such as streptokinase and tissue plasminogen activator (TPA). The constructed term *thrombolytic* is made up of the combining form that means "clot" (*thromb/o*) and the suffix that means "pertaining to loosen or dissolve" (*-lytic*).

treadmill stress test

8.87 If a heart condition is suspected, a cardiologist will often require the patient to undergo exercise during echocardiography or electrocardiography (or both) in an effort to examine heart function under stress. The most common term for this procedure is _____ _____ _____.

valvuloplasty
VAL vyoo loh plass tee

8.88 The surgical repair of a heart valve is called _____. The constructed form of this term is written valvul/o/plasty. If repair is not possible due to the extent of the damage or defect, valve replacement may be required using an artificial valve or a porcine (pig) valve.

PRACTICE: Treatments, Procedures, and Devices of the Cardiovascular System

The Right Match

Match the term on the left with the correct definition on the right.

_____ 1. cardiac pacemaker

_____ 2. defibrillation

_____ 3. phlebotomy

_____ 4. Holter monitor

_____ 5. coronary stent

_____ 6. PET scan

_____ 7. treadmill stress test

_____ 8. nitroglycerin

_____ 9. auscultation

_____ 10. Doppler sonography

a. an artificial metallic scaffold that is implanted to prevent closure of a coronary artery

b. a drug that is commonly used as an emergency vasodilator

c. patient undergoes exercise during echocardiography or electro-cardiography to examine heart function under stress

d. a battery-powered device that is implanted under the skin and wired to the wall of the heart

e. puncture into a vein, usually to remove blood for sampling or donation

f. a portable electrocardiograph worn by the patient

g. an electric charge applied to the chest wall to stop the heart conduction system momentarily, then restart it with a more normal heart rhythm

h. a noninvasive procedure that provides blood flow images using positron emission tomography (PET) techniques combined with radioactive isotope labeling

i. an ultrasound procedure that evaluates blood flow

j. a physical examination that involves listening to internal sounds

Break the Chain

Analyze these medical terms:

    a) Separate each term into its word parts; each word part is labeled for you (**p** = prefix, **r** = root, **cf** = combining form, and **s** = suffix).

    b) For the Bonus Question, write the requested definition in the blank that follows.

---

1. a) arteriogram   _____ / ___ / _____
                                                     cf   s

    b) *Bonus Question:* What is the definition of the suffix? _____

---

2. a) echocardiography   _____ / ___ / _____ / ___ / _____
                                             cf   cf   s

    b) *Bonus Question:* What is the definition of the first combining form? _____

---

3. a) embolectomy   _____ / _____
                                        r   s

    b) *Bonus Question:* What is the definition of the word root? _____

---

4. a) sphygmomanometry   _____ / ___ / _____ / ___ / _____
                                           cf   cf   s

    b) *Bonus Question:* What is the definition of the suffix? _____

---

5. a) phlebotomist   _____ / ___ / _____ / _____
                                         cf   r   s

    b) *Bonus Question:* What is the definition of the combining form? _____

---

6. a) electrocardiography   _____ / ___ / _____ / ___ / _____
                                           cf   cf   s

    b) *Bonus Question:* What is the definition of the suffix? _____

---

7. a) cardiopulmonary resuscitation _____ / ___ / _____ / _____
                                           cf   r   s

    b) *Bonus Question:* What is the definition of the word root in the first word? _____

---

8. a) endarterectomy   _____ / _____ / _____
                                        p   r   s

    b) *Bonus Question:* What is the definition of the prefix? _____

---

9. a) valvuloplasty   _____ / ___ / _____
                                        cf   s

    b) *Bonus Question:* What is the definition of the suffix? _____

Abbreviations of the Cardiovascular System

The abbreviations that are associated with the cardiovascular system are summarized here. Study these abbreviations, and review them in the exercise that follows.

Abbreviation	Definition
AED	automated external defibrillator
AI	aortic insufficiency
AS	aortic stenosis
ASD	atrial septal defect
ASHD	arteriosclerotic heart disease
AV	atrioventricular
CABG	coronary artery bypass graft
CAD	coronary artery disease
CHF	congestive heart failure
CP	chest pain
CPR	cardiopulmonary resuscitation
ECG, EKG	electrocardiogram

Abbreviation	Definition
ICD	implantable cardioverter defibrillator
LA	left atrium
LV	left ventricle
MI	myocardial infarction
MVP	mitral valve prolapse
PET	positron emission tomography
RA	right atrium
RV	right ventricle
SCA	sudden cardiac arrest
VSD	ventricular septal defect

PRACTICE: Abbreviations

Fill in the blanks with the abbreviation or the complete medical term.

Abbreviation		Medical Term
1.	_____	congestive heart failure
2.	ASD	_____
3.	_____	coronary artery bypass graft
4.	MI	_____
5.	_____	positron emission tomography
6.	CPR	_____
7.	_____	arteriosclerotic heart disease
8.	AV	_____
9.	_____	electrocardiogram
10.	CAD	_____
11.	_____	automated external defibrillator
12.	RV	_____
13.	_____	ventricular septal defect
14.	MVP	_____

▶▶▶▶ Chapter Review

Word Building _____

Construct medical terms from the following meanings. (Some are built from word parts, some are not.) The first question has been completed as an example.

1.   generalized disease of the heart muscle   *cardiomyo*pathy

2.   inflammation of the heart and blood vessels   angio_____

3.   narrowing of a blood vessel   angio_____

4.   tumor arising from a blood vessel   angi_____

5.   hardening of the arteries   _____sclerosis

6.   abnormally slow heart rate   _____cardia

7.   a sensation of pain in the heart   cardio_____

8.   incision into an artery to remove plaque   end_____ectomy

9.   abnormal hypertrophy of the heart   cardio_____

10. inflammation of the inner heart membrane   endo_____

11. an abnormal heart rhythm   dys_____

12. high blood pressure that is persistent   _____tension

13. death of a portion of the myocardium   _____cardial in_____

14. inflammation of the myocardium   myo_____

15. a process of recording heart electrical activity   _____cardiography

16. inflammation of a vein   _____itis

17. a recording of an X-ray of an artery   angio_____

18. general surgical repair of a blood vessel   _____plasty

19. use of an endoscope to evaluate a blood vessel   angio_____

20. an incision into an artery   arterio_____

21. listening to heart sounds with a stethoscope   aus_____

22. use of sound waves to diagnose a heart condition   _____cardiography

▶▶▶▶ **Medical Report Exercises**

Robert Gorman _____

Read the following medical report, then answer the questions that follow.

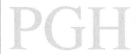

PEARSON GENERAL HOSPITAL

5500 University Avenue Metropolis, ID
Phone: (211) 594-4000 • Fax: (211) 594-4001

Medical Consultation: Cardiology

Date: 11/16/2011

Patient: Robert Gorman

Patient Complaint: Chest pain, lack of energy, reduced appetite.

History: 62-year-old Caucasian male with a recent history of mild chest pain, shortness of breath, and malaise. No murmur reported. Dental tooth extractions were performed recently and no follow-up treatment with antibiotics was reported.

Family History: Father deceased at 79 years with CHF following bypass surgery. Mother, 89 years, with complete hysterectomy following diagnosis of stage 1 cervical cancer; no reported conditions otherwise.

Allergies: Penicillin

Physical Examination: Vital signs include slightly elevated bp, 135/90; slightly elevated pulse, 78/min, no fever. Auscultation revealed possible murmur during systole (ventricular contraction). ECG and stress ECHO not abnormal.

Diagnosis: Endocarditis and possible chronic valvular infection.

Treatment: Begin antibiotic therapy using IV drip STAT with frequent follow-up. If chest pain continues after several weeks, reevaluate for consideration of valvuloplasty.

Richard Freemann, M.D.
_____
Richard Freeman, M.D.

Photo Source: Yuri Arcurs/Shutterstock

Comprehension Questions

1. What complaints support the diagnosis? _____

_____

_____

2. Why is the patient history an important part of this diagnosis? _____

_____

_____

3. What is the meaning of the abbreviation CHF? _____

_____

_____

Case Study Questions

The following Case Study provides further discussion regarding the patient in the medical report. Fill in the blanks with the correct terms. Choose your answers from the following list of terms. (Note that some terms may be used more than once.)

angina pectoris	cardiologist	endocarditis
angiostenosis	cardiology	myocardial infarction
atherosclerosis	cardiovalvulitis	stress ECHO
block	electrocardiography	valvuloplasty

A patient named Robert Gorman complained of pain in the heart area of the chest, or (a) _____,

and was subsequently referred to (b) _____ for immediate diagnosis and treatment. The specialist, a

(c) _____, diagnosed the pain as having a cause from insufficient blood supply to the heart. The patient

was given medication and educated about heart disease management. Several weeks later, the patient was readmitted

due to continued complaints of chest pain. After evaluating heart electrical events with (d) _____,

the physician performed a technique using sound waves to evaluate heart activity during physical exercise, known as

a(n) (e) _____ _____. The ECG showed a normal conduction system, thereby ruling

out damage to the conduction system, or a heart (f) _____. The stress ECHO also showed mostly

normal results, ruling out damage to the heart muscle, or a(n) (g) _____ _____

because the heart muscle was receiving sufficient levels of oxygen. Because blood flow was normal, the narrowing of

a coronary artery, generally called a(n) (h) _____, was eliminated as a cause, which also eliminated

the common plaque-forming disease that causes a stenosis, known as (i) _____. However, the stress

ECHO did reveal an abnormal valvular activity during ventricular contraction, or systole, indicating a valvular disorder

called (j) _____. A course of treatment was ordered that included a long-term, non-penicillin antibiotic

therapy with an IV drip. If the patient did not improve, consideration for a surgical operation to repair a damaged valve,

called (k) _____, would be made.

Danika Price

For a greater challenge, read the following medical report and answer the critical thinking questions that follow from the information in the chapter.

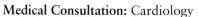

PEARSON GENERAL HOSPITAL

PGH

5500 University Avenue Metropolis, NY
Phone: (211) 594-4000 • Fax: (211) 594-4001

Medical Consultation: Cardiology

Date: 08/15/2011

Patient: Danika Price

Patient Complaint: Intermittent pain in the upper abdomen

History: 42-year-old female. Essential hypertension diagnosed 4 years ago at age 38 following second childbirth.

Family History: Essential hypertension in father, negative in mother. Both parents are in their 60s with no heart disease recorded.

Allergies: None

Physical Examination: Vital signs include no fever, slightly elevated bp of 130/95, slightly elevated pulse of 82/min. Aortogram revealed aortic aneurysm, confirmed by MRI.

Diagnosis: Aortic aneurysm in upper abdominal aorta inferior to celiac trunk.

Treatment: Angioplasty of abdominal aorta.

Donald H. Surley, M.D.

Donald H. Surley, M.D.

Photo Source: Monkey Business Images/Shutterstock

Comprehension Questions

1. What is the actual cause of the abdominal pain reported by the patient? _____

_____

_____

2. What procedure provided the evidence for the diagnosis? _____

_____

_____

3. What is an angioplasty and how might it correct an aortic aneurysm? _____

_____

_____

Case Study Questions

The following case study provides additional discussion of the patient's condition in the medical report. Fill in the blanks with the correct terms from your readings in this chapter.

Danika Price, a 42-year-old female patient with a history of persistently high blood pressure, or

(l) _____, complained of intermittent pain sensations in the upper abdomen. Upon evaluation during

which an X-ray was taken of the aorta, called a(n) (m) _____, it became apparent that the source of the

pain was from abdominal spasms of the aorta wall, called (n) _____, due to an abnormal dilation of the

vessel wall known as a(n) (o) _____. To prevent a possible rupture of the wall of the aorta, a surgical

repair called a(n) (p) _____ was scheduled. During the repair, an incision was made into the wall of the

vessel in a procedure called a(n) (q) _____ and the vessel wall received a stent to strengthen it. The

patient made a complete recovery, and received education on ways to control her essential hypertension.

The Respiratory System

LEARNING OBJECTIVES

After completing this chapter, you will be able to:

1 Define and spell the word parts used to create terms for the respiratory system.

2 Break down and define common medical terms used for symptoms, diseases, disorders, procedures, treatments, and devices associated with the respiratory system.

3 Build medical terms from the word parts associated with the respiratory system.

4 Pronounce and spell common medical terms associated with the respiratory system.

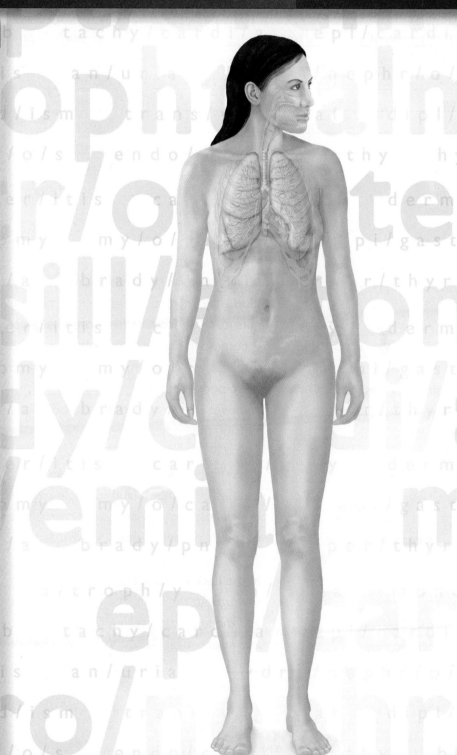

Anatomy and Physiology Terms ▶▶▶▶▶

The following table provides the combining forms that specifically apply to the anatomy and physiology of the respiratory system. Note that the combining forms are colored red to help you identify them when you see them again later in the chapter.

Combining Form	Definition	Combining Form	Definition
alveol/o	air sac, alveolus	phragm/o, phragmat/o	partition
bronch/o	airway, bronchus	pleur/o	pleura, rib
hem/o, hemat/o	blood	pneum/o, pneumon/o	air, lung
laryng/o	voice box, larynx	pulmon/o	lung
lob/o	a rounded part, lobe	rhin/o	nose
muc/o	mucus	sept/o	putrefying; wall, partition
nas/o	nose	sinus/o	cavity
ox/i	oxygen	thorac/o	chest, thorax
pharyng/o	throat, pharynx	trache/o	windpipe, trachea

respiratory system	**9.1** The **respiratory** (RESS pih rah tor ee) **system** brings oxygen into the bloodstream, through which it is transported to all body cells. The system gets its name from its function: The process of providing cells with oxygen is commonly known as **respiration.** This term is derived from the word *respiratio*, which means "to breathe again." In addition to bringing oxygen into the bloodstream, the _____ _____ also removes the waste product, carbon dioxide, from the blood and channels it outside the body.
lower respiratory tract **carbon dioxide**	**9.2** When you inhale, oxygen flows into the lungs after traveling through a series of chambers and tubes, known as the upper respiratory tract. It includes the nasal cavity, pharynx, and larynx. The lower portion of the respiratory system, known as the _____ _____ _____, consists of the trachea in the neck and chest, the bronchial tree, which branches extensively throughout the lungs, the tiny air sacs within the lungs known as alveoli, and the lungs themselves. Gas exchange occurs across the walls of alveoli and adjacent capillaries. When you exhale, _____ _____ flows out of the lungs through the same route but in the opposite direction.

9.3 The functions of the respiratory system may be summarized as follows:

- Provides a stream of _____ into the blood through the process of inhalation, followed by diffusion.

- Removes _____ from the blood through the process of diffusion, followed by exhalation.

oxygen

carbon dioxide

9.4 Use the anatomy terms that appear in the left column to fill in the corresponding blanks in Figures 9.1a■ and 9.1b■.

1. palate
2. tonsil
3. epiglottis
4. thyroid
5. pharynx
6. trachea
7. lung
8. main bronchus

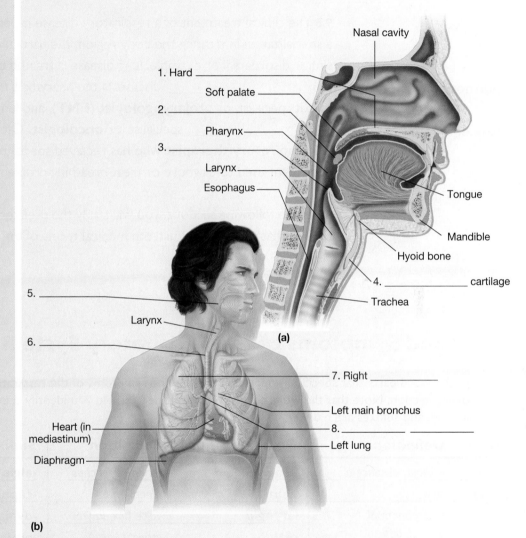

Figure 9.1 ■
The respiratory system. (a) Sagittal section of the head and neck, revealing the organs of the upper respiratory tract: the nose, pharynx, and larynx.
(b) The organs of the lower respiratory tract, which includes the trachea, right and left primary bronchi, bronchial tree, and lungs.

Medical Terms of the Respiratory System ▶▶▶▶▶

respiratory	**9.5** Diseases of the respiratory system reduce the amount of oxygen that is normally supplied to body cells and increase the levels of carbon dioxide in the blood and other tissues. Severe respiratory disease can lead to a failure of oxygen delivery and may result in death. The most common symptoms of respiratory disease are breathing problems. If these problems are not identified and treated early, additional complications may arise. In general, _____ disease may be caused by congenital conditions, infections, allergies, tumors, heart disease, or injury.
pulmonologist **cancer**	**9.6** The clinical treatment of a respiratory disease is performed by a physician with a specialization in treating the body region, the particular disorder, or a set of similar disorders. For example, lung disease is treated by a pulmonary specialist, or _____, disease of the pharynx is treated by a nose and throat specialist, or **otolaryngologist** (**ENT**), and lung cancer is treated by a _____ specialist, or **oncologist.** Often assisting the physician is a **respiratory therapist** who has received special training in the operation of equipment used to diagnose or treat breathing problems.
	9.7 In the following sections, you will study the prefixes, combining forms, and suffixes that combine to build the medical terms of the respiratory system.

Signs and Symptoms of the Respiratory System

Here are the word parts that specifically apply to the signs and symptoms of the respiratory system that are covered in the following section. Note that the word parts are color-coded to help you identify them: prefixes are green, combining forms are red, and suffixes are blue.

Prefix	Definition
a-, an-	without, absence of
brady-	slow
dys-	bad, abnormal, painful, difficult
epi-	upon, over, above, on top
eu-	normal, good
hyper-	excessive, abnormally high, above
hypo-	deficient, abnormally low, below
tachy-	rapid, fast

Combining Form	Definition
bronch/o	airway, bronchus
hem/o	blood
laryng/o	voice box, larynx
orth/o	straight
ox/i	oxygen
rhin/o	nose
thorac/o	chest, thorax

Suffix	Definition
-algia	condition of pain
-capnia	condition of carbon dioxide
-dynia	condition of pain
-emia	condition of blood
-oxia	condition of oxygen
-phonia	condition of sound or voice
-pnea	breath
-ptysis	to cough up
-rrhagia	abnormal discharge
-spasm	sudden, involuntary muscle contraction
-staxis	dripping

KEY TERMS A–Z

acapnia
ah KAP nee ah

9.8 The suffix *-capnia* means "condition of carbon dioxide." When the prefix that means "without, absence of" is added, the term _____ is constructed, which is the absence of carbon dioxide. The constructed form of this term is a/capnia. A sign of reduced carbon dioxide in an expiration (exhaled air) sample indicates hyperventilation has been occurring, and an absence of this waste product of metabolism indicates metabolic failure.

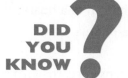

DID YOU KNOW

▶▶▶▶▶ *-capnia*

The suffix *-capnia* is derived from the Greek word *kapnos,* which means "smoke," referring to exhaled air. It refers specifically to the gas, carbon dioxide.

anoxia
ah NOK see ah

9.9 The suffix meaning "condition of oxygen" is *-oxia*. When the prefix that means "without, absence of" is added, the term _____ is made, which is the absence of oxygen. The constructed form of **anoxia** is written an/oxia.

aphonia
ah FOH nee ah

9.10 The suffix *-phonia* means "condition of sound or voice." Adding the prefix that means "without, absence of" forms the term _____, which is the absence of voice. The constructed form of this term is written a/phonia.

apnea
AP nee ah

a/pnea

apnea

9.11 The suffix *-pnea* means "breath." Adding the prefix that means "without, absence of" forms the term _____, which is a longer-than-normal pause between breaths. This constructed term is written ____/_____. A common form of apnea is known as **sleep** _____, in which one or more pauses in breathing or shallow breaths occur while sleeping. The pauses may last for a few seconds to several minutes, usually anywhere from 5 to 30 or more times per minute. When normal breathing resumes, a choking or snorting sound is often made.

bradypnea
brad ip NEE ah

9.12 Adding the prefix *brady-*, which means "slow," to the suffix that means "breath" produces the term for an abnormal slowing of the breathing rhythm, _____. The constructed form of **bradypnea** is written brady/pnea.

bronchospasm
BRONG koh spazm

9.13 A narrowing of the airway caused by the contraction of smooth muscles in the walls of the tiny tubes known as bronchioles within the lungs is called **bronchospasm.** The constructed form of this term is bronch/o/spasm. A _____ is a common sign of the respiratory disease asthma (Frame 9.32) and may lead to the additional symptom of apnea (Frame 9.11).

Cheyne-Stokes respiration
chain stohks * ress pih RAY shun

9.14 The sign known as **Cheyne-Stokes respiration** is a repeated pattern of distressed breathing marked by a gradual increase of deep breathing, followed by shallow breathing, and apnea. _____-_____ _____ is a sign of brain dysfunction or congestive heart failure.

dysphonia
diss FOH nee ah

9.15 The prefix *dys-* means "bad, abnormal, painful, or difficult." When used with the suffix that means "condition of sound or voice," the term _____ is formed. It is the symptom of a hoarse voice. The constructed form of **dysphonia** is written dys/phonia.

dyspnea
DISP nee ah

9.16 Adding the prefix *dys-* to the suffix that means "breath" forms the term _____. It is the symptom of difficult breathing, usually caused by a respiratory disease or cardiac disorder. In contrast, a normal breathing rhythm is called **eupnea** (yoop NEE ah). The constructed form of dyspnea is written dys/pnea, and eupnea is eu/pnea.

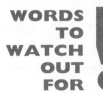

WORDS TO WATCH OUT FOR ▶▶▶▶▶ **Terms with No Word Roots**

Many terms related to the respiratory system contain no word root (or combining form), such as *dysphonia, dyspnea, epistaxis, hyperpnea,* and *hypopnea.* Don't let those terms confuse you when you're interpreting their meanings.

epistaxis
ep ih STAK siss

9.17 A nosebleed is clinically called **epistaxis.** It is a constructed term that literally means "dripping upon" and is written epi/staxis. An _____ can be a sign of high blood pressure, a nasal sinus infection, inhalation of a toxic irritant or particle, or a blow to the face. It is also called **rhinorrhagia** (rye noh RAH jee ah), another constructed term. The constructed form is written rhin/o/rrhagia and literally means "abnormal discharge of nose."

hemoptysis
hee MOP tih siss

9.18 The symptom of coughing up and spitting out blood is called _____, which combines the combining form *hem/o* that means "blood" and the suffix *-ptysis* that means "to cough up." The constructed form of this term is written hem/o/ptysis.

hemothorax
hee moh THOH raks

9.19 A term composed of two word parts, which literally means "chest blood" is _____. It is the pooling of blood within the pleural cavity surrounding the lungs. The term is written hem/o/thorax. Note that this term has no prefix or suffix; it is constructed of a combining form (*hem/o*) and a noun (*thorax*).

hypercapnia
HIGH per KAP nee ah

9.20 The prefixes *hyper-* and *hypo-* have opposite meanings. For example, excessive levels of carbon dioxide in the blood is a sign called _____. The opposite sign, in which carbon dioxide blood levels are deficient, or abnormally low, is **hypocapnia** (HIGH poh KAP nee ah).

hyperpnea
HIGH perp NEE ah

9.21 The sign of abnormally deep breathing or an abnormally high rate of breathing is called _____ and is common among patients suffering from the respiratory disease emphysema (Frame 9.43). Hyperpnea is also a common symptom of heart failure and anxiety (panic) attacks. By contrast, the sign of abnormally rapid breathing is more common among patients experiencing asthma (Frame 9.32) and is called **hyperventilation** (HIGH per vent ih LAY shun). The constructed form of **hyperpnea** is written hyper/pnea, and that of hyperventilation is hyper/ventilation.

WORDS TO WATCH OUT FOR

▶▶▶▶▶ *-pnea* and *-capnia*

Two suffixes pertaining to the respiratory system sound similar but have very different meanings: *-pnea* means "breath" and is found in numerous medical terms such as *apnea, tachypnea,* and *orthopnea.* The suffix *-capnia,* meaning "condition of carbon dioxide" and appearing in terms such as *hypocapnia* and *hypercapnia,* sounds similar but is spelled with an *i* instead of an *e.*

hypopnea
high POPP nee ah

9.22 The opposite sign of hyperpnea is abnormally shallow breathing and is called _____. This constructed term is written hypo/pnea.

hypoventilation
HIGH poh vent ih LAY shun

9.23 A reduced breathing rhythm that fails to meet the body's gas exchange demands is called _____. The constructed form of this term is hypo/ventilation. It is opposite to an accelerated breathing rhythm, which you learned is called hyperventilation (Frame 9.21).

hypoxemia
high pahk SEE mee ah

hypoxia
high PAHK see ah

9.24 Abnormally low levels of oxygen in the blood is a sign of a respiratory deficiency called **hypoxemia.** This constructed term is written hyp/ox/emia. Notice that the letter o in *hypo-* is dropped to make _____ easier to pronounce. This technique is also used to form the term **hypoxia,** which is written as hyp/oxia. _____ is the sign of abnormally low levels of oxygen throughout the body.

laryngospasm
lair ING goh spazm

9.25 A **laryngospasm** is the closure of the glottis, the opening into the larynx, due to muscular contractions of the throat. _____ is a constructed term written laryng/o/spasm.

orthopnea or THAHP nee ah	**9.26** The combining form *orth/o* means "straight." When the suffix for breath is added, the term **orthopnea** is formed. _____ is the limited ability to breathe when lying down and becomes relieved when sitting upright. The constructed form of this term is *orth/o/pnea*.
paroxysm pahr AHK sizm	**9.27** The term **paroxysm** refers to a sudden onset of symptomatic sharp pain or a convulsion. _____ is derived from the Greek word *paroxysmos,* which means "to sharpen or to irritate."
sputum SPYOO tum	**9.28** Respiratory diseases often include the symptom of **sputum,** which is an expectorated (coughed out from the lungs) matter. _____ contains mucus, inhaled particulates, and sometimes pus or blood.
tachypnea tak ihp NEE ah	**9.29** The prefix *tachy-* means "rapid or fast." When combined with the suffix that means "breath," it forms the term _____. The constructed form of this term for rapid breathing is written *tachy/pnea*.
thoracalgia thor ah KAL jee ah	**9.30** The symptom of pain in the chest region is called _____. The constructed form of this term is written *thorac/algia*. An alternate term with the same meaning is **thoracodynia** (thor AH koh DIN ee ah).

PRACTICE: Signs and Symptoms of the Respiratory System

The Right Match

Match the term on the left with the correct definition on the right.

_____ 1. thoracalgia

_____ 2. apnea

_____ 3. eupnea

_____ 4. bradypnea

_____ 5. paroxysm

_____ 6. hemoptysis

_____ 7. sputum

_____ 8. hemothorax

_____ 9. hypercapnia

_____ 10. hypoxemia

_____ 11. Cheyne-Stokes respiration

a. reoccurrence of a symptom or a convulsion

b. coughing up and spitting out blood

c. expectorated (spit out) matter that contains mucus, inhaled particulates, and sometimes pus and blood

d. normal breathing

e. slow breathing

f. pause in breathing

g. excessive carbon dioxide blood levels

h. deficient levels of oxygen in the blood

i. pain in the chest region

j. blood in the pleural cavity

k. pattern of repeated distressed breathing marked by a gradual increase of deep breathing, followed by shallow breathing, and apnea

Break the Chain

Analyze these medical terms:

    a)   Separate each term into its word parts; each word part is labeled for you (**p** = prefix, **r** = root, **cf** = combining form, and **s** = suffix).

    b)   For the Bonus Question, write the requested definition in the blank that follows.

The first set has been completed for you as an example.

1. a)   bronchospasm   *bronch/o/spasm*
                                             cf   s

    b)   *Bonus Question:* What is the definition of the suffix? *sudden involuntary muscle contraction*

2. a)   dysphonia   _____/_____
                                         p   s

    b)   *Bonus Question:* What is the definition of the suffix? _____

3. a)   dyspnea   _____/_____
                                         p   s

    b)   *Bonus Question:* What is the definition of the prefix? _____

4. a)   epistaxis   _____/_____
                                         p   s

    b)   *Bonus Question:* What is the definition of the suffix? _____

5. a)   hyperpnea   _____/_____
                                         p   s

    b)   *Bonus Question:* What is the definition of the suffix? _____

6. a)   laryngospasm   _____/___/_____
                                         cf   s

    b)   *Bonus Question:* What is the definition of the combining form? _____

Diseases and Disorders of the Respiratory System

Here are the word parts that specifically apply to the diseases and disorders of the respiratory system that are covered in the following section. Note that the word parts are color-coded to help you identify them: prefixes are green, combining forms are red, and suffixes are blue.

Prefix	Definition
a-	without, absence of
epi-	upon, over, above, on top

Combining Form	Definition
atel/o	incomplete
bronch/o, bronch/i	airway, bronchus
carcin/o	cancer
coccidioid/o	Coccidioides immitis (a fungus)
coni/o	dust
cyst/o	bladder, sac
embol/o	plug
fibr/o	fiber
glott/o	opening into the windpipe
laryng/o	voice box, larynx
myc/o	fungus
nas/o	nose
pharyng/o	throat, pharynx
pleur/o	pleura, rib
pneum/o, pneumon/o	air, lung
pulmon/o	lung
py/o	pus
rhin/o	nose
sinus/o	cavity
sphyx/o	pulse
sten/o	narrow
thorac/o	chest, thorax
tonsill/o	almond, tonsil
trache/o	windpipe, trachea
tubercul/o	little swelling

Suffix	Definition
-al	pertaining to
-ary	pertaining to
-ectasis	expansion, dilation
-genic	pertaining to producing, forming
-ia	condition of
-ic	pertaining to
-ism	condition or disease
-itis	inflammation
-oma	tumor
-osis	condition of

KEY TERMS A–Z

asphyxia
ass FIK see ah

9.31 The word root meaning "pulse" is *sphyx.* It is included in the term **asphyxia,** which is the absence of respiratory ventilation, or suffocation. The constructed form of _____ is written a/sphyx/ia and literally means "condition of without pulse."

asthma
AZ mah

9.32 A condition of the lungs that is characterized by widespread narrowing of the bronchioles and formation of mucous plugs is known as **asthma.** The term is derived from the Greek word *astma,* which means "to pant." Illustrated in Figure 9.2■, _____ produces the symptoms of wheezing, shortness of breath, chest pain, and frequent coughing during an episode, the frequency of which varies with every patient. It is regarded as an inflammatory response to an allergic substance by the lungs. According to the American Academy of Allergy, roughly 20 million Americans suffer from this chronic disease, nine million of whom are under the age of 18 years. When asthma is complicated with bronchitis (see Frame 9.35), it is referred to as **asthmatic bronchitis** (az MAHT ik * brong KYE tiss).

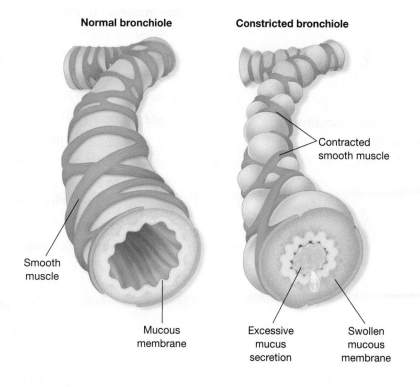

Figure 9.2 ■
Asthma. (a) A normal bronchiole. (b) An asthmatic bronchiole. During an asthma "attack," the bronchioles constrict to reduce the airway. In addition, the mucous membrane lining the bronchioles swells, and thickened mucous secretions form plugs that further reduce the airway.

Normal bronchiole

Constricted bronchiole

Contracted smooth muscle

Smooth muscle

Mucous membrane

Excessive mucus secretion

Swollen mucous membrane

atelectasis
at eh LEK tah siss

9.33 The alveoli in the lungs normally retain a small amount of air even during a forced expiration, which prevents them from collapsing. In the condition called **atelectasis,** trauma or disease disables this protective mechanism and causes the alveoli to collapse, preventing air from entering (see Frame 9.60). _____ is a constructed term composed of two word parts, *atel,* which means "incomplete," and *-ectasis,* which means "expansion, dilation." Its constructed form is written atel/ectasis. The common term for this condition is **collapsed lung.**

bronchiectasis
BRONG kee EK tah siss

9.34 Another term that uses the suffix -*ectasis* is _____, which is a chronic, abnormal dilation (widening) of the bronchi. The constructed form of this term is written bronchi/ectasis. It is often caused by a recurrent inflammation or infection of the airways, and is usually accompanied with an abundant, purulent sputum. If the condition is present at birth it is called congenital bronchiectasis, and if it develops later in life it is known as acquired bronchiectasis.

bronchitis
brong KYE tiss

9.35 Recall that the suffix that means "inflammation" is -*itis*. This will be used in many terms in this section. Inflammation of the bronchi is called _____. The constructed form of this term is bronch/itis. Acute bronchitis is usually associated with a respiratory tract infection. Chronic bronchitis is usually caused by smoking, although allergies may cause this condition in some people.

bronchogenic carcinoma
brong koh JENN ik *
kar sih NOH mah

9.36 An aggressive form of cancer arising from cells within the bronchi is known as **bronchogenic carcinoma** (Figure 9.3■). The constructed form of this term is written bronch/o/genic carcin/oma. In 2011, there were approximately 110,000 cases of _____ _____ in men and 90,000 cases in women in the United States, making it the most common form of any type of cancer. Although it is commonly referred to as lung cancer, it is different than other forms of lung cancer because the cells arise from the bronchi rather than the soft tissues of the lung. It is well established that smoking tobacco products is the cause of at least 90% of all cases of bronchogenic carcinoma.

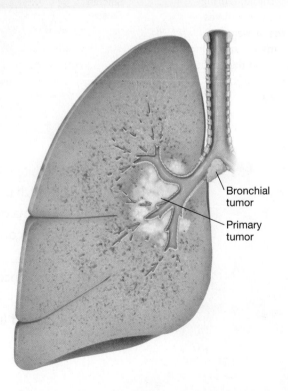

Bronchial tumor

Primary tumor

Figure 9.3 ■
Bronchogenic carcinoma. An illustration of a sectioned lung that contains tumors associated with a bronchial wall.

bronchopneumonia
BRONG koh noo MOH nee ah

9.37 An acute inflammatory disease involving the bronchioles and the alveoli is called **bronchopneumonia.** This constructed term is written bronch/o/pneumon/ia. It is usually caused by a bacterial infection that involves the bronchi and the soft tissue of the lungs, causing the alveoli to fill with fluid, leading to the loss of air space. _____ often occurs in a lobe of a lung, lending it the alternate name of **lobar pneumonia.**

chronic obstructive pulmonary disease

9.38 An obstruction of air flow to and from the lungs may be a consequence of chronic bronchitis and emphysema. When the two conditions appear simultaneously, the diagnosis is given as **chronic obstructive pulmonary disease,** abbreviated **COPD.** _____ _____ _____ _____ is usually persistent until death.

coccidioidomycosis
kok SIDD ee oy doh mye KOH siss

9.39 The combining form *myc/o* means "fungus." A fungal infection of the upper respiratory tract, which often spreads to the lungs and other organs, is called **coccidioidomycosis.** This constructed term is written coccidioid/o/myc/osis and is based on the name of the causative fungus, *Coccidioides immitis.* Also called **valley fever** due to its place of origin in the San Joaquin Valley of California, _____ is caused by inhaling spores of the fungal pathogen.

coryza
koh RYE zah

9.40 The common cold is caused by a virus that infects the upper respiratory tract causing local inflammation. It is clinically called **coryza,** which is derived from the Greek word for runny nose, *koryza.* Because a cold is an acute illness, it is often called acute _____. It is also called **rhinitis** (rye NYE tiss), due to the inflammation.

croup
kroop

9.41 A viral infectious disease that is relatively common among infants and young children produces a characteristic hoarse cough with a sound resembling the bark of a dog. Commonly known as **croup,** the cough results from a swelling of the larynx in response to a viral infection. The clinical term for _____ is **laryngotracheobronchitis** (lair RING goh TRAY kee oh brong KYE tiss), abbreviated **LTB.** The constructed form of this term reveals six word parts and is written laryng/o/trache/o/bronch/itis.

cystic fibrosis
SISS tik * fye BROH siss

9.42 A severe hereditary disease that is characterized by excess mucus production in the respiratory tract, digestive tract, and elsewhere is called **cystic fibrosis** and is abbreviated **CF.** This constructed term is written cyst/ic fibr/osis. _____ _____ literally means "condition of fibrous cysts (bladders)." CF causes difficulty breathing because of the dense mucus that obstructs the airways. It strikes roughly 1 in 2,500 children and is commonly fatal before the age of 30 years.

9.43 A chronic lung disease characterized by the symptoms of dyspnea (Frame 9.16), a chronic cough, formation of a barrel chest due to labored breathing, and a gradual deterioration caused by chronic hypoxemia (Frame 9.24) and hypercapnia (Frame 9.20) is called **emphysema.** It is a Greek word that means "to inflate." The symptoms arise when the alveolar walls deteriorate, resulting in a loss of elasticity that causes an inability to exhale normally, making breathing extremely difficult. Smoking is the leading cause of _____, and when it is combined with chronic bronchitis, they are diagnosed as chronic obstructive pulmonary disease (COPD), described in Frame 9.38. Emphysema is illustrated in Figure 9.4■.

emphysema
em fih SEE mah

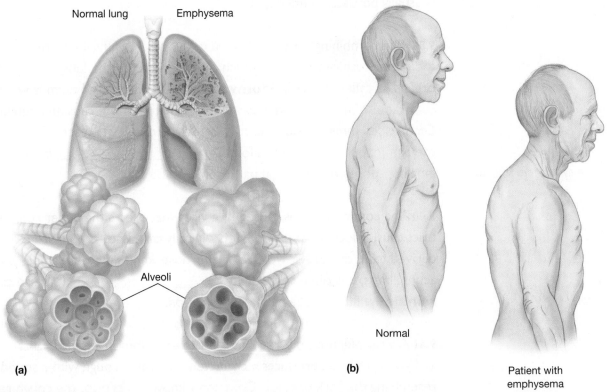

Normal lung   Emphysema

Alveoli

(a)

Normal

(b)

Patient with emphysema

Figure 9.4 ■
Emphysema. (a) Illustration comparing normal lungs and emphysemic lungs. The inserts illustrate how alveolar walls deteriorate in emphysema, reducing their surface area by convergence.
(b) Common appearance of a patient with emphysema. Characteristic signs include reduced weight, a barrel chest, and a drawn facial appearance, all due to the need to inhale deeply and forcibly exhale with nearly every breath.

epiglottitis
ep ih glah TYE tiss

9.44 Inflammation of the epiglottis is called **epiglottitis.** This constructed term is written epi/glott/itis. _____ is usually caused by a bacterial infection that spreads from the throat to the epiglottis and can be very serious in children due to the danger of airway obstruction.

laryngitis
LAIR in JYE tiss

9.45 Inflammation of the larynx is called _____. The constructed form of this term is written laryng/itis. It is characterized by the symptom of dysphonia (Frame 9.15).

9.46 A form of pneumonia (Frame 9.54) that is caused by the bacterium *Legionella pneumophilia* is called **Legionnaires' disease,** or _____.

legionellosis
lee juh nell OH siss

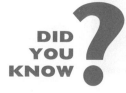

▶▶▶▶▶ **Legionnaires' Disease**

Legionellosis was first identified in 1976, when many members at an American Legion convention became afflicted with an infection that caused 21 deaths. It took intensive research to reveal the causative bacteria and why it spread so quickly: it was delivered throughout the hotel ventilation system under ideal conditions for the bacteria to proliferate.

lung cancer

9.47 More people die from _____ _____ than any other type of cancer each year, roughly 88,000 men and 70,000 women (according to the Centers for Disease Control in the year 2007, the last year statistics were made available). There are three primary types of lung cancer: bronchogenic carcinoma (described in Frame 9.36), small-cell lung carcinoma, and non-small cell lung carcinoma. Also known as **adenocarcinoma of the lung,** lung cancer arises from cells lining the bronchi or from the soft tissues of the lung (Figure 9.5■). In all three types of lung cancer, smoking accounts for at least 90% of all cases. Smoking increases the risk of lung cancer significantly, but it also increases the risk of developing cancer of the lip, mouth, tongue, pharynx, and other organs as well. The American Cancer Society predicts that, worldwide, three million people will die of smoking-caused cancers in 2012 and 500,000 from inhaling secondhand smoke.

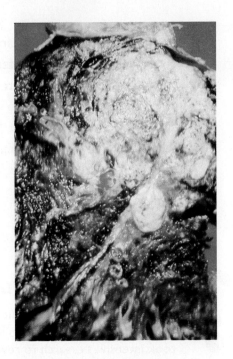

Figure 9.5 ■
Lung cancer. Photograph of part of a lung removed after death. The yellow area is a large tumor and the blackened area below it indicates the patient was a heavy smoker.
Source: Courtesy of National Institutes of Health, National Cancer Institute Visuals Online, Bethesda, MD.

nasopharyngitis nay zoh FAIR in JYE tiss	**9.48** Recall again the suffix that means "inflammation," which is *-itis*. Inflammation of the nose and pharynx is called _____. The constructed form of this term is written nas/o/pharyng/itis. It may be caused by an allergic reaction or bacterial or viral infection.
pertussis per TUSS siss	**9.49** An acute infectious disease characterized by inflammation of the larynx, trachea, and bronchi that produces spasmodic coughing is called **pertussis.** The term is a Latin word that means "intense cough." _____ is commonly known as **whooping cough** because of the noise produced at the end of a cough when the larynx spasms, producing a long inspirational noise. If not treated, it can become fatal due to the exhaustive coughing and obstructed airflow.
pharyngitis FAIR in JYE tiss	**9.50** Inflammation of the pharynx is called _____. The constructed form of this term is written pharyng/itis. Pharyngitis is commonly called "sore throat."
pleural effusion PLOO ral * eh FYOO zhun	**9.51** Effusion refers to the leakage of fluid. In the disease _____ _____, fluid leaks into the pleural cavity. It usually occurs as a response by the body to injury or infection of the pleural membranes. Pleural is a constructed term that is written pleur/al.

pleuritis
ploo RYE tiss

9.52 Inflammation of the pleural membranes is called _____. This constructed term is written pleur/itis. It is also called **pleurisy.** Inflammation of the pleural membranes and the lungs is a disease called **pleuropneumonia** (PLOO roh noo MOH nee ah).

pneumoconiosis
noo moh KOH nee OH siss

9.53 Inflammation of the lungs, when caused by the chronic inhalation of fine particles, is called **pneumoconiosis.** The constructed form of this term is pneum/o/coni/osis, which literally means "condition of dusty lungs." The term arose because the disease is usually caused by mining and manufacturing activities. The inflammation leads to the formation of a fibrotic tissue around alveoli, reducing their ability to stretch with incoming air, which impedes the efficiency of gas exchange. The most common forms of _____ are **asbestosis** (az bess TOH siss), caused by inhalation of asbestos fibers, and **silicosis** (sill ih KOH siss), caused by inhalation of fine silicone dust.

pneumonia
noo MOH nee ah

9.54 Inflammation of soft lung tissue (excluding the bronchi) that results in the formation of an exudate (fluid) within alveoli is the general condition known as **pneumonia.** The constructed form of this term is pneumon/ia. The exudate fills the alveoli, which impedes the efficiency of gas exchange (Figure 9.6■). The filling of alveoli with exudate has the same effect as drowning, so _____ is sometimes referred to as "drowning in your own fluids." Pneumonia is usually caused by bacterial, viral, or fungal pathogens, which trigger the inflammatory response, although it can also be caused by smoke inhalation. Viral and bacterial pneumonia are leading causes of death worldwide. Fungal pneumonia is relatively rare, although infection by the fungus *Pneumocystis jiroveci* is a common sign of AIDS.

Figure 9.6 ■
Pneumonia. This common lung inflammation may be caused by bacteria, viruses, or fungi and is often diagnosed with a chest X-ray. In this chest X-ray of infected lungs, the inflammation appears as the hazy area.
Source: Courtesy of Dr. Thomas Hooten and the Centers for Disease Control Public Health Image Library, Atlanta, GA.

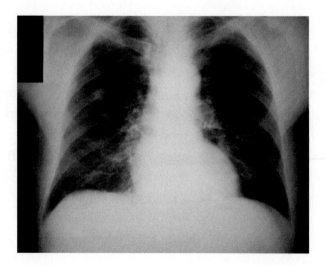

pneumonitis
NOO moh NYE tiss

9.55 An inflammatory condition of the lungs that is independent of a particular cause is called _____. The constructed form of this term is written pneumon/itis. Pneumonitis is often associated with pulmonary edema (Frame 9.57), which is the accumulation of fluid within the lungs outside the alveoli.

pneumothorax
NOO moh THOH raks

9.56 A **pneumothorax** is the abnormal presence of air or gas within the pleural cavity (Figure 9.7■). It is caused by a penetrating injury to the chest or severe coughing and leads to atelectasis (Frame 9.33). _____ is a constructed term that is written pneum/o/thorax.

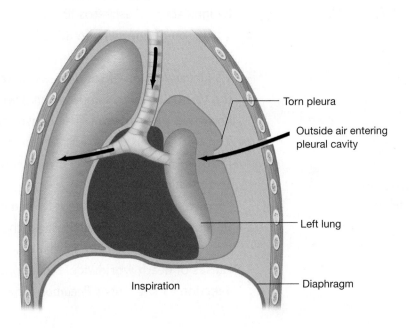

Torn pleura

Outside air entering pleural cavity

Left lung

Inspiration

Diaphragm

Figure 9.7 ■
Pneumothorax, caused by a penetrating chest wound.

pulmonary edema
PULL mon air ee * eh DEE mah

9.57 The accumulation of fluid within the tiny air sacs within the lungs (the alveoli) is a response to infection or injury and is called **pulmonary edema.** The most common cause of _____ _____ is cardiovascular disease, including congestive heart failure. Pulmonary edema may also arise from adult respiratory distress syndrome (ARDS), which you will learn about soon in Frame 9.60. Pulmonary edema is often associated with pneumonia (Frame 9.54) and pneumonitis (Frame 9.55). *Pulmonary* is a constructed term that is written as pulmon/ary, and *edema* means "swelling."

pulmonary embolism
PULL mon air ee * EM boh lizm

9.58 A blood clot that moves along with the bloodstream is called an **embolus** (EM boh lus). It is derived from the Greek word *embolos,* which means "a plug." An embolus can become dangerous if it lodges in a blood vessel, causing an occlusion that blocks the flow of blood to form an **embolism.** A blockage in the pulmonary circulation by a blood clot is called a _____ _____. Abbreviated **PE,** it is a complication to an injury or surgery elsewhere in the body. Pulmonary embolism is a constructed term that is written as pulmon/ary embol/ism.

pyothorax
pye oh THOH raks

9.59 The presence of pus in the pleural cavity is called **pyothorax.** This constructed term is written py/o/thorax. _____ is also known as **empyema** (em pye EE mah).

respiratory distress syndrome

9.60 A severe respiratory disease that is characterized by rapid respiratory failure is known as **respiratory distress syndrome (RDS).** It occurs in two different forms. One form affects newborns and is called **neonatal** _____ _____ _____ **(NRDS).** It is caused by insufficient surfactant, a substance produced by alveolar cells that prevents atelectasis (lung collapse). It mainly strikes premature infants because they have not yet developed the ability to produce surfactant. The second form affects adults and is called **adult** (or **acute**) **respiratory distress syndrome (ARDS).** It is caused by severe lung infections or injury that result in damage to lung capillary walls and bronchioles, causing a rapid accumulation of purulent fluid into alveoli and bronchioles that places the patient in immediate danger of "drowning in their own fluids." Thus, ARDS often involves pneumonia (Frame 9.54) and pulmonary edema (Frame 9.57). It requires swift medical intervention with blood transfusions, anti-inflammatory drugs, and antibiotics to save the patient's life.

rhinitis
rye NYE tiss

9.61 Inflammation of the mucous membrane lining the nasal cavity is called **rhinitis.** The constructed form of this term is written rhin/itis. Acute _____ is one of the clinical terms for the common cold (Frame 9.40).

severe acute respiratory syndrome

9.62 A severe, rapid-onset viral infection resulting in respiratory distress that includes acute lung inflammation, alveolar damage, and atelectasis (Frame 9.33) is often referred to by its abbreviation, **SARS.** The long form is _____ _____ _____ _____. It is usually caused by the influenza virus and can become fatal due to the aggressive immunological response that injures alveoli and bronchioles.

sinusitis sigh nuss EYE tiss	**9.63** Similar to rhinitis (Frame 9.61), the condition known as _____ is an inflammation of the mucous membranes. It affects the nasal cavity and also the paranasal sinuses that are located within the frontal, sphenoid, ethmoid, and maxillary bones of the skull. The constructed form of this term is written sinus/itis.
tonsillitis TAHN sill EYE tiss	**9.64** Inflammation of one or more tonsils is called _____. This constructed term is written tonsill/itis.
tracheitis tray kee EYE tiss **tracheostenosis** TRAY kee oh steh NOH siss	**9.65** Inflammation of the trachea is called _____. The constructed form of this term is written trache/itis. It is usually caused by a bacterial infection that travels downward from the larynx. The combining form that means "narrow" is sten/o. Inflammation leads to a narrowing of the trachea, known as _____. Also constructed of word parts, it can be written trache/o/sten/osis.
tuberculosis too BER kyoo LOH siss	**9.66** Infection of the lungs by the bacterium *Mycobacterium tuberculosis* causes the disease _____, abbreviated **TB** (Figure 9.8■). This term is constructed of two word parts, tubercul/osis, and literally means "condition of a little swelling." The little swelling, or tubercle, is a colony of bacteria within the soft tissue of the lung that forms a hardened barrier, preventing white blood cells from entering and destroying the bacteria. In time, the bacterial colonies multiply throughout the lung until necrosis and inflammation overwhelm the function of gas exchange.

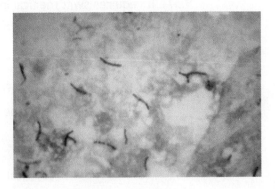

Figure 9.8 ■
Tuberculosis. Microphotograph of the
Mycobacterium tuberculosis, the cause of
the disease TB.
*Source: Courtesy of Dr. George P. Kubica
and the Centers for Disease Control.*

upper respiratory infection	**9.67** A generalized infection of the upper respiratory tract (nasal cavity, pharynx, and larynx) is called a(n) _____ _____ _____, or **URI.**

PRACTICE: Diseases and Disorders of the Respiratory System

Linkup

Link the word parts in the list to create the terms that match the definitions. You may use word parts more than once. Remember to add combining vowels when needed—and that some terms do not use any combining vowel. The first one is completed as an example.

Prefix	Combining Form	Suffix
a-	bronch/o	-ary
dia-	coni/o	-cele
neo-	embol/o	-ectasis
	legionell/o	-ia
	phragmat/o	-ism
	pleur/o	-itis
	pneum/o	-osis
	pulmon/o	-plasm
	py/o	
	sinus/o	
	sphyx/o	
	sten/o	
	thorac/o	
	tonsill/o	
	trache/o	
	tubercul/o	

	Definition	Term
1.	inflammation of the pleurae; also called pleurisy	*pleuritis*
2.	inflammation of the mucous membranes of the nasal cavity and also the paranasal sinuses	
3.	dilation of the bronchi	
4.	narrowing of the trachea	
5.	the absence of respiratory ventilation, or suffocation	
6.	inflammation of a tonsil	
7.	tumor of the lung	
8.	inflammation of the lungs caused by the chronic inhalation of fine particles, which leads to the formation of a fibrotic tissue around the alveoli	
9.	infection of the lungs by the bacterium *Mycobacterium tuberculosis*	
10.	pneumonia caused by the bacterium *Legionella pneumophilia*	
11.	blockage in the pulmonary circulation by a mobile blood clot	

The Right Match

Match the term on the left with the correct definition on the right.

_____ 1. emphysema

_____ 2. pertussis

_____ 3. asthma

_____ 4. severe acute respiratory syndrome

_____ 5. croup

_____ 6. atelectasis

_____ 7. tracheitis

_____ 8. tuberculosis

_____ 9. coryza

_____ 10. pyothorax

a. severe viral infection resulting in respiratory distress that includes lung inflammation, alveolar damage, and atelectasis

b. condition of pus in the pleural cavity

c. inflammation of the trachea

d. collapsed lung

e. also known as whooping cough

f. clinical term for the common cold

g. condition of the lungs that is characterized by widespread narrowing of the bronchioles and formation of mucous plugs

h. chronic lung disease named by a Greek word that means "to inflate"

i. a barking cough caused by an acute obstruction in the larynx among children

j. a highly contagious bacterial disease

Treatments, Procedures, and Devices of the Respiratory System

Here are the word parts that specifically apply to the treatments, procedures, and devices of the respiratory system that are covered in the following section. Note that the word parts are color-coded to help you identify them: prefixes are green, combining forms are red, and suffixes are blue.

Prefix	Definition
anti-	against, opposite of
endo-	within

Combining Form	Definition
aden/o	gland
angi/o	blood vessel
bronch/o	airway, bronchus
dilat/o	to widen
laryng/o	voice box, larynx
lob/o	a rounded part, lobe
ot/o	ear
ox/i	oxygen
pleur/o	pleura, rib
pneum/o, pneumon/o	lung, air
pulmon/o	lung
rhin/o	nose
spir/o	breathe
thorac/o	chest, thorax
trache/o	windpipe, trachea

Suffix	Definition
-al	pertaining to
-ary	pertaining to
-centesis	surgical puncture
-ectomy	surgical excision, removal
-gram	a record or image
-graphy	recording process
-ion	process
-logist	one who studies
-meter	measure, measuring instrument
-metry	measurement, process of measuring
-oid	resembling
-plasty	surgical repair
-scopy	process of viewing
-stomy	surgical creation of an opening
-tomy	incision, to cut

KEY TERMS A–Z

acid-fast bacilli smear

9.68 A clinical test performed on sputum to identify the presence of bacteria that react to acid is called **acid-fast bacilli smear,** abbreviated **AFB.** An _____-_____ _____ _____ is frequently used with chest X-rays to confirm a diagnosis of tuberculosis.

adenoidectomy
ADD eh noyd EK toh mee

9.69 A pharyngeal tonsil is called an **adenoid** (ADD eh noyd). This constructed term, written aden/oid, means "resembling a gland." In some cases, a chronically inflamed adenoid must be surgically removed to avoid complications, including obstruction of the nasopharynx. Remember that the suffix *-ectomy* means "surgical excision, removal." So, combine that with the term *adenoid,* and it creates the name for this procedure, _____. The constructed form of this term reveals three word parts and is written aden/oid/ectomy.

antihistamine
an tih HISS tah meen

9.70 A histamine is a compound released by certain cells in response to allergens that cause bronchial constriction and blood vessel dilation. The dilation of blood vessels increases the movement of plasma out of capillaries and into the interstitial space, resulting in the swelling of tissues with fluid, or **edema.** A therapeutic drug that inhibits the effects of histamines is called an _____, which uses the prefix that means "against, opposite of."

arterial blood gases

9.71 A clinical test on arterial blood to identify the levels of oxygen and carbon dioxide is called _____ _____ _____. It is abbreviated **ABGs.**

aspiration
ass pih RAY shun

9.72 The removal of fluid, air, or foreign bodies with suction is a procedure called **aspiration.** _____ is derived from the Latin word *aspiratus,* which means "to breathe on."

auscultation
aw skull TAY shun

9.73 A procedure that involves listening to sounds within the body as part of a physical examination, often with the aid of a stethoscope, is called **auscultation.** The term _____ is derived from the Latin word *ausculto,* which means "to listen to." As part of a physical examination that addresses the respiratory system, auscultation involves listening to chest sounds during inhalation and exhalation (Figure 9.9■). Abnormal sounds include wheezing, a sign of asthma (Frame 9.32); rales, a sign of pulmonary edema (Frame 9.57) or atelectasis (Frame 9.33); and gurgles, a sign of pneumonia (Frame 9.54).

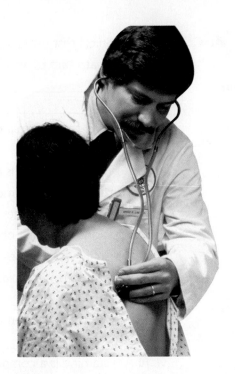

Figure 9.9 ■
Auscultation. The stethoscope is pressed against the body wall to listen for sound waves associated with breathing.
Source: Courtesy of National Institutes of Health, National Cancer Institute Visuals Online, Bethesda, MD.

bronchodilation
BRONG koh dye LAY shun

9.74 A procedure that uses a bronchodilating agent to relax the smooth muscles of the airways in an effort to stop bronchial constriction, thereby allowing the patient to breathe easier, is called _____. The constructed form of this term is written bronch/o/dilat/ion, which means "process of widening the airway."

bronchography
brong KOG rah fee

9.75 The suffix -*graphy* means "recording process." The X-ray imaging of the bronchi is called _____. This procedure produces an X-ray image of the bronchi called a **bronchogram** (BRONG koh gram) and uses a contrast medium to highlight the bronchial tree. In many respiratory clinics, bronchography is being replaced by bronchoscopy (Frame 9.76) and CT scans.

bronchoscopy
brong KOSS koh pee

9.76 Remember that the suffix -*scopy* means "process of viewing." The evaluation of the bronchi using a flexible fiber-optic tube mounted with a small lens at one end and attached to an eyepiece and computer monitor at the other end is called _____. This constructed term is written bronch/o/scopy. The instrument is a modified endoscope, known as a **bronchoscope** (BRONG koh skope), which is inserted through the nose to observe the trachea and bronchi (Figure 9.10■).

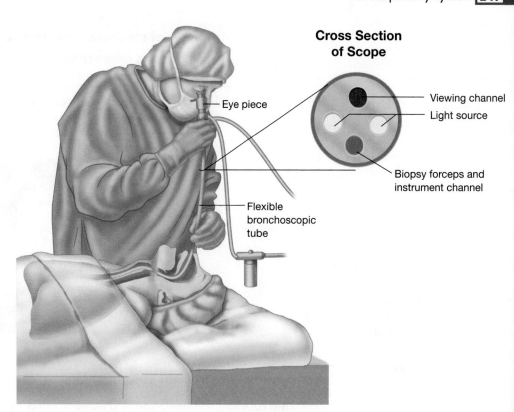

Cross Section
of Scope

Eye piece

Viewing channel

Light source

Biopsy forceps and
instrument channel

Flexible
bronchoscopic
tube

Figure 9.10 ■
Bronchoscopy.

chest CT scan

9.77 Diagnostic imaging of the chest by a computed tomography (CT) instrument is called _____ _____ _____ (Figure 9.11■). The procedure is used to diagnose respiratory tumors, pleural effusion, pleuritis, and other diseases by providing 3-D images of the thoracic cavity.

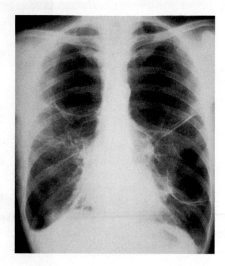

Figure 9.11 ■
Chest CT scan. The stringy, cobweb-like area indicates lung damage from smoking that has resulted in emphysema.
Source: Courtesy of National Institutes of Health Image Bank, Bethesda, MD.

chest X-ray

9.78 An X-ray image of the thoracic cavity that is used to diagnose tuberculosis, tumors, and other conditions of the lungs is called a

_____ _____ (Figure 9.12■).

Abbreviated **CXR,** it is also called a **chest radiograph.**

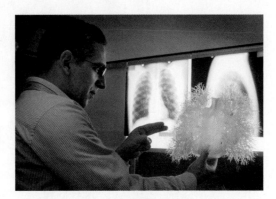

Figure 9.12 ■
Chest X-ray. A physician is examining chest X-rays with the aid of a plastic model of the bronchial tree.
Source: Courtesy of National Institutes of Health Image Bank, Bethesda, MD.

CPAP

9.79 A device that is commonly used to regulate breathing during sleep as a treatment for sleep apnea (Frame 9.11) is called **continuous positive airway pressure,** abbreviated _____. The CPAP machine includes a mask that fits over the mouth and nose, or just the nose, and gently blows air to encourage rhythmic breathing (Figure 9.13■).

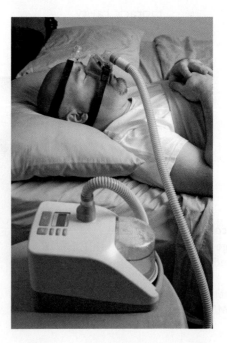

Figure 9.13 ■
Continuous positive airway pressure (CPAP) device. The sleeping subject is receiving the benefits of the flow of air generated by the CPAP device.
Source: © Amy Walters/Fotolia.

ears, nose, and throat specialist	**9.80** A physician specializing in the treatment of upper respiratory tract disease is called an **ENT,** which is the abbreviation of _____ _____ _____ _____. Alternate terms include **otolaryngologist** (OH toh LAIR in GAHL oh jist), **otonasolaryngologist** (OH toh NAY so LAIR in GAHL oh jist), and **otorhinolaryngologist** (oh toh RYE no LAIR in GAHL oh jist). The constructed form of otorhinolaryngologist is ot/o/rhin/o/laryng/o/logist.
endotracheal	**9.81** Insertion of a noncollapsible breathing tube into the trachea through the nose or mouth is called **endotracheal intubation** (EHN doh TRAY kee al * in too BAY shun). It is performed to open the airway or, if the patient is comatose, to keep the airway open. _____ is a constructed term written endo/trache/al, which means "pertaining to within the trachea."
expectorant ek SPEK toh rant	**9.82** A drug that breaks up mucus and promotes the coughing reflex to expel the mucus is called an **expectorant.** The term _____ is derived from the Latin word *expectoro,* which means "spit out of the chest."
incentive spirometry in SEHN tiv * spy RAH meh tree	**9.83** A valuable postoperative breathing therapy is called **incentive spirometry** (Figure 9.14■). It involves the use of a portable **spirometer** (Frame 9.94) to promote deeper breathing to improve lung expansion after an operation. Usually self-administered, _____ _____ reduces pulmonary complications and helps to correct atelectasis.

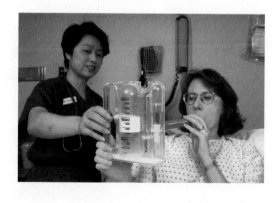

Figure 9.14 ■
Incentive spirometry. A portable incentive spirometer is useful for encouraging patients to exercise their breathing function following an operation.

laryngectomy lair in JEK toh mee	**9.84** Surgical removal of the larynx is performed during a _____. The constructed form of this term is written laryng/ectomy. It is often required as a treatment for laryngeal cancer and is usually followed by training or insertion of a device to enable the patient to communicate orally. Laryngectomy patients have a permanent tracheostomy (Frame 9.103).

laryngoscopy
lair ring GOSS koh pee

9.85 A diagnostic procedure that uses a modified endoscope, called a **laryngoscope** (lair RING goh skope), to visually examine the larynx is called _____.

laryngotracheotomy
lair ring goh TRAY kee OTT oh mee

9.86 A surgical incision into the larynx and trachea is usually performed to provide a secondary opening for inspiration and expiration, allowing air to bypass the upper respiratory tract. Remember that the suffix -tomy means "incision, to cut." Combine that with the combining forms for larynx and trachea, and you form the term for this procedure, _____. The constructed form of this term reveals five word parts and is written laryng/o/trache/o/tomy.

lobectomy
loh BEK toh mee

9.87 Surgical removal of a single lobe of a lung is sometimes required as a treatment for lung cancer, if the tumor is isolated in one lobe. The procedure is called _____. It may involve the removal of more than one lobe if required. Lobectomy is a constructed term, written lob/ectomy.

mechanical ventilation

9.88 A medical treatment to provide supplemental oxygen to patients in respiratory distress is called **mechanical ventilation.** It provides assisted breathing using a **ventilator,** which pushes air into the patient's airway (Figure 9.15■). _____ _____ is often used by a respiratory therapist in a clinical setting or by an emergency medical technician at the site of injury and in transit to a hospital.

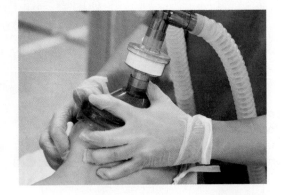

Figure 9.15 ■
Mechanical ventilation. The photograph shows a patient receiving breathing assistance by the use of a portable mechanical ventilator.
Source: beerkoff/Shutterstock.

nebulizer
NEBB yoo lye zer

9.89 A device used to convert a liquid medication to a mist and deliver it to the lungs with the aid of deep inhalation is called a **nebulizer** (Figure 9.16■). The term _____ is derived from the Latin word *nebula*, which means "fog."

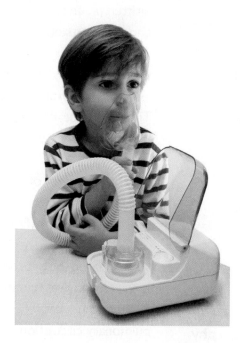

Figure 9.16 ■
Nebulizer. The nebulizer converts a liquid medication to a mist that is easily inhaled. A face mask, such as the one shown here, is often included to direct the mist.
Source: © g215/Fotolia.

oximetry
ok SIM eh tree

9.90 The suffix *-metry* means "measurement, process of measuring," and the combining form that means "oxygen" is *ox/i*. Therefore, the procedure that measures oxygen levels in the blood using an instrument called an **oximeter** (ok SIM eh ter) is called _____. The constructed form of this term is *ox/i/metry*. A small, handheld oximeter that provides a digital readout of oxygen levels by noninvasive physical contact with a finger is called a **pulse oximeter** (Figure 9.17■).

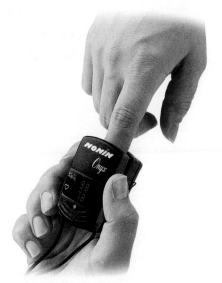

Figure 9.17 ■
Pulse oximetry. The small device provides a digital readout of oxygen levels in the blood.
Source: Courtesy of Nonin Medical, Inc.

pleurocentesis ploor oh sehn TEE siss	**9.91** The suffix *-centesis* means "surgical puncture." The surgical puncture and aspiration of fluid from the pleural cavity is a diagnostic procedure called _____. After aspiration, the fluid is analyzed for the presence of bacteria and white blood cells, the presence of which indicates pleuritis (Frame 9.52). Pleurocentesis is a constructed term, written pleur/o/centesis. It is also called **thoracentesis** (Frame 9.99) or **thoracocentesis.**
pneumonectomy NOO moh NEK toh mee	**9.92** Many terms in this section have used the suffix that means "surgical excision, removal," *-ectomy*. A word root that means "lung" is *pneumon*. Therefore, surgical removal of a lung is called _____, or **pneumectomy** (noo MEK toh mee). It is performed as a radical treatment for lung cancer, in which tumors have progressed throughout one lung. The constructed form of **pneumonectomy** is written pneumon/ectomy. If the surgery is limited to the removal of a single lobe, recall that the procedure is called a lobectomy (Frame 9.87).
pulmonary angiography PULL mon air ee * AN jee OG rah fee	**9.93** A diagnostic procedure that evaluates the blood circulation of the lungs is called **pulmonary angiography.** In this procedure, X-ray images are taken of the lungs following the injection of a contrast medium into the pulmonary circulation. _____ _____ is a constructed term represented as pulmon/ary angi/o/graphy, which literally means "recording of blood vessel pertaining to lung."
pulmonary function tests	**9.94** A series of diagnostic tests performed to determine the cause of lung disease by evaluating lung capacity through the use of spirometry (Frame 9.83) is called _____ _____ _____. Spirometry involves breathing into a tube connected to an instrument, called a **spirometer.** Both are terms that use the combining form that means "breathe," *spir/o*. The spirometer measures the amount of air inhaled and exhaled after a normal breathing cycle, called tidal volume (TV), the amount of air inhaled and exhaled during a forced expiration, called vital capacity (VC), and other values shown in Figure 9.18■.

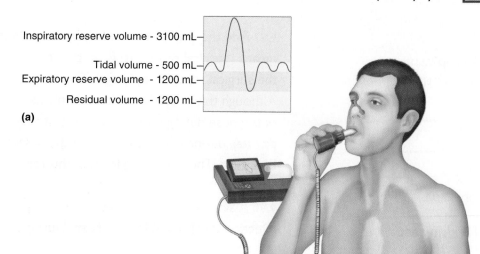

Inspiratory reserve volume - 3100 mL—
Tidal volume - 500 mL—
Expiratory reserve volume - 1200 mL—
Residual volume - 1200 mL—

(a)

(b)

Figure 9.18 ■
Pulmonary function test: spirometry. (a) Normal respiratory volumes, as measured during spirometry. A patient's spirometry data is compared to this chart to identify breathing deficiencies. (b) Illustration of a patient exhaling into a spirometer, which measures air volume.

pulmonologist
PUL moh NAHL oh jist

9.95 A physician specializing in the treatment of diseases affecting the lower respiratory tract, particularly the lungs, is called a pulmonary specialist or

_____.

resuscitation
ree SUSS ih TAY shun

9.96 An emergency procedure that is used to restore breathing is known as pulmonary **resuscitation.** The most common form is cardiopulmonary

_____, or **CPR,** which combines chest compressions with artificial breathing.

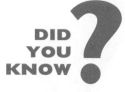

DID YOU KNOW ?

▶▶▶▶▶ **Resuscitation**

The term *resuscitation* is derived from the Latin word *resuscito,* which means "to rise up again" or "revive." Its present meaning refers to any procedure that involves a restoration of breathing and includes the popular technique of compressing the chest and heart called cardiopulmonary resuscitation (CPR). It also includes mouth-to-mouth resuscitation, in which air is blown into the patient's mouth while holding the nose, and the Heimlich maneuver, during which an obstruction (usually food) may be dislodged by reaching around a standing patient and pushing upward on the diaphragm to force an expulsion of air.

rhinoplasty
RYE noh plass tee

9.97 Add the combining form that means "nose" (*rhin/o*) to the suffix that means "surgical repair" to form the term _____, which is the surgical repair of the nose. This constructed term is written rhin/o/plasty. Although this procedure is commonly used to modify the external appearance of the nose during cosmetic surgery, it may include **septoplasty** (SEP toh plass tee), during which deviation of the nasal septum is corrected to improve breathing. The combining form in this term, *sept/o*, means "wall, partition."

TB skin test

9.98 A simple skin test to determine the presence of a tuberculosis infection is called a **TB skin test.** During a _____ _____ _____, a purified protein derivative (PPD) sample of the TB bacillus is injected beneath the epidermis of the skin (called an intradermal injection). A reddened, swollen skin lesion at the injection site a few days later indicates a previous exposure (Figure 9.19■) and requires follow-up with a chest X-ray. It is also called **PPD skin test** and **Mantoux skin test** (after the French physician Charles Mantoux).

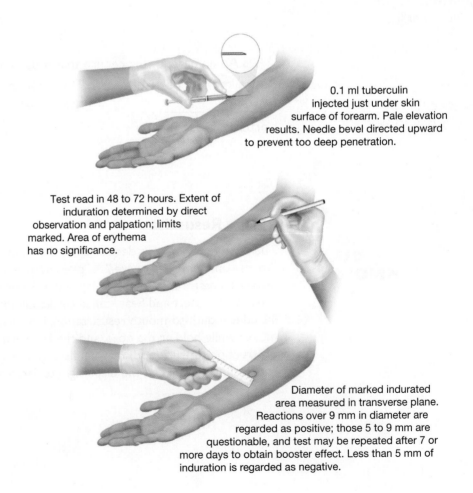

0.1 ml tuberculin injected just under skin surface of forearm. Pale elevation results. Needle bevel directed upward to prevent too deep penetration.

Test read in 48 to 72 hours. Extent of induration determined by direct observation and palpation; limits marked. Area of erythema has no significance.

Diameter of marked indurated area measured in transverse plane. Reactions over 9 mm in diameter are regarded as positive; those 5 to 9 mm are questionable, and test may be repeated after 7 or more days to obtain booster effect. Less than 5 mm of induration is regarded as negative.

Figure 9.19 ■
TB skin test.

thoracentesis
THOR ah sehn TEE siss

9.99 The suffix that means "surgical puncture" is *-centesis*. Surgical puncture using a needle and syringe into the thoracic cavity to aspirate pleural fluid for diagnosis or treatment is called a _____. It is also called **thoracocentesis** (THOR ah koh sehn TEE siss) or **pleurocentesis** (Frame 9.91). Thoracentesis is a constructed term written thora/centesis; note that, in this term, the syllable *co* is removed from the combining form *thoraclo* for ease of pronunciation. The procedure is often used to treat pleural effusion (Frame 9.51) by draining the excess fluid from the pleural cavity.

thoracostomy
THOR ah KOSS toh mee

9.100 The suffix *-stomy* means "surgical creation of an opening." Surgical puncture into the chest cavity, usually for the insertion of a drainage or air tube, is called a _____. The constructed form of this term is written thorac/o/stomy. The procedure is often termed "placing a chest tube."

thoracotomy
THOR ah KOTT oh mee

9.101 Recall the suffix that means "incision, to cut." Add this to the combining form that means "chest, thorax," and you form the term _____, which is a surgical incision into the chest wall. The constructed form of this term is thorac/o/tomy.

tracheoplasty
TRAY kee oh PLASS tee

9.102 The suffix *-plasty* means "surgical repair." Surgical repair of the trachea is called _____. The constructed form of this term reveals three word parts and is written trache/o/plasty.

tracheostomy
TRAY kee OSS toh mee

9.103 Recall the suffix that means "surgical creation of an opening." Surgical creation of an opening into the trachea, usually for the insertion of a breathing tube, is called _____. This constructed term is written trache/o/stomy. The procedure is shown in Figure 9.20■.

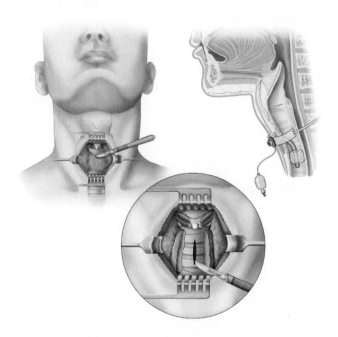

Figure 9.20
Tracheostomy. A tracheotomy, or incision into the trachea, is performed to create an opening into the trachea as shown in this series of illustrations.

tracheotomy TRAY kee OTT oh mee	**9.104** Surgical incision into the trachea is a required part of a tracheostomy (Frame 9.103). The incision is called a _____. The constructed form of this term is written trache/o/tomy.
ventilation-perfusion scanning	**9.105** A diagnostic tool that uses nuclear medicine, or the use of radioactive material, to evaluate pulmonary function is called **ventilation-perfusion scanning.** Abbreviated **VPS,** it can identify pulmonary embolism (Frame 9.58) and pulmonary edema (Frame 9.57). _____-_____ _____ is also called **lung scan** and **V/Q scan.**

PRACTICE: Treatments, Procedures, and Devices of the Respiratory System

The Right Match

Match the term on the left with the correct definition on the right.

_____ 1. pulmonary function tests

_____ 2. pulse oximeter

_____ 3. bronchodilation

_____ 4. arterial blood gases

_____ 5. TB skin test

_____ 6. auscultation

_____ 7. ventilation-perfusion scanning

_____ 8. nebulizer

_____ 9. pulmonary angiography

_____ 10. expectorant

a. breaks up mucus and promotes coughing

b. also called PPD skin test and Mantoux skin test

c. oxygen and carbon dioxide blood levels

d. device used to convert a liquid medication to a mist and deliver it to the lungs

e. physical examination that includes listening to sounds within the body

f. a blood oxygen measuring device that reads oxygen levels by noninvasive physical contact with a finger

g. procedure that uses a bronchodilating agent in an inhaler to reduce bronchial constriction

h. X-ray of lung blood vessels

i. diagnostic tool that uses nuclear medicine, or the use of radioactive material, to evaluate pulmonary function

j. use of spirometry to evaluate lung function

Break the Chain

Analyze these medical terms:

   a) Separate each term into its word parts; each word part is labeled for you (**p** = prefix, **r** = root, **cf** = combining form, and **s** = suffix).

   b) For the Bonus Question, write the requested definition in the blank that follows.

1. a) tracheotomy   _____/___/_____
                              cf   s

   b) *Bonus Question:* What is the definition of the suffix? _____

2. a) thoracentesis   _____/_____
                              r   s

   b) *Bonus Question:* What is the definition of the word root? _____

3. a) pneumonectomy   _____/_____
                              r   s

   b) *Bonus Question:* What is the definition of the word root? _____

4. a) bronchoscopy   _____/___/_____
                              cf   s

   b) *Bonus Question:* What is the definition of the suffix? _____

5. a) adenoidectomy   _____/_____/_____
                              r   s   s

   b) *Bonus Question:* What is the definition of the first suffix? _____

6. a) bronchodilation   _____/___/_____/_____
                              cf   r   s

   b) *Bonus Question:* What is the definition of the suffix? _____

7. a) lobectomy   _____/_____
                              r   s

   b) *Bonus Question:* What is the definition of the word root? _____

8. a) rhinoplasty   _____/___/_____
                              cf   s

   b) *Bonus Question:* What is the definition of the combining form? _____

9. a) septoplasty   _____/___/_____
                              cf   s

   b) *Bonus Question:* What is the definition of the suffix? _____

Abbreviations of the Respiratory System

The abbreviations that are associated with the respiratory system are summarized here. Study these abbreviations, and review them in the exercise that follows.

Abbreviation	Definition
ABGs	arterial blood gases
AFB	acid-fast bacilli
ARDS	adult (acute) respiratory distress syndrome
CF	cystic fibrosis
COPD	chronic obstructive pulmonary disease
CPAP	continuous positive airway pressure device
CPR	cardiopulmonary resuscitation
CXR	chest X-ray
LTB	laryngotracheobronchitis

Abbreviation	Definition
NRDS	neonatal respiratory distress syndrome
PE	pulmonary embolism
PPD	purified protein derivative
RDS	respiratory distress syndrome
SARS	severe acute respiratory syndrome
TB	tuberculosis
URI	upper respiratory infection
VPS or V/Q scan	ventilation-perfusion scanning

PRACTICE: Abbreviations

Fill in the blanks with the abbreviation or the complete medical term.

Abbreviation

1. _____
2. _____
3. ARDS
4. _____
5. CPR
6. _____
7. URI

Medical Term

laryngotracheobronchitis

tuberculosis

_____

chest X-ray

_____

cystic fibrosis

_____

▶▶▶▶ Chapter Review

Word Building

Construct medical terms from the following meanings. (Some are built from word parts, some are not.) The first question has been completed as an example.

1. inflammation of the larynx   _____*laryng*itis

2. absence of oxygen   _____oxia

3. inflammation of the bronchi   bronch_____

4. respiratory failure characterized by atelectasis   respiratory _____

5. physical exam that includes listening to body sounds   _____ (do this one on your own!)

6. deficient oxygen levels in the blood   hyp_____

7. difficulty breathing   _____pnea

8. excessive carbon dioxide levels in the blood   hyper_____

9. abnormal dilation of the bronchi   bronchi _____

10. lung inflammation due to dust inhalation   _____coniosis

11. cancer in the cells within the bronchi   bronchogenic _____

12. an inherited disease of excessive mucus production   cystic _____

13. inflammation of the trachea   trache_____

14. the absence of respiratory ventilation   _____sphyxia

15. X-ray image of the bronchi   broncho_____

16. surgical puncture and aspiration of fluid from the pleural cavity   thorac_____

17. measurement of oxygen levels in the blood   oxi_____

▶▶▶▶ Medical Report Exercises

Geoffrey Piscotti _____

Read the following medical report, then answer the questions that follow.

PGH **PEARSON GENERAL HOSPITAL**

5500 University Avenue Metropolis, WI
Phone: (211) 594-4000 • Fax: (211) 594-4001

Medical Consultation: ENT

Date: 2/15/2011

Patient: Geoffrey Piscotti

Patient Complaint: Difficulty breathing, sometimes with chest pain. Tired much of the time, with stuffy nose that sometimes bleeds.

History: 6-year-old male with no prior medical history.

Family History: Father, 37 years, 9th-grade teacher in public school system. Mother, 32 years, respiratory therapist in downtown clinic. No surgeries or major medical concerns.

Allergies: None.

Physical examination: Vital signs normal, except slight fever of 99.6°F and labored breathing. Minor laryngo-tracheobronchitis and sinusitis apparent on X-rays. TB skin test positive; sputum test positive for TB. Active TB confirmed with chest scan.

Diagnosis: Tuberculosis, active form.

Treatment: Inpatient care with oxygen assist and antibiotic cocktail IV drip. Follow with long-term oral antibiotic cocktail. Inform County Health and CDC of incident and potential exposures.

Maria S. Zayas, M.D.
Maria S. Zayas, M.D.

Photo Source: Losevsky Pavel/Shutterstock

Comprehension Questions

1. What complaints support the diagnosis? _____

_____

_____

2. Based on the family history, how do you think the TB infection originated? _____

_____

_____

3. What is the meaning of the abbreviation TB? _____

_____

_____

Case Study Questions

The following Case Study provides further discussion regarding the patient in the medical report. Fill in the blanks with the correct terms. Choose your answers from the following list of terms. (Note that some terms may be used more than once.)

acid-fast	chest X-rays	laryngotracheobronchitis
bronchodilating	coryza (or acute rhinitis)	tuberculosis (TB)

Geoffrey Piscotti, a 6-year-old boy with a previous healthy history, was admitted into an emergency clinic when his mother became concerned about his respiratory function. She explained that he had come home from school three weeks ago with a common cold, or (a) _____. He began coughing violently shortly afterward, preventing him from sleeping. Physical exams showed an acute inflammation of the larynx, trachea, and bronchi, indicating the acute condition known as (b) _____, which was bacterial in origin. Following the prescribed use of antibiotic therapy and the use of inhaled (c) _____ agents to reduce bronchial constriction, the patient recovered initially. Several months passed and then the coughing returned and the boy complained of low energy. Following a (d) _____ skin test and a sputum test that included (e) _____-_____ bacilli, positive results indicated an active lung infection known as (f) _____. TB was confirmed with the use of radiographic images of the thorax, or (g) _____ _____. The course of treatment included a cocktail of antibiotics administered over a six-month period.

Shareena Mushreen _____

For a greater challenge, read the following medical report, then answer the critical thinking questions that follow.

PEARSON GENERAL HOSPITAL

PGH

5500 University Avenue Metropolis, CA
Phone: (211) 594-4000 • Fax: (211) 594-4001

Medical Consultation: ENT

Date: 6/16/2011

Patient: Shareena Mushreen

Patient Complaint: Difficulty breathing, often with chest pain.

History: 65-year-old female. Recent immigrant with no prior medical history available.

Family History: Parents deceased 25 years; no siblings reported.

Allergies: None

Physical Examination: Vital signs abnormal: bp 132/95, pulse 81/min., temp. 99.7°F. Pulse oximetry and pulmonary function test indicate hypoxemia. Auscultation positive for pneumonia. Acid-fast bacilli negative. HIV test negative. Blood culture positive for *Pneumocystis jiroveci*.

Diagnosis: Pneumonia with HIV negative.

Treatment: Antibiotic therapy to defeat pneumonia with inpatient oxygen-tent treatment. Further testing recommended to explore the source of the pneumonia infection.

George T. Cohn, M.D.
George T. Cohn, M.D.

Comprehension Questions

1. Why would the diagnosed condition of pneumonia cause the patient complaint? _____

   _____

   _____

2. Why is additional testing recommended to explore the source of the infection? _____

   _____

   _____

3. What is the source of the infection causing the pneumonia? _____

   _____

   _____

Case Study Questions

The following case study provides additional consideration of the patient in the medical report. Recall the terms from this chapter to fill in the blanks with the correct terms.

A 65-year-old female, Shareen Mushareen, complained of difficulty breathing and chest pain, two symptoms

called (h) _____ and (i) _____. Her personal physician began with a chest (j)

_____ using a stethoscope, followed by fingertip assessment of oxygen levels in the blood using

a (k) _____ and a measurement of breathing volumes, using a (l) _____. The

tests indicated reduced oxygen levels in the blood, called (m) _____, in combination with reduced

lung capacity. Breathing sounds suggested labored breathing with some gurgling sounds. The physician diagnosed

the condition as a lung inflammation with alveolar fluids, called (n) _____, caused by an unknown

infectious agent. To identify the source of the infectious agent, sputum and blood tests were performed that included

(o) _____ _____ bacilli, HIV testing, and histological blood tests. The tests

showed the infectious agent as a fungus that is an opportunistic pathogen in immune-suppressed patients, known as

(p) _____ _____. This disease, called (q) _____, is a common

diagnostic indicator of patients suffering from HIV infection. An antibody test for HIV was administered, with negative

results. The patient was admitted for continual monitoring during antibiotic therapy and was kept within an oxygen tent

to improve oxygen blood levels. After the treatment, blood tests confirmed the pathogen had been defeated.

10

The Digestive System

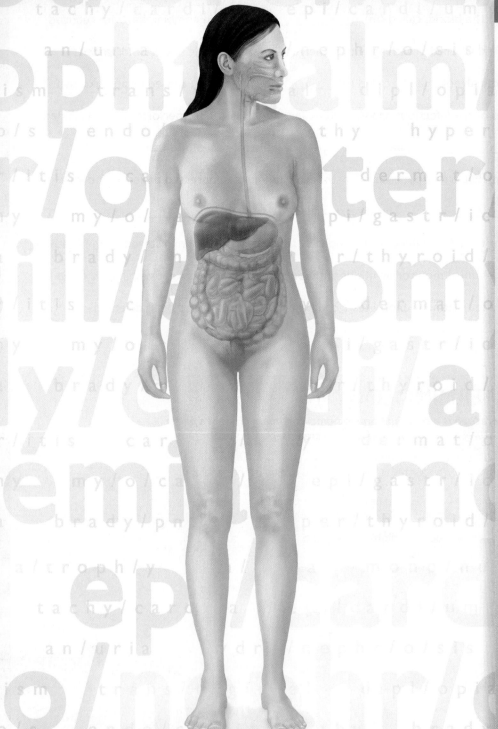

After completing this chapter, you will be able to:

1 Define and spell the word parts used to create terms for the digestive system.

2 Break down and define common medical terms used for symptoms, diseases, disorders, procedures, treatments, and devices associated with the digestive system.

3 Build medical terms from the word parts associated with the digestive system.

4 Pronounce and spell common medical terms associated with the digestive system.

Anatomy and Physiology Terms ▶▶▶▶▶

The following table provides the combining forms that specifically apply to the anatomy and physiology of the digestive system. Note that the combining forms are colored red to help you identify them when you see them again later in the chapter.

Combining Form	Definition	Combining Form	Definition
abdomin/o	abdomen	gloss/o	tongue
an/o	anus	hepat/o	liver
append/o, appendic/o	appendix	ile/o	to roll, ileum
bil/i	bile	jejun/o	empty, jejunum
cec/o	blind intestine, cecum	lingu/o	tongue
chol/e	bile, gall	or/o	mouth
choledoch/o	common bile duct	pancreat/o	sweetbread, pancreas
col/o, colon/o	colon	peps/o, pept/o	digestion
cyst/o	bladder, sac	peritone/o	to stretch over, peritoneum
dent/o	teeth	proct/o	rectum or anus
duoden/o	twelve, duodenum	pylor/o	pylorus
enter/o	small intestine	rect/o	rectum
esophag/e, esophag/o	gullet, esophagus	sial/o	saliva
gastr/o	stomach	sigm/o	the letter s, sigmoid colon
gingiv/o	gums	stomat/o	mouth

digestive
dye JEST iv

GI

10.1 The _____ system converts food into a form the body can use for energy, growth, and repair. It derives its name from its primary function, **digestion**. The term is from the Latin word *digestus,* which means "to divide, dissolve, or set in order." The digestive system performs all three: When the body digests food, it divides and dissolves it into simpler parts, setting the food parts in order for powering other body functions. Digestion occurs gradually, as food is passed from one organ to the next through the digestive tract, or gastrointestinal (GI) tract. The organs of the _____ tract form a long continuous tube that includes the mouth, pharynx, esophagus, stomach, small intestine, and large intestine. The small intestine includes three segments: the duodenum, jejunum, and ileum. The large intestine also includes three segments, called the cecum, colon, and rectum. Accessory organs contribute to digestion, mainly by secreting enzymes and other chemicals into the GI tract. They include the salivary glands, liver, gallbladder, and pancreas.

digestion

10.2 You have just learned that _____, which is the breakdown of food particles into their small subunits, is the primary function of the digestive system. Chemical digestion is performed by enzymes, and mechanical digestion is achieved by chewing in the mouth and mixing and churning actions produced by muscles in the walls of the stomach. Other important functions of the digestive system include

- Absorption of nutrients, which occurs across the wall of the small intestine
- Regulation of sugar levels in the blood, which is achieved by endocrine cells of the pancreas and by liver cells
- Conservation of water, which occurs as water is absorbed across the walls of the small and large intestines

10.3 Use the anatomy terms that appear in the left column to fill in the corresponding blanks in Figures 10.1■ and 10.2■.

1. **pharynx**
2. **esophagus**
3. **stomach**
4. **pancreas**
5. **small intestine**
6. **large intestine**
7. **gallbladder**
8. **liver**

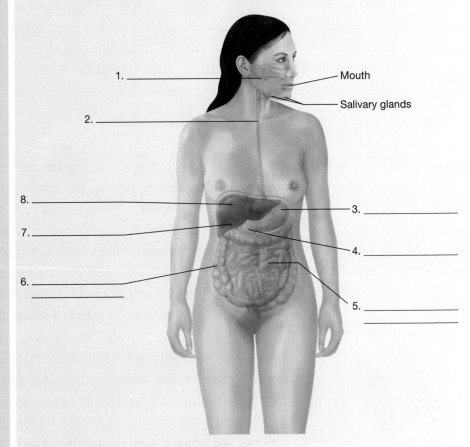

Figure 10.1 ■
Organs of the digestive system.

9. teeth
10. palate
11. uvula
12. pharynx
13. tongue

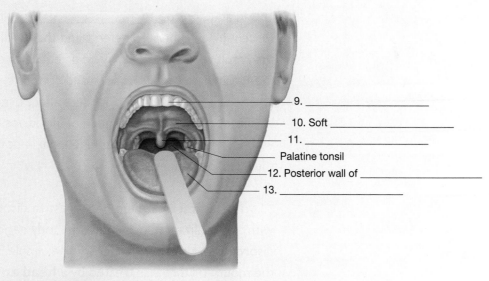

9. _____
10. Soft _____
11. _____
Palatine tonsil
12. Posterior wall of _____
13. _____

Figure 10.2 ■
The oral cavity. Anterior view of the open mouth.

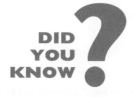

DID YOU KNOW?

▶▶▶▶▶ **Duodenum, Jejunum, and Ileum**

The three segments of the small intestine are the duodenum, jejunum, and ileum. The term *duodenum* is derived from the Medieval Latin word, *duodeni,* which means "twelve." This word first appeared in the anatomical texts in 1050 AD, taken from a monk's description of it as the "first part of the small intestine, about 12 fingerbreadths in length." *Ileum* means "to roll" in Greek and is named after its peristaltic waves of muscle contraction that roll through the organ like ocean waves. The term *jejunum* is named from the Latin word *jejunus,* meaning "empty."

Medical Terms of the Digestive System ▶▶▶▶▶

digestive flora

10.4 The digestive system is under a constant risk of infection because food and other substances that often contain pathogens are introduced into the body through the mouth every day. To make matters even more risky, the GI tract normally contains an enormous number of bacteria. Known as the digestive flora, most of these organisms are beneficial when their populations are contained within the tract. For example, *E. coli* assists in the breakdown of indigestible plant materials and synthesizes vitamin K. But if the _____ _____ is allowed to increase in density or spread to other body areas, severe infections can result.

infections	**10.5** In addition to _____, the GI tract organs are also susceptible to inherited defects and the development of tumors. In each case, the result of the disease may be a reduction of the body's ability to digest food, eliminate wastes, absorb and conserve water, or perform other specific functions. Most digestive disorders affect overall health rather than remain localized, due to the abundance of blood vessels and lymphatics associated with GI tract organs and the functional importance of accessory organs like the liver and pancreas.
disease	**10.6** The clinical treatment of a digestive disorder is performed by a physician with a specialization in treating the body region or organ, the particular disorder, or a set of disorders. For example, a _____ of the mouth or throat is treated by a **head and neck specialist,** stomach or intestinal disease is treated by a **gastroenterologist** (GAS troh EN ter AL oh jist), a disease of the rectum is treated by a **proctologist** (prok TALL oh jist), and a disease of the liver is treated by a **hepatobiliary** (heh PAT oh BIL ee air ee) **specialist.** Cancer is treated by an **oncologist,** often in association with a regional specialist. The area within a hospital that treats digestive disorders is often called **internal medicine.**
digestive **eating**	**10.7** Because most digestive organs are located deep within the body, the diagnosis of _____ disorders can benefit from noninvasive imaging procedures. Consequently, magnetic resonance imaging (MRI), computed tomography (CT) scans, and specialized X-ray techniques are often used. Once diagnosed, most disorders may be treated with therapeutic agents or by surgery. Some disorders, such as _____ disorders, are treated with psychological counseling and a strict diet regimen.
	10.8 In the following sections, you will study the prefixes, combining forms, and suffixes that combine to build the medical terms of the digestive system.

Signs and Symptoms of the Digestive System

Here are the word parts that specifically apply to the signs and symptoms of the digestive system that are covered in the following section. Note that the word parts are color-coded to help you identify them: prefixes are green, combining forms are red, and suffixes are blue.

Prefix	Definition
a-	without, absence of
dia-	through
dys-	bad, abnormal, painful, difficult
re-	back

Combining Form	Definition
bil/i	bile
flux/o	flow
gastr/o	stomach
halit/o	breath
hemat/o	blood
hepat/o	liver
peps/o, pept/o	digestion
phag/o	eat, swallow
steat/o	fat

Suffix	Definition
-algia	condition of pain
-dynia	condition of pain
-emesis	vomiting
-emia	condition of blood
-ia	condition of
-megaly	abnormally large
-osis	condition of
-rrhea	discharge

KEY TERMS A–Z

aphagia
ah FAY jee ah

10.9 The prefix *a-* means "without, absence of," and the combining form *phag/o* means "eat, swallow." Combining these word parts forms the term _____, which is the inability to swallow. This constructed term contains three word parts, as shown when it is written a/phag/ia. Although the literal meaning is "without eating or swallowing," clinical use of the term has changed its meaning to "inability to swallow."

ascites
ah SIGH teez

10.10 The Greek word that means "bag" is *askos*. It is used to create the term **ascites,** which is an accumulation of fluid within the peritoneal cavity that produces an enlarged abdomen. _____ is a sign of liver disease, congestive heart failure, or irritation to the peritoneum.

constipation
kon stih PAY shun

10.11 Infrequent or incomplete bowel movements are characteristic of **constipation.** It is a sign of an intestinal disorder. The term _____ is derived from the Latin word *constipatus*, which means "to press together."

diarrhea dye ah REE ah	**10.12** An opposite condition to constipation is **diarrhea,** in which a frequent discharge of watery fecal material occurs. It is a constructed term, written dia/rrhea. _____ literally means "discharge through" and may be caused by an improper diet, but it is more commonly a sign of infection by virus, bacteria, or protozoa. It is particularly dangerous to infants, who are in danger of severe dehydration. Approximately two million children die across the world each year from dehydration resulting from diarrhea.
dyspepsia diss PEPP see ah	**10.13** A common symptom of digestive difficulty that literally translates to "condition of difficult digestion" is _____. This constructed term contains three word parts, as shown in dys/peps/ia. Commonly called indigestion, it is accompanied by stomach or esophageal pain or discomfort.
dysphagia diss FAY jee ah	**10.14** Difficulty in swallowing is called **dysphagia.** It often accompanies a sore throat, although its chronic form can be a sign of oral or pharyngeal cancer. _____ is a constructed term and is written dys/phag/ia.
flatus FLAY tuss	**10.15** The term *flatus* is a Latin word that means "a blowing." It is used to describe the presence of gas, or air, in the GI tract, which is simply called _____. Gas is expelled through the anus as **flatulence** (FLAT yoo lens).
gastrodynia GAS troh DINN ee ah	**10.16** The combining form for stomach is *gastr/o,* and a suffix that means "condition of pain" is *-dynia.* Therefore, the symptom of stomach pain is known as _____. This constructed term includes three word parts and is written gastr/o/dynia. It is also known as **gastralgia** (gast RAL jee ah).
halitosis hal ih TOH siss	**10.17** The word root *halit* means "breath." It is derived from the Latin word for breath, *halitus.* Adding the suffix *-osis* forms the term **halitosis.** Although there is no word part included to give the term a negative meaning, nonetheless _____ means "bad breath." The constructed form is written halit/osis.
hematemesis HEE mah TEM eh siss	**10.18** Vomiting blood is a sign of a severe digestive disorder, such as a bleeding peptic ulcer (Frame 10.61) or stomach cancer (Frame 10.42). It is called **hematemesis,** which is a constructed term written hemat/emesis. The literal meaning of _____ is "vomiting blood."

hepatomegaly
HEPP ah toh MEG ah lee

10.19 A sign of liver disease is abnormal enlargement of the liver, called _____. This constructed term is written hepat/o/megaly, which literally means "abnormally large liver."

jaundice
JAWN diss

10.20 A yellowish-orange coloration of the skin, sclera of the eyes, and deeper tissues is a collective sign of liver disease called **jaundice** (Figure 10.3■). The condition of _____ results from the accumulation of bile pigments in the bloodstream that are normally removed by the liver.

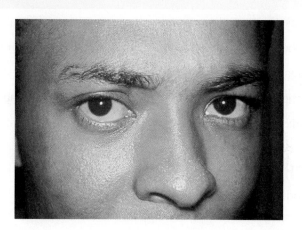

Figure 10.3 ■
Jaundice. Photograph of an individual with liver disease, evidenced by the yellowing of the sclera of the eyes and the skin.
Source: Courtesy of Dr. Thomas F. Sellers and Emory University, Centers for Disease Control Public Health Image Library, Atlanta, GA.

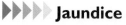

DID YOU KNOW?

▶▶▶▶▶ **Jaundice**

The term *jaundice* is derived from the French word for yellow, *jaune,* to describe the yellowing appearance of the skin and sclera. An alternate term for this symptom is *icterus,* which is the Greek word meaning "yellow bird."

nausea
NAW see ah

10.21 A symptom of dizziness that includes an urge to vomit is called **nausea.** When _____ is accompanied by vomiting, it is abbreviated **N&V.** Nausea is derived from the Latin and Greek words for seasickness, *nausia.*

reflux
REE fluks

10.22 A backward flow of material in the GI tract, or regurgitation, is called **reflux.** This constructed term is written re/flux. The literal meaning of _____ is "back flow."

steatorrhea
STEE at oh REE ah

10.23 Abnormal levels of fat in the feces is a sign of digestive malfunction. It is called **steatorrhea,** which is a constructed term written steat/o/rrhea. Because *steat/o* is the combining form for fat, _____ literally means "discharge of fat."

PRACTICE: Signs and Symptoms of the Digestive System

The Right Match

Match the term on the left with the correct definition on the right.

_____ 1. dysphagia   a. backward flow of material in the GI tract

_____ 2. reflux   b. gas trapped in the GI tract

_____ 3. flatus   c. difficulty in swallowing

_____ 4. halitosis   d. infrequent or incomplete bowel movements

_____ 5. ascites   e. frequent discharge of watery fecal material

_____ 6. diarrhea   f. bad breath

_____ 7. nausea   g. from the French word for yellow

_____ 8. constipation   h. a symptomatic urge to vomit

_____ 9. jaundice   i. accumulation of fluid in the peritoneal cavity

Break the Chain

Analyze these medical terms:

    a) Separate each term into its word parts; each word part is labeled for you (**p** = prefix, **r** = root, **cf** = combining form, and **s** = suffix).

    b) For the Bonus Question, write the requested definition in the blank that follows.

The first set has been completed for you as an example.

1. a) aphagia   _a/phag/ia_
                               p   r   s

    b) *Bonus Question:* What is the definition of the suffix? _condition of_ _____

2. a) dyspepsia   _____/_____/_____
                                  p   r   s

    b. *Bonus Question:* What is the definition of the word root? _____

3. a) gastrodynia   _____/___/_____
                                  cf   s

    b) *Bonus Question:* What is the definition of the combining form? _____

4. a) hematemesis   _____/_____
                                  r   s

    b) *Bonus Question:* What is the definition of the suffix? _____

5. a) steatorrhea   _____/___/_____
                                  cf   s

    b) *Bonus Question:* What is the definition of the combining form? _____

6. a) hepatomegaly   _____/___/_____
                                  cf   s

    b) *Bonus Question:* What is the definition of the combining form? _____

Diseases and Disorders of the Digestive System

Here are the word parts that specifically apply to the diseases and disorders of the digestive system that are covered in the following section. Note that the word parts are color-coded to help you identify them: prefixes are green, combining forms are red, and suffixes are blue.

Prefix	Definition
an-	without, absence of
dys-	bad, abnormal, painful, difficult
mal-	bad

Combining Form	Definition
aden/o	gland
appendic/o	appendix
cheil/o	lip
chol/e	bile, gall
cholecyst/o	gallbladder
choledoch/o	common bile duct
cirrh/o	orange
col/o	colon
diverticul/o	diverticulum
duoden/o	twelve, duodenum
enter/o	small intestine
esophag/e, esophag/o	gullet, esophagus
gastr/o	stomach
gingiv/o	gums
gloss/o	tongue
hem/o	blood
hepat/o	liver
lip/o	fat
lith/o	stone
orex/o	appetite
pancreat/o	sweetbread, pancreas
parot/o	parotid gland
pept/o	digestion
peritone/o	to stretch over, peritoneum
polyp/o	small growth
proct/o	rectum or anus
rect/o	rectum
sial/o	saliva
volv/o	to roll

Suffix	definition
-al	pertaining to
-ectasis	expansion, dilation
-ia	condition of
-iasis	condition of
-ic	pertaining to
-itis	inflammation
-malacia	softening
-megaly	abnormally large
-oid	resembling
-oma	tumor
-osis	condition of
-pathy	disease
-penia	abnormal reduction in number, deficiency
-ptosis	drooping
-sis	state of
-y	process of

anorexia nervosa
  AN or EKS ee ah * nerv OH sah

10.24 An emotional eating disorder in which the patient avoids food due to a compulsion to become thin in appearance is known as **anorexia nervosa.** The medical term _____ _____ is a constructed term written an/orex/ia nervosa and literally means "nervous condition of absence of appetite." It results in extreme weight loss and nutritional deficiencies and can become fatal if left untreated.

appendicitis
  ah pen dih SIGH tiss

10.25 Inflammation of the appendix is called _____. It is a constructed term written appendic/itis and is illustrated in Figure 10.4■.

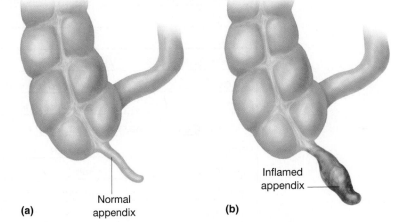

(a) Normal appendix

Inflamed appendix

(b)

Figure 10.4 ■
Appendicitis. (a) A normal appendix. (b) An inflamed appendix in appendicitis.

bulimia
  boo LEEM ee ah

10.26 A common eating disorder involving repeated gorging with food followed by induced vomiting or laxative abuse is known as **bulimia.** Commonly known as "binging and purging," the term _____ is derived from the Greek word that means "ravenous hunger," *boulimia.*

cheilitis
  kye LYE tiss

10.27 Because the combining form for lip is *cheil/o*, inflammation of the lip is called _____, a constructed term written cheil/itis. Another term using this combining form is **cheilosis** (kye LOH siss). It is a general condition of the lip, which often includes splitting of the lips and corners of the mouth, usually resulting from vitamin B deficiency.

cholecystitis
  koh lee siss TYE tiss

10.28 The combining form for gallbladder is *cholecyst/o*, which literally means "bladder of gall." Inflammation of the gallbladder is therefore called _____, which can be written cholecyst/itis. It is usually caused by stones lodged within the gallbladder, which are commonly called gallstones.

choledochitis
KOH leh dok EYE tiss

choledoch/o/lith/iasis

10.29 The combining form for common bile duct, which is a tube that carries bile from the liver to the small intestine, is *choledoch/o*. Thus, inflammation of the common bile duct is called _____. Adding the term *lithiasis* to the word root to describe the presence of stones within the common bile duct forms the term **choledocholithiasis** (KOH leh doh koh lith EYE ah siss). This constructed term is written _____/__/_____/____.

cholelithiasis
KOH lee lith EYE ah siss

10.30 A generalized condition of stones lodged within the gallbladder or bile ducts is called _____. It is illustrated in Figure 10.5■. This constructed term includes four word parts, as shown when it is written chol/e/lith/iasis.

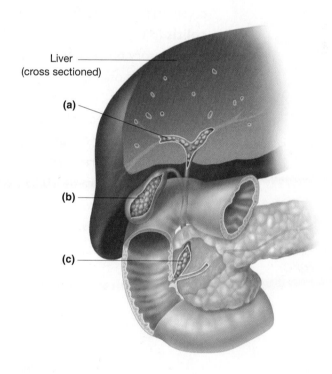

Liver
(cross sectioned)

(a)

(b)

(c)

Figure 10.5 ■
Cholelithiasis. Common sites of gallstones in the generalized condition.
(a) Stones in the hepatic duct.
(b) Stones in the gallbladder.
(c) Stones in the common bile duct.

cirrhosis
ser ROH siss

10.31 A chronic, progressive liver disease characterized by the gradual loss of liver cells and their replacement by fat and other forms of connective tissue is known as **cirrhosis**. It is shown in Figure 10.6■. The constructed form of _____ is written cirrh/osis. It literally means "condition of orange," referring to the common symptom of a yellowish-orange coloration of the skin (jaundice, Frame 10.20). Chronic alcoholism is responsible for about 75% of cirrhosis cases. The remainder are usually caused by viral infections, such as hepatitis B and C.

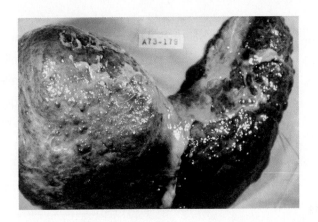

Figure 10.6 ■
Cirrhosis. Cirrhosis is characterized by a chronic deterioration of the liver, replacing healthy cells with connective tissue that causes a mottled appearance. In this photograph, the liver was removed from a deceased patient in an advanced state of cirrhosis.
Source: Pearson Education

colitis
   koh LYE tiss

10.32 Inflammation of the segment of the large intestine known as the colon is called _____. Colitis often includes excessive peristaltic contractions, mucus production, and cramping pain. If chronic bleeding of the colon wall occurs to form bloody diarrhea, the condition is called **ulcerative colitis** (UHL ser ah tiv * koh LYE tiss). Ulcerative colitis is a form of chronic inflammatory bowel disease, or IBD (Frame 10.54). *Colitis* is a constructed term, written col/itis.

colorectal cancer
   kohl oh REK tal * KAN ser

10.33 Cancer of the colon often includes cancer of the rectum, forming the life-threatening disease known as **colorectal cancer.** *Colorectal* is a constructed term written col/o/rect/al. This form of cancer often arises as a polyp (Frame 10.63), which is an abnormal mass of tissue that projects from the wall of the organ into the interior like a mushroom, to become an aggressive, metastatic tumor. The most common sites of _____ _____ are illustrated in Figure 10.7■.

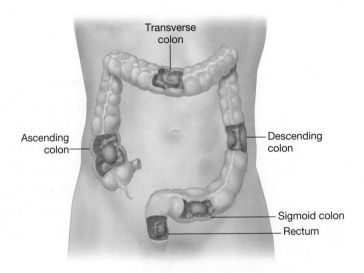

Figure 10.7 ■
Colorectal cancer. The most common sites of tumor development are shown.

Crohn disease
KRON * dih ZEEZ

10.34 A chronic inflammation of any part of the GI tract, most commonly the ileum of the small intestine, that involves ulcerations, scar tissue formation, and thickening adhesions of the organ wall, is called **Crohn disease.** Also known as **regional ileitis** or **regional enteritis,** it is believed to be an inherited condition. _____ _____ is a form of chronic inflammatory bowel disease, or IBD (Frame 10.54).

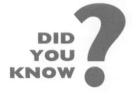

DID YOU KNOW ?

▶▶▶▶▶ **Crohn Disease**

Dr. B. B. Crohn first described the disease that bears his name in 1932. At the time, he believed this chronic form of IBD was caused by a pathogen. New evidence suggests that he may have been correct, although the causative organism has not yet been identified.

diverticulosis
DYE ver tik yoo LOH siss

diverticul/itis

10.35 In some individuals, small pouches called **diverticula** form on the wall of the colon (Figure 10.8■). The presence of diverticula is often without symptoms or with mild bowel discomfort and is called _____. This constructed term is written diverticul/osis. If the pouches become inflamed, it produces a more painful condition known as **diverticulitis** (DYE ver tik yoo LYE tiss), which increases the risk of developing colorectal cancer (Frame 10.33). The constructed form of this term is _____/____.

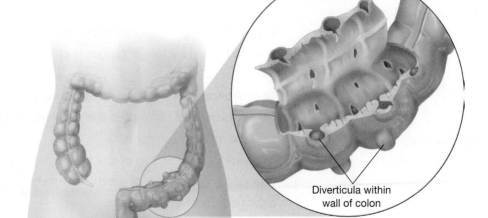

Diverticula within wall of colon

Figure 10.8 ■
Diverticulosis. It is the presence of abnormal pouches in the wall of the large intestine (diverticula). If the pouches become inflamed to produce diverticulitis, the risk of developing colorectal cancer is elevated.

duodenal ulcer doo ODD eh nal * UL ser	**10.36** An ulcer, or erosion, in the wall of the duodenum of the small intestine is called a _____ _____. The constructed form of *duodenal* is written duoden/al.
dysentery DIS en tair ee	**10.37** An acute inflammation of the GI tract that is caused by bacteria, protozoa, or chemical irritants is called **dysentery.** This constructed term is written dys/enter/y and literally means "difficult intestine." _____ is characterized by severe diarrhea and can become a life-threatening disease by causing dehydration.
enteritis EHN ter EYE tiss	**10.38** The word root for intestine is *enter*. Thus, inflammation of the small or large intestine is called _____, which can be written enter/itis to show the word parts.
esophagitis eh soff ah JYE tiss **esophag/o/malacia**	**10.39** Inflammation of the esophagus is called **esophagitis.** This constructed term is written esophag/itis. It is often caused by acid reflux (Frame 10.22) from the stomach, which burns the esophageal lining to produce the inflammation. Chronic _____ may lead to either a morbid softening of the esophageal wall, called **esophagomalacia** (eh soff ah go mah LAY shee ah), or the development of **esophageal cancer.** The constructed form of *esophagomalacia* is written _____/__/_____.
food-borne illness	**10.40** Ingestion of food contaminated with harmful bacteria can cause symptoms of diarrhea and vomiting, even in otherwise healthy people, but in the very young, elderly, and immunosuppressed it can become life threatening. Common causes of **food-borne illness,** or food poisoning, include *E. coli, Salmonella,* and *Staphylococci.* In addition, the extremely toxic anaerobic bacterium, *Clostridium botulinum,* causes a severe form of _____-_____ _____, especially in improperly prepared home-canned foods. The life-threatening disease caused by this organism is called **botulism** (BOTT yoo lizm).
gastrectasis gas TREK tah siss	**10.41** Abnormal stretching, or dilation, of the stomach is called **gastrectasis.** This constructed term uses the suffix *-ectasis* (meaning "expansion, dilation") and is written gastr/ectasis. _____ may be caused by overeating, obstruction of the pyloric opening, or hiatal hernia (Frame 10.53). The related condition of **gastromegaly** (GAS troh MEG ah lee) is an abnormal enlargement of the stomach.

gastric cancer
GAS trik * KAN ser

10.42 Commonly known as stomach cancer, _____ _____ is an aggressive, metastatic cancer arising from cells lining the stomach (Figure 10.9■). Risk of developing gastric cancer increases with chronic infection of the stomach by the bacterium *Helicobacter pylori*.

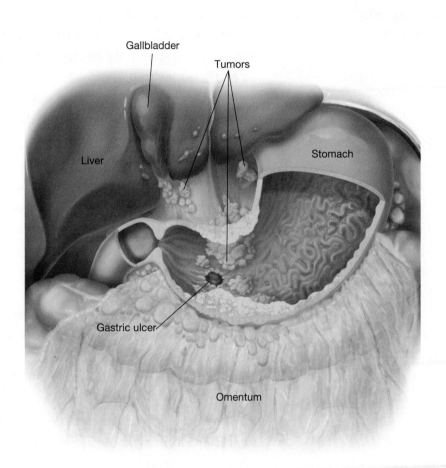

Gallbladder

Tumors

Liver

Stomach

Gastric ulcer

Omentum

Figure 10.9 ■
Gastric cancer. In advanced stages of gastric cancer, malignant cells spread to form tumors in the lymph nodes, liver, omentum, pancreas, and bile ducts.

gastric ulcer
GAS trik * UL ser

10.43 An ulcer, or erosion, in the wall of the stomach is commonly called a _____ _____. It is often caused by an imbalance between the secretion of the protective mucous layer and the secretion of hydrochloric acid in the stomach, which is often the result of infection by the bacterium *Helicobacter pylori* (*H. pylori*).

gastritis
gas TRY tiss

gastroenteritis
GAS troh en ter EYE tiss

gastr/o/enter/o/col/**itis**

gastroesophageal
GAS troh eh SOFF ah JEE al

gastromalacia
GAS troh mah LAY shee ah

giardiasis
jee ahr DYE ah siss

10.44 Inflammation of the stomach is called **gastritis.** The constructed form of this term is written gastr/itis. The acute form of _____ is usually caused by an improper diet or an infection, and the chronic form may be caused by a chronic bacterial infection, peptic ulcers (Frame 10.61), or gastric cancer (Frame 10.42). If the small intestine is involved in the inflammation, it is called _____. This constructed term is written gastr/o/enter/itis. If the first segment of the small intestine, the duodenum, is specifically involved, it is called **gastroduodenitis** (GAS troh doo oh den EYE tiss), written gastr/o/duoden/itis. Inflammation of the stomach, small intestine, and colon all at once is called **gastroenterocolitis** (GAS troh EN ter oh koh LYE tiss). The constructed form of this term reveals six word parts and is written _____/__/_____/__/_____/_____

10.45 A recurring backflow, or reflux, of stomach contents into the esophagus is a condition called **gastroesophageal reflux disease,** or **GERD.** It is usually the result of a weakened esophageal sphincter and produces the burning pain of indigestion. The term _____ is constructed of word parts and is written gastr/o/esophag/e/al.

10.46 The suffix -*malacia* means "softening." The softening of the stomach wall may occur during advanced stages of stomach cancer and other chronic diseases of the stomach. It is called _____. The constructed form of this term is written gastr/o/malacia.

10.47 Infection by the intestinal protozoa *Giardia intestinalis* or *Giardia lamblia* produces symptoms of diarrhea, cramps, nausea, and vomiting (Figure 10.10■). The disease is usually contracted by drinking contaminated water and is known as _____. This constructed term is written giardia/sis.

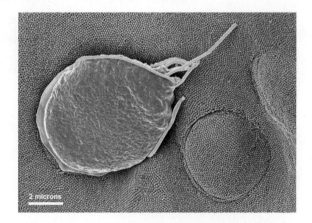

Figure 10.10 ■
Giardiasis. Colorized electron micrograph of a *Giardia* protozoan adhering to the surface of an epithelial cell lining the small intestine. The tiny red circles are microvilli, which number roughly 3,000 on a single intestinal cell.
Source: Courtesy of Dr. Stan Erlandsen, Centers for Disease Control Public Health Image Library, Atlanta, GA.

gingivitis jin jih VYE tiss	**10.48** Inflammation of the gums, or gingivae, is called _____. It is usually caused by chronic bacterial activity at the junction of the teeth and gums. The constructed form of this term is gingiv/itis.
glossitis gloss EYE tiss **gloss/itis**	**10.49** A combining form for tongue, *gloss/o,* is derived from the Greek word *glossa.* Any disease of the tongue is called a **glossopathy** (gloss AH path ee). This constructed term is written gloss/o/pathy. An example of a glossopathy is _____, which is an inflammation of the tongue often caused by exposure to allergens, toxic substances, or extreme heat or cold. The constructed form of glossitis is _____/_____.
hemorrhoids HEM oh roydz	**10.50** A varicose, or swollen, condition of the veins in the anus produces painful swellings that may break open and bleed, known as **hemorrhoids.** This term literally means "resembling leakage of blood." _____ are commonly called "piles."
hepatitis	**10.51** A viral-induced inflammation of the liver is called viral _____. This constructed term is written hepat/itis. There are five known forms of hepatitis, which are categorized with the letters *A* through *E* and described in the Did You Know? box.

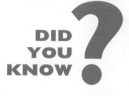

▶▶▶▶▶ Hepatitis Types

DID YOU KNOW ?

There are five main categories of hepatitis, all caused by related forms of a virus. Type A (infectious hepatitis) is transmitted by eating contaminated food. Type B (serum hepatitis) is transmitted via body fluids, such as blood or semen. Type C is mainly transmitted through the blood and often causes permanent liver damage. Type D is similar to type B and may combine with it to severely damage the liver. Type E is similar to type A and is the most common form in countries that have contaminated water supplies.

hepatoma hepp ah TOH mah	**10.52** The suffix that means "tumor" is *-oma.* A tumor arising from cells within the liver is called a **malignant** _____. The constructed form of this term is hepat/oma. The disease is also called **hepatocellular carcinoma,** or **HCC.** This form of liver cancer accounts for about 85% of the cases and is often associated with alcoholic cirrhosis or hepatitis B.

hiatal hernia
high A tahl * HER nee ah

10.53 Protrusion of the cardiac portion of the stomach through the hiatus of the diaphragm to enter the thoracic cavity is called a _____ _____. It causes the symptom of heartburn that results from the movement of stomach acids into the esophagus and is illustrated in Figure 10.11■. Another type of digestive system hernia, called **inguinal hernia,** is a protrusion of a small intestinal segment through the abdominal wall in the inguinal region. A **direct inguinal hernia** occurs in males and is a protrusion into the scrotal cavity. Also, an **umbilical hernia** occurs when a small intestinal segment enters through a tear in the membrane covering the abdominal wall at the umbilical (navel) region. In each of these cases, the hernia may become strangulated, which restricts blood flow to the protruding organ. A **strangulated hernia** requires medical intervention to avoid loss of the affected organ.

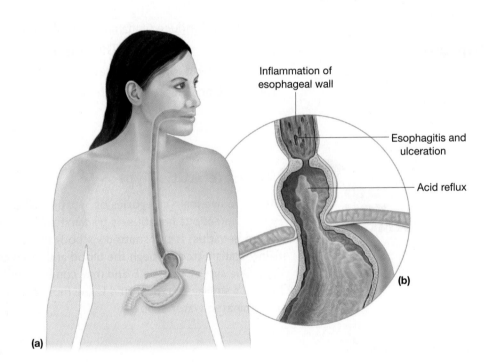

Inflammation of esophageal wall

Esophagitis and ulceration

Acid reflux

(b)

(a)

Figure 10.11 ■
Hiatal hernia. (a) The hernia occurs when the stomach protrudes through the diaphragm and into the thoracic cavity, often leading to the movement of stomach fluids into the esophagus that creates esophageal reflux and esophagitis.
(b) A close-up of a hiatal hernia.

inflammatory bowel disease

10.54 You have learned from Frames 10.32 and 10.34 that _____ _____ _____, or **IBD,** is a general term that includes the conditions ulcerative colitis and Crohn disease. IBD is a syndrome affecting different patients in different ways. It includes a wide spectrum of conditions and symptoms that range from chronic diarrhea and enteritis to ulcerative colitis and Crohn disease.

intussusception
IN tuh suh SEP shun

10.55 Although the small intestine is anchored to the abdominal wall by the peritoneal membranes, it is subject to infolding. Infolding of a segment of the small intestine within another segment is a condition called **intussusception** and results in a reduction of intestinal motility. It is illustrated in Figure 10.12■. The term _____ is a combination of Latin words that collectively mean "to take within."

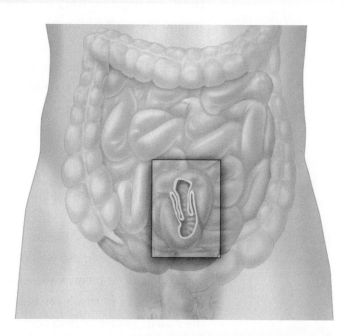

Figure 10.12 ■
Intussusception. The condition is caused by an infolding of the small intestine, which often causes a reduction of intestinal motility.

irritable bowel syndrome

10.56 A chronic disease characterized by periodic disturbances of large intestinal (bowel) function without clear physical damage is called **irritable bowel syndrome, or IBS.** Episodes of _____ _____ _____ include abdominal pain caused by intestinal muscle spasms and flatus and are often associated with fluctuations between diarrhea and constipation.

lactose intolerance
LAHK tos * in TOHL er ans

10.57 Most people produce an enzyme in the small intestine that breaks down lactose, the primary sugar in milk and milk products. A lack of this enzyme results in the uncomfortable symptoms of flatus and diarrhea when dairy foods are consumed. This condition is called _____ _____, and is abbreviated **LI.**

malabsorption syndrome
MAL ab sorp shun * SIN drom

10.58 The prefix *mal-* means "bad." A disorder that is characterized by difficulty absorbing one or more nutrients is called **malabsorption syndrome.** It can have severe consequences, depending on the nutrients that cannot be absorbed. An example of _____ _____ is the inability to absorb fat molecules, resulting in a life-threatening disease called **lipopenia** (LYE poh PEE nee ah). This is a constructed term written as lip/o/penia.

pancreatitis
PAN kree ah TYE tiss

10.59 Inflammation of the pancreas is called **pancreatitis.** This constructed term is written pancreat/itis. Possible causes include tumor development and bacterial infection. If pancreatic functions are affected, the complications of acute _____ can become life threatening.

parotitis
pahr oh TYE tiss

10.60 The largest salivary glands are called parotid glands and are located around the angle of the jaw. Inflammation of one or both parotid glands is called _____. If caused by a virus, it is usually referred to as **mumps.** The term *parotitis* is a constructed term, written parot/itis. It may also be referred to as **sialoadenitis** (sigh AL oh add eh NYE tiss). The constructed form of this term, written sial/o/aden/itis, literally means "inflammation of saliva gland."

peptic ulcer
PEPP tik * UL ser

10.61 The term **peptic** is a constructed term, pept/ic, that means "pertaining to digestion." An erosion into the inner wall of an organ along the GI tract is generally called a _____ _____. Usually, a peptic ulcer occurs in the wall of the stomach as a gastric ulcer (Frame 10.43), or in the wall of the duodenum as a duodenal ulcer (Frame 10.36). A gastric ulcer is shown in Figure 10.13■. The ulcer is formed when the protective mucus layer becomes eroded, exposing the inner lining to the caustic effects of hydrochloric acid. Roughly 80% of peptic ulcers are associated with an infection of *Helicobacter pylori (H. pylori),* which triggers an immune response that reduces mucus production.

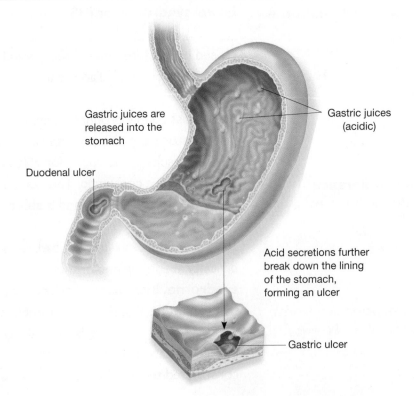

Gastric juices are released into the stomach

Gastric juices (acidic)

Duodenal ulcer

Acid secretions further break down the lining of the stomach, forming an ulcer

Gastric ulcer

Figure 10.13 ■
Peptic ulcer. A peptic ulcer may occur in the stomach (gastric ulcer), as shown here, or in the duodenum (duodenal ulcer). The most common cause is associated with infection by *H. pylori.*

peritonitis
pair ih toh NYE tiss

10.62 The peritoneum is the extensive membrane that lines the inner wall of the abdominopelvic cavity and covers most of its organs. Inflammation of this membrane is called _____. This constructed term is written periton/itis (the e on the end of the word root is dropped in this case). The inflammation is the body's response to an infection of the peritoneum, usually bacterial, that can become life threatening without medical intervention.

polyposis
pall ee POH siss

10.63 Any abnormal mass of tissue that projects inward from the wall of a hollow organ is called a **polyp** (PALL ip). The term means "small growth." It is usually a benign growth that may occur in the nose, throat, or large intestine. The presence of many polyps is called _____ and is illustrated in Figure 10.14■. The constructed form of this term is polyp/osis, which literally means "condition of small growths." Polyposis usually occurs in the colon or rectum of the large intestine, where it increases the risk for colorectal cancer (Frame 10.33).

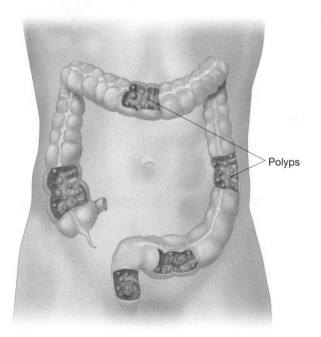
Polyps

Figure 10.14 ■
Polyps and polyposis. A polyp is a protruding growth from a mucous membrane lining a hollow organ. In the disease polyposis, multiple polyps develop, usually along the inner wall of the large intestine.

proctitis
prok TYE tiss

10.64 A combining form meaning "rectum" or "anus" is _proct/o_. Inflammation of the anus, and usually the rectum as well, is called _____. This constructed term is written proct/itis.

proctoptosis
PROK top TOH siss

10.65 Recall that the suffix _-ptosis_ means "drooping." A drooping, or prolapse, of the rectum is a condition called _____. The constructed form of this term is proct/o/ptosis.

volvulus

VOLL vyoo lus

10.66 A severe twisting of the intestine that leads to obstruction is called **volvulus.** The term is derived from the Latin word that means "to roll." A _____ that has caused a severe obstruction is illustrated in Figure 10.15■.

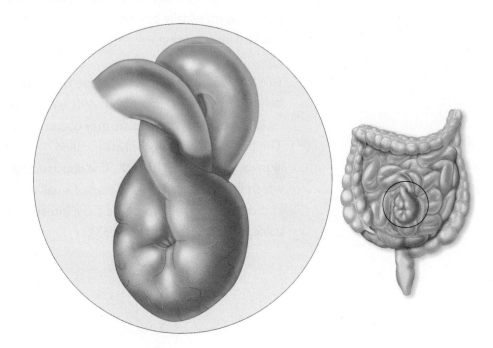

Figure 10.15 ■
Volvulus. A volvulus results when the small intestine twists, causing an obstruction that can lead to severe complications.

PRACTICE: Diseases and Disorders of the Digestive System

The Right Match

Match the term on the left with the correct definition on the right.

_____ 1. gastrectasis

_____ 2. polyp

_____ 3. gingivitis

_____ 4. giardiasis

_____ 5. bulimia

_____ 6. duodenal ulcer

_____ 7. volvulus

_____ 8. intussusception

_____ 9. cirrhosis

_____ 10. Crohn disease

_____ 11. irritable bowel syndrome

_____ 12. hernia

_____ 13. gastroenterocolitis

_____ 14. cheilitis

_____ 15. choledocholithiasis

_____ 16. colitis

_____ 17. diverticulitis

_____ 18. gastroesophageal reflux disease

a. infolding of a segment of the small intestine within another segment

b. a chronic inflammation of any part of the GI tract, usually of the ileum

c. intestinal infection by the protozoa *Giardia intestinalis* or *Giardia lamblia*

d. inflammation of abnormal pouches in the colon

e. twisting of the intestine causing an obstruction

f. a protrusion of intestine through connective tissue or a wall of the cavity in which it is normally enclosed

g. characterized by periodic bowel disturbances

h. a chronic liver disease

i. abnormal stretching of the stomach

j. an abnormal mass projecting inward

k. an eating disorder of binging and purging

l. an erosion in the wall of the duodenum of the small intestine

m. inflammation of the colon

n. inflammation of the gums

o. inflammation of the stomach and intestines

p. presence of stones in the common bile duct

q. recurring backflow of stomach contents into the esophagus

r. inflammation of the lips

Linkup

Link the word parts in the list to create the terms that match the definitions. You may use word parts more than once. Remember to add combining vowels when needed—and that some terms do not use any combining vowel. The first one is completed as an example.

Prefix	Combining Form	Suffix
an-	appendic/o	-ia
dys-	chol/e	-itis
	enter/o	-malacia
	esophag/e, esophag/o	-oma
	gastr/o	-osis
	gloss/o	-sis
	hepat/o	-y
	lith/o	
	orex/o	
	pancreat/o	
	polyp/o	
	proct/o	

Definition

Term

1. inflammation of the appendix — *appendicitis*

2. inflammation of the tongue — _____

3. condition of stones lodged within the gallbladder or bile ducts — _____

4. condition of prolapse of the rectum — _____

5. tumor within the liver — _____

6. softening of the stomach wall — _____

7. inflammation of the esophagus — _____

8. inflammation of the stomach and small intestine — _____

9. inflammation of the pancreas — _____

10. acute inflammation of the GI tract caused by bacteria, protozoa, or chemical irritants — _____

11. eating disorder in which the patient refuses food due to a compulsion to become thin — _____

12. condition of many polyps — _____

Treatments, Procedures, and Devices of the Digestive System

Here are the word parts that specifically apply to the treatments, procedures, and devices of the digestive system that are covered in the following section. Note that the word parts are color-coded to help you identify them: prefixes are green, combining forms are red, and suffixes are blue.

Prefix	Definition
an-	without, absence of
anti-	against, opposite of
dia-	through
endo-	within

Combining Form	Definition
abdomin/o	abdomen
acid/o	a solution or substance with a pH less than 7
append/o	appendix
cheil/o	lip
cholecyst/o	gallbladder
choledoch/o	common bile duct
col/o	colon
duoden/o	twelve, duodenum
esophag/e, esophag/o	gullet, esophagus
fec/o	feces
gastr/o	stomach
gingiv/o	gums
gloss/o	tongue
ile/o	to roll, ileum
lapar/o	abdomen
lith/o	stone
nas/o	nose
polyp/o	small growth
pylor/o	pylorus
vag/o	vagus nerve

Suffix	Definition
-al	pertaining to
-centesis	surgical puncture
-ectomy	surgical excision, removal
-emetic	pertaining to vomiting
-gram	a record or image
-graphy	recording process
-ic	pertaining to
-plasty	surgical repair
-rrhaphy	suturing
-rrhea	discharge
-scopy	process of viewing
-spasmodic	pertaining to a sudden, involuntary muscle contraction
-stomy	surgical creation of an opening
-tomy	incision, to cut

KEY TERMS A–Z

abdominocentesis
ab DOM ih noh sehn TEE siss

10.67 Because the suffix *-centesis* means "surgical puncture," a surgical puncture through the abdominal wall to remove fluid is a procedure called _____. This constructed term is written abdomin/o/centesis. An alternate term for this procedure is **paracentesis** (pair ah sehn TEE siss).

WORDS TO WATCH OUT FOR ▶▶▶▶▶ **abdomen and *abdomin/o***

The combining form meaning "abdomen" is *abdomin/o*, which is found in terms such as abdominocentesis. Notice that the combining form uses a letter *i* and not an *e*, as in *abdomen*.

antacid
ant ASS id

10.68 An agent that reduces the acidity of the stomach cavity is called an **antacid.** Note that the letter *i* is deleted from the prefix *anti-* to make _____ easier to pronounce. Most mild medications neutralize the acid pH of the stomach, whereas stronger medications inhibit the amount of acid produced and are called proton pump inhibitors. *Antacid* is a constructed term, written as ant/acid.

antiemetic
an tye ee MEH tik

10.69 An **antiemetic** is a drug that prevents or stops the vomiting reflex. This constructed term is written anti/emetic. _____ literally means "pertaining to against vomiting."

antispasmodic
an tye spaz MOH dik

anti/dia/rrhe/al

10.70 A drug that reduces peristalsis activity in the GI tract, which arrests the muscular spasms involved in diarrhea, is called an **antispasmodic.** The constructed form of _____ is written anti/spasmodic. An **antidiarrheal** (an tye dye ah REE al) may also be used to treat the symptoms of diarrhea (Frame 10.12), but usually by increasing water absorption in the colon while decreasing spasms. This constructed term is written _____/_____/_____/___.

appendectomy
app ehn DEK toh mee

10.71 The surgical removal of the appendix is called _____. It is performed to treat the acute condition of appendicitis (Frame 10.25).

cathartic
kah THAHR tik

10.72 An agent that stimulates strong waves of peristalsis of the colon is called a **cathartic.** Derived from the Greek word *katharos,* which means "purging, cleansing," a _____ is used to treat the symptom of constipation. An agent that causes mild waves of peristalsis is called a **laxative.**

cheilorrhaphy
kye LOR ah fee

10.73 Because the combining form of lip is *cheil/o* and the suffix *-rrhaphy* means "suturing," the procedure of suturing a lip is called _____. The constructed form of this term is cheil/o/rrhaphy.

cholecystectomy
KOH lee siss TEK toh mee

10.74 The word root for gallbladder is *cholecyst*, which literally means "bladder of gall." The surgical removal of the gallbladder is called _____. The constructed form of this term is cholecyst/ectomy.

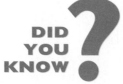 **Cholecystectomy**

Due to the prevalence of cholecystitis, cholecystectomy is the most common surgery of the abdomen performed in the United States, numbering about 500,000 each year. To reduce the invasiveness of the procedure, laparoscopic surgery using a specialized endoscope is increasing in popularity, replacing the more traditional form of cholecystectomy.

cholecystogram
KOH lee SISS toh gram

10.75 The procedure of producing an X-ray image of the gallbladder is known as **cholecystography** (KOH lee siss TOG rah fee). This constructed term is written cholecyst/o/graphy. The X-ray image of the gallbladder is called a _____.

choledocholithotomy
koh lee doh koh lih THOTT oh mee

10.76 The combining form for the common bile duct is *choledoch/o*, and the combining form for stone is *lith/o*. The surgery that involves the removal of one or more obstructive gallstones from the common bile duct is called _____. This constructed term has five word parts and is written choledoch/o/lith/o/tomy.

cleft palate

10.77 A **cleft palate** is a congenital defect in which the bones supporting the roof of the mouth, or hard palate, fail to fuse during fetal development, leaving a space between the oral cavity and nasal cavity. A _____ _____ is often accompanied by an opening in the upper lip, called a **cleft lip.**

colectomy
koh LEK toh mee

10.78 Surgical removal of a segment of the colon is called a _____. The constructed form of this term is col/ectomy.

colostomy
koh LAH stom ee

10.79 The suffix *-stomy* means "surgical creation of an opening." When this procedure is performed on the colon, it is called a _____. The artificial opening that is created serves as an artificial anus, usually following the excision of the distal part of the colon. The new opening is referred to as a **stoma** (STOE mah). Variations of colostomy are illustrated in Figure 10.16■. *Colostomy* is a constructed term, written col/o/stomy.

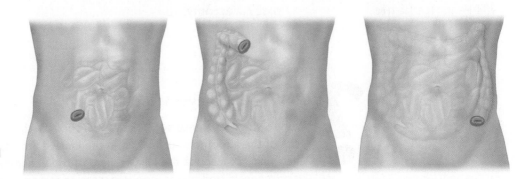

Figure 10.16 ■
Colostomy. Alternate versions of colostomy are illustrated, each of which creates one or more new openings that serve as an artificial anus.

fecal occult blood test
FEE kal * uh kult

10.80 A clinical lab test performed to detect blood in the feces is called a **fecal occult blood test,** abbreviated **FOBT.** The word *occult* means "hidden, concealed," indicating that the presence of blood is often hidden in the feces and requires a lab procedure to identify it. A positive

_____ _____ _____

_____ may indicate polyposis or colorectal cancer if hemorrhoids have been ruled out. *Fecal* is a constructed term that is written as fec/al.

gastrectomy
gas TREK toh mee

10.81 Surgical removal of part of the stomach or, in extreme cases, the entire organ, is called _____. This constructed term is written gastr/ectomy. A part of the stomach may be removed to treat peptic ulcers (Frame 10.61). The entire organ may be removed as a method to treat gastric cancer (Frame 10.42).

gastric lavage
GAS trik * lah VAHZH

10.82 A cleansing procedure in which the stomach is irrigated with a prescribed solution is known as **gastric lavage.** A _____

_____ is performed after ingestion of a toxic substance or drug overdose or to remove irritants before or after surgery. A similar irrigation procedure may be performed on the colon to remove unwanted substances and is called **colonic irrigation.** If the unwanted material is a fecal blockage in the colon or rectum, an **enema** (EN eh mah) is used instead.

gavage
gah VAHZH

10.83 The process of feeding a patient through a tube inserted into the nose that extends through the esophagus to enter the stomach is called **gavage**. The term _____ is derived from the French word, *gaver*, which means "to force-feed." The tube used in this procedure is called a **nasogastric tube.** The term *nasogastric* is constructed of four word parts and is written nas/o/gastr/ic.

GI endoscopy
en DAH sko pee

10.84 Visual examination of the GI tract that is made possible by the use of an endoscope is called _____ _____ and is shown in Figure 10.17■. The endoscope is a long, flexible tube with fiber optics, a camera, and surgical tools at one end and an eyepiece tube that can be connected to a viewing monitor at the other end. The endoscope may undergo modifications for insertion into each organ of the GI tract. Procedures using modified endoscopes to examine upper GI tract organs include **esophagoscopy** (eh SOFF ah GOSS koh pee), which examines the esophagus, **gastroscopy** (gas TROSS koh pee), which views the stomach, **esophagogastroduodenoscopy** (eh SOFF ah goh GAS troh DOO oh dehn OSS koh pee), which examines the esophagus, stomach, and duodenum, and **laparoscopy** (lap ahr OSS koh pee), which examines the abdominal cavity. Endoscopic procedures examining the lower GI tract include **colonoscopy** (kohl on OSS koh pee), which views the colon, **sigmoidoscopy** (SIG moyd OSS koh pee), which examines the sigmoid colon, and **proctoscopy** (prokt OSS koh pee), which observes the rectum. Notice that all of these are constructed terms that are formed by adding the combining form of the organ (or organs) to the suffix *-scopy*, which means "process of viewing." For example, the constructed form of esophagogastroduodenoscopy is written esophag/o/gastr/o/duoden/o/scopy.

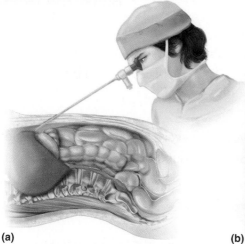

(a)

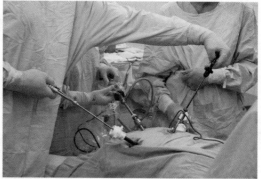

(b)

Figure 10.17 ■
GI endoscopy. (a) Similar to other forms of GI endoscopy, laparoscopy involves the insertion of a specialized endoscope through the abdominal wall by way of a small incision. (b) In this photograph of an abdominal (laparoscopic) surgery, several endoscopes have been inserted into the patient. *Source: © Cosmic/Fotolia.*

GI series

10.85 A **GI series** is a common term applied to several diagnostic techniques that provide radiographic examination of the GI tract. In most cases, the radiographic substance barium sulfate is administered to highlight the GI tract organ or organs within a series of X-ray photographs. The X-rays expose abnormalities in the organs, such as ulcers or tumors. In an **upper _____ _____ (UGI)**, a **barium swallow, barium shake,** or **barium meal** is ingested to provide X-ray images of the esophagus, stomach, and duodenum (Figure 10.18a■). An enema is the introduction of a substance into the colon or rectum to prepare for an evaluation, to evacuate the bowel, to administer drugs, or to introduce nutrients. A **barium enema (BE)** is the administration of barium sulfate into the colon or rectum for a **lower GI series (LGI)** of X-rays (Figure 10.18b■).

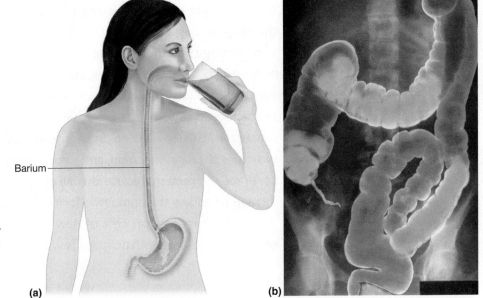

Figure 10.18 ■
GI series. (a) Upper GI series begins with a barium swallow, barium shake, or barium meal.
(b) Lower GI series begins with administration of a barium enema to provide the color-enhanced X-ray of the large intestine shown here.
Source: CNRI/Phto Researchers, Inc.

Barium

(a)   (b)

gingivectomy
JIN jih VEK toh mee

10.86 Surgical removal of diseased tissue in the gums, or gingivae, is called _____. This constructed term is written gingiv/ectomy.

glossorrhaphy
gloss OR ah fee

10.87 An injury that involves a severe bite through the tongue often requires surgery to close the wound with sutures. This surgery is called _____, which is a constructed term written gloss/o/rrhaphy.

hemorrhoidectomy
HEM oh royd EK toh mee

10.88 Surgical removal of hemorrhoids is performed during a _____. The constructed form of this term is hemorrhoid/ectomy.

ileostomy
ILL ee OSS toh mee

10.89 A surgical creation of an opening through the abdominal wall and into the ileum of the small intestine is called an **ileostomy.** The new opening is called a **stoma** (STOE mah). An _____ is performed to establish an alternative anus for the passage of feces, usually following a radical colectomy in which the entire colon is removed (Frame 10.78). *Ileostomy* is a constructed term written as ile/o/stomy.

WORDS TO WATCH OUT FOR

▶▶▶▶ **Ilium and Ileum**

Spelling medical terms correctly is very important for proper understanding and communication. Two terms, *ilium* and *ileum,* sound identical and look almost the same, but they refer to two different body parts. The *ilium* is the upper, wing-shaped bone of the pelvic girdle. The *ileum* is the third segment of the small intestine that delivers digestive waste material to the cecum of the large intestine. You might remember that *ileum* has an e if you think of the combining form for small intestine: *enter/o,* with an e.

---

laparotomy
lap ah ROTT oh mee

10.90 The Greek word for the soft abdomen is *lapara,* which serves as the origin for the combining form for abdomen, *lapar/o.* The surgical procedure that involves an incision through the abdominal wall, often from the base of the sternum to the pubic bone, is called a _____. The constructed form of this term is lapar/o/tomy.

polypectomy
pall ih PEK toh mee

10.91 Because polyps (Frame 10.63) represent benign tumors that can become inflamed and change form to become metastatic, surgical removal is sometimes necessary. The surgical removal of polyps is known as _____. The constructed form of this term is polyp/ectomy.

pyloroplasty
pye LOR oh plass tee

10.92 Surgical repair of the pylorus region of the stomach, which may include repair of the pyloric valve, is known as a _____. This constructed term is written pylor/o/plasty.

stool culture and sensitivity

10.93 If a pathogen is a suspected cause of a disease that affects the GI tract, a test may be performed called a **stool culture and sensitivity.** Abbreviated **C&S,** the _____ _____ _____ _____ includes obtaining stool (fecal) samples, using the samples to grow microorganisms in culture, and identifying the microorganisms to determine which antibiotics will effectively kill the pathogens.

vagotomy
vay GOTT oh mee

10.94 The vagus nerve is a cranial nerve that innervates much of the GI tract, providing sensory information to the brain relating to digestion and stimulating peristalsis of GI tract organs. The surgical dissection of branches of the vagus nerve may be performed in an effort to reduce gastric juice secretion as a treatment for chronic **gastric ulcers** (Frame 10.43). This procedure is called _____. The constructed form of this term is vag/o/tomy.

PRACTICE: Treatments, Procedures, and Devices of the Digestive System

The Right Match

Match the term on the left with the correct definition on the right.

_____ 1. colonoscopy

_____ 2. abdominocentesis

_____ 3. antacid

_____ 4. gastric lavage

_____ 5. cholecystography

_____ 6. cheilorrhaphy

_____ 7. ileostomy

_____ 8. stool culture and sensitivity

_____ 9. upper GI series

_____ 10. gavage

a. test that uses a stool sample to grow and identify microorganisms in a culture

b. process of feeding a patient through a tube inserted into the nose that descends into the stomach

c. also known as paracentesis

d. procedure of suturing a lip

e. procedure of producing an X-ray image of the gallbladder

f. endoscopy of the colon

g. cleansing procedure in which the stomach is irrigated with a prescribed solution

h. an agent that neutralizes stomach acid

i. surgical creation of an opening through the abdominal wall and into the ileum of the small intestine

j. a barium substance is ingested to provide X-ray images of the esophagus, stomach, and duodenum

Break the Chain

Analyze these medical terms:

    a)   Separate each term into its word parts; each word part is labeled for you (**p** = prefix, **r** = root, **cf** = combining form, and **s** = suffix).

    b)   For the Bonus Question, write the requested definition in the blank that follows.

1. a.   antiemetic   _____ / _____
                                             p   s

      b.   *Bonus Question:* What is the definition of the suffix? _____

2. a.   glossorrhaphy   _____ / ___ / _____
                                             cf   s

      b.   *Bonus Question:* What is the definition of the combining form? _____

3. a.   sigmoidoscopy   _____ / ___ / _____
                                             cf   s

      b.   *Bonus Question:* What is the definition of the combining form? _____

4. a.   hemorrhoidectomy   _____ / _____
                                         (noun)   s

      b.   *Bonus Question:* What is the definition of the second suffix? _____

5. a.   laparotomy   _____ / ___ / _____
                                             cf   s

      b.   *Bonus Question:* What is the definition of the combining form? _____

6. a.   pyloroplasty   _____ / ___ / _____
                                             cf   s

      b.   *Bonus Question:* What is the definition of the suffix? _____

7. a.   antidiarrheal   _____ / _____ / _____ / _____
                                           p   p   s   s

      b.   *Bonus Question:* What is the definition of the prefix? _____

8. a.   gingivectomy   _____ / _____
                                         r   s

      b.   *Bonus Question:* What is the definition of the word root? _____

9. a.   vagotomy   _____ / ___ / _____
                                         cf   s

      b.   *Bonus Question:* What is the definition of the suffix? _____

Abbreviations of the Digestive System

The abbreviations that are associated with the digestive system are summarized here. Study these abbreviations, and review them in the exercise that follows.

Abbreviation	Definition
BE	barium enema
C&S	stool culture and sensitivity
EGD	esophagogastroduodenoscopy
FOBT	fecal occult blood test
GERD	gastroesophageal reflux disease
GI	gastrointestinal

Abbreviation	Definition
IBD	inflammatory bowel disease
IBS	irritable bowel syndrome
LGI	lower GI series
LI	lactose intolerance
N&V	nausea and vomiting
UGI	upper GI series

PRACTICE: Abbreviations

Fill in the blanks with the abbreviation or the complete medical term.

Abbreviation

1. BE
2. _____
3. UGI
4. _____
5. N&V
6. _____
7. IBS
8. _____
9. C&S
10. _____
11. FOBT
12. _____
13. LI

Medical Term

_____

inflammatory bowel disease

_____

gastroesophageal reflux disease

_____

upper GI series

_____

lower GI series

_____

gastrointestinal

_____

esophagogastroduodenoscopy

_____

Chapter Review

Word Building

Construct medical terms from the following meanings. (Some are built from word parts, some are not.) The first question has been completed as an example.

1. indigestion   _____*dys*pepsia

2. enlargement of the liver   _____y

3. difficulty swallowing   _____phag_____

4. inflammation of the lip   _____itis

5. inflammation of the gallbladder   cholecyst_____

6. condition of gallstones   chole_____

7. inflammation of the colon   _____itis

8. cancer of the colon and rectum   _____al cancer

9. inflammation of the small intestine   enter_____

10. softening of the stomach wall   gastro_____

11. condition of diverticula   diverticul_____

12. tumor of the liver   _____oma

13. inflammation of a salivary gland   _____itis

14. surgical removal of hemorrhoids   _____ectomy

15. surgical creation of an opening into the colon   _____ostomy

16. endoscopic evaluation of the rectum   proct_____

17. endoscopic evaluation of the abdominal cavity   _____oscopy

18. surgical repair of the tongue with sutures   gloss_____

19. surgical removal of a polyp   polyp_____

▶▶▶▶ Medical Report Exercises

Maria Nguygen _____

Read the following medical report, then answer the questions that follow.

PEARSON GENERAL HOSPITAL

PGH

5500 University Avenue Metropolis, SD
Phone: (211) 594-4000 • Fax: (211) 594-4001

Medical Consultation: Internal Medicine

Date: 4/05/2011

Patient: Maria Nguygen

Patient Complaint: Diarrhea, flatus, abdominal cramping, with occasional vomiting for approximately four weeks prior to initial office visit.

History: 10-year-old female, showing normal height but underweight by 15 pounds; otherwise no prior medical concerns.

Family History: Father of Asian descent, 42 years old, with food allergies to milk products; suspect ulcer tested positive for *H. pylori* but declined treatment. Mother of Hispanic descent, 38 years old, with no reported medical concerns.

Allergies: Suspected lactose intolerance.

Physical Examination: Vital signs normal. Progressive intestinal pain with diarrhea and cramping. Colonoscopy positive for inflamed diverticula of colon; BE test reveals inflammation of ileum.

Diagnosis: Crohn disease with intussusception of ileum, confirmed with laparoscopy.

Treatment: Treat with antispasmotics and anti-inflammatories. Educate patient's parents about management of Crohn disease. Prep patient for laparoscopic correction of intusssusception in one week while monitoring patient daily.

Joanne M. Mergenthaler, M.D.
Joanne M. Mergenthaler, M.D.

Photo Source: © Alptraum/Dreamstime.com

Comprehension Questions

1. What is the diagnosis? _____

_____

_____

2. Which findings support the diagnosis? _____

_____

_____

3. What is a laparoscopy? _____

_____

_____

Case Study Questions

The following Case Study provides further discussion regarding the patient in the medical report. Fill in the blanks with the correct terms. Choose your answers from the following list of terms. (Note that some terms may be used more than once.)

barium enema	diarrhea	irritable bowel syndrome
constipation	flatus	lactose intolerance
Crohn disease	inflammatory bowel	laparoscopy

A 10-year-old female named Maria Nguygen was admitted following a history of four weeks of intermittent

watery stools, or (a) _____, accompanied with trapped gas, or (b) _____,

occasional reduced peristalsis of the large intestine, or (c) _____, abdominal pain,

and vomiting. Initial diagnosis by her personal GP was the lack of the digestive enzyme lactase, known

as (d) _____ _____, although IBS, or (e) _____

_____ _____, was ruled as another possibility. With time, symptoms of pain

and bowel irregularity increased, raising the concern that the child might be suffering from a chronic inflammation

of the ileum, or (f) _____ _____, a type of IBD, or (g) _____

_____ disease. Once admitted, thorough testing, including a lactase enzyme test, BE (also known as

(h) _____ _____), a UGI series, and an endoscopy into the abdomen, called a

(i) _____, ensued. The laparoscopy confirmed the initial diagnosis of Crohn disease. Because of the

patient's age, her parents were educated about managing this chronic disorder.

Mark Swanson

For a greater challenge, read the following medical report, then answer the critical thinking questions that follow.

PEARSON GENERAL HOSPITAL

PGH

5500 University Avenue Metropolis, NH
Phone: (211) 594-4000 • Fax: (211) 594-4001

Medical Consultation: Internal Medicine

Date: 4/05/2011

Patient: Mark Swanson

Patient Complaint: Abdominal cramping, pain, intermittent constipation and diarrhea, pain during defecation.

History: 21-year-old male with complaints of abdominal discomfort on file in pediatrics since age 8; treated with OTC medications. Weight loss of 10% during the past 2 years, suspected anorexia nervosa (not confirmed).

Family History: Father is lactose-intolerant with chronic colitis and hemorrhoidal complaints. Mother has no digestive complaints, although her father died at age 45 years of primary gastric carcinoma.

Allergies: Lactose intolerant since age of 8 years.

Physical Examination: Vital signs are normal. Colonoscopy shows three ulcerations in ileum near ileocecal valve, diverticulosis in the ascending colon, and three internal perforated hemorrhoids; stool culture and sensitivity is negative.

Diagnosis: Crohn disease with diverticulosis complicated with three internal perforated hemorrhoids.

Treatment: Right hemicolectomy with temporary ileostomy and hemorrhoidectomy, followed by dietary consult with staff nutritionist.

Arthur Broward, M.D.

Arthur Broward, M.D.

Photo Source: Diego Cervo/Shutterstock

Comprehension Questions

1. Which parent's genes had more likely contributed to the diagnosed disease? _____

   _____

   _____

2. Why do you think a temporary ileostomy is part of the treatment? _____

   _____

   _____

3. What is a hemicolectomy? _____

   _____

   _____

Case Study Questions

The following case study provides additional discussion regarding the patient in the medical report. Fill in the blanks from information provided in the chapter.

Mark Swanson, a 21-year-old male patient with a pediatric history of abdominal discomfort, had experienced

recent weight loss and was suspected of suffering from the mental disorder, (m) _____

_____. However, a gastroenterologist examined him further and initially found evidence of chronic

inflammation of the colon, called (n) _____ _____. Additional tests were ordered

that included endoscopy of the colon, or (o) _____, an abdominal CT scan, and a test for bacterial

infection called a (p) _____ and sensitivity test. The results of the test revealed ulcerations of the

ileum near its union with the (q) _____ at the ileocecal valve, a condition of numerous small pouches

in the large intestinal wall known as (r) _____, and three internal perforated hemorrhoids. These

findings indicated a diagnosis of Crohn disease. The treatment program for this chronic disease included a partial

excision of the ascending colon, called a right (s) _____; surgical creation of an artificial opening

through the abdominal wall and into the ileum to serve as a temporary anus, called an (t) _____; and

surgical removal of the hemorrhoids in a procedure called (u) _____.

MEDICAL TERMINOLOGY INTERACTIVE

Medical Terminology Interactive is a premium online homework management system that includes a host of features to help you study. Registered users will find:

- Fun games and activities built within a virtual hospital
- Powerful tools that track and analyze your results—allowing you to create a personalized learning experience
- Videos, flashcards, and audio pronunciations to help enrich your progress
- Streaming video lesson presentations and self-paced learning modules

www.pearsonhighered.com/mti

11

The Urinary System

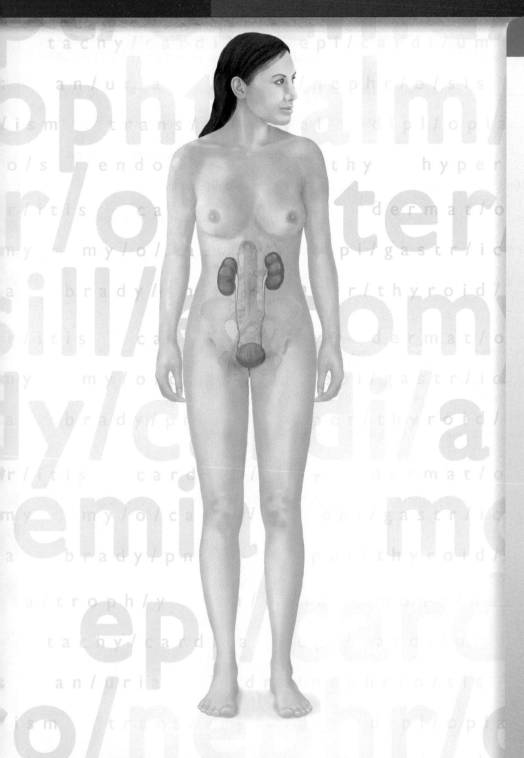

After completing this chapter, you will be able to:

1 Define and spell the word parts used to create terms for the urinary system.

2 Break down and define common medical terms used for symptoms, diseases, disorders, procedures, treatments, and devices associated with the urinary system.

3 Build medical terms from the word parts associated with the urinary system.

4 Pronounce and spell common medical terms associated with the urinary system.

Anatomy and Physiology Terms ▶▶▶▶▶

The following table provides the combining forms that specifically apply to the anatomy and physiology of the urinary system. Note that the combining forms are colored red to help you identify them when you see them again later in the chapter.

Combining Form	Definition	Combining Form	Definition
albumin/o	albumin (a protein)	nephr/o	kidney
blast/o	germ, bud, developing cell	pyel/o	renal pelvis
glomerul/o	little ball, glomerulus	ren/o	kidney
gluc/o	sweet, sugar	ureter/o	ureter
glyc/o, glycos/o	sweet, sugar	urethr/o	urethra
meat/o	opening, passage	ur/o, urin/o	urine

urinary
YOU rih nair ee

kidneys

11.1 The _____ system functions as the sanitation engineer of the body, maintaining the purity and health of the body's fluids by removing unwanted waste materials and recycling other materials. The kidneys are its most important organs. They filter gallons of fluids from the bloodstream every day, removing metabolic wastes, toxins, excess ions, and water that leave the body as urine, while returning needed materials back into the blood. Because waste removal is essential for your survival, the kidneys are vital organs; a loss of both _____ requires medical intervention to sustain life. Other organs of the urinary system transport urine or store it before it can be released to the exterior of the body. They are the paired ureters, the urinary bladder, and the urethra.

urine

11.2 You have just learned that the primary function of the kidneys is the removal of metabolic wastes, toxins, excess ions, and water from the bloodstream. This function is performed by the formation of urine as a watery waste. _____ is formed by three processes occurring in the kidneys: filtration of the blood to produce a filtrate, reabsorption of excess water, ions, and nutrients in the filtrate to return them to the bloodstream, and secretion of excess ions as waste into the filtrate. In addition to forming urine, the kidneys also perform other vital functions:

- Regulation of blood pressure

- Regulation of pH within body fluids

- Regulation of water and salt concentrations

- Regulation of red blood cell production

11.3 Use the anatomy terms that appear in the left column to fill in the corresponding blanks in Figures 11.1■ through 11.3■.

1. **kidney**
2. **renal artery and vein**
3. **ureter**
4. **bladder**
5. **urethra**

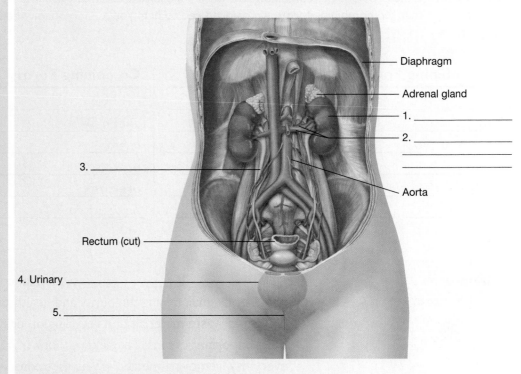

Diaphragm

Adrenal gland

1. _____

2. _____

_____

_____

3. _____

Aorta

Rectum (cut) _____

4. Urinary _____

5. _____

Figure 11.1 ■
Organs of the urinary system. This illustration is an anterior view of a female with the abdominal wall and digestive organs removed.

6. **renal**
7. **pelvis**
8. **ureter**

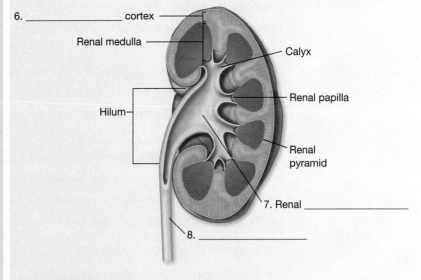

6. _____ cortex

Renal medulla

Calyx

Renal papilla

Hilum

Renal pyramid

7. Renal _____

8. _____

Figure 11.2 ■
The kidney. Illustration of a sectioned kidney, which reveals its internal features.

9. **distal convoluted**
10. **duct**
11. **glomerulus**

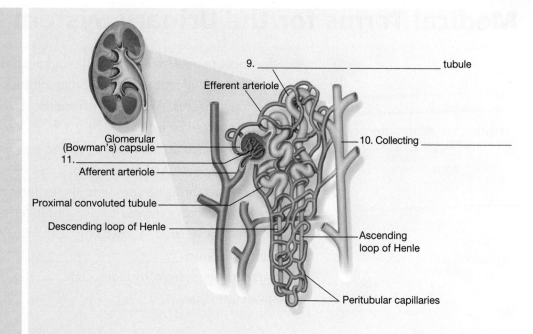

9. _____ _____ tubule

Efferent arteriole

Glomerular
(Bowman's) capsule

11. _____

Afferent arteriole

Proximal convoluted tubule

Descending loop of Henle

10. Collecting _____

Ascending
loop of Henle

Peritubular capillaries

Figure 11.3 ■
The nephron. The nephron is the basic subunit of each kidney.

Medical Terms for the Urinary System ▶▶▶▶▶

mucous membrane

infections

11.4 For most people, the major pathological challenge to the health of the urinary system is infection, due to communication to the exterior by way of the urinary meatus. Although the urethra, urinary bladder, and ureters are each protected by a _____ _____, bacteria and viruses are sometimes able to gain entry into the internal organs through the meatus. Once established, they are capable of spreading through the urinary tract, bringing disease to the kidneys and beyond. Also, the close location of the urinary meatus to the anus in females enables some bacterial populations that normally form the intestinal flora to infect the urinary tract. In addition to _____, other sources of disease may afflict the urinary system, including tumors, stones, inherited disorders, and cardiovascular disease.

urine

11.5 Because _____ originates from the bloodstream and the urinary system releases urine on a regular basis, urine testing provides a convenient means for testing general health. Many diseases can be diagnosed from a urine sample that contains abnormal contents, such as blood cells, bacteria, albumin (a protein normally found in blood), glucose, and high levels of creatinine (a protein product of metabolism).

urology

nephrology
neh FROL oh jee

11.6 The clinical treatment of urinary disease is a medical discipline known as **urology** (yoo RAHL oh jee). In most hospitals and clinics, the unit specializing in the treatment of urinary diseases is simply called _____. A physician specializing in this field of medicine is called a **urologist.** The field that specializes in the treatment of kidney disease is _____. A physician specializing in this field is a **nephrologist.**

11.7 In the following sections, you will study the prefixes, combining forms, and suffixes that combine to build the medical terms of the urinary system.

Signs and Symptoms of the Urinary System

Here are the word parts that specifically apply to the signs and symptoms of the urinary system that are covered in the following section. Note that the word parts are color-coded to help you identify them: prefixes are green, combining forms are red, and suffixes are blue.

Prefix	Definition
an-	without, absence of
dia-	through
dys-	bad, abnormal, painful, difficult
poly-	excessive, over, many

Combining Form	Definition
albumin/o	albumin (a protein)
azot/o	urea, nitrogen
bacteri/o	bacteria
glycos/o	sweet, sugar
hem/o, hemat/o	blood
ket/o, keton/o	ketone
noct/o	night
olig/o	few in number
protein/o	protein
py/o	pus

Suffix	Definition
-emia	condition of blood
-urea	urine
-uresis	urination
-uria	pertaining to urine, urination

KEY TERMS A–Z

albuminuria
AL byoo men YOO ree ah

11.8 A **urinalysis** (Frame 11.82) is a clinical procedure that examines the composition of urine using a variety of tests, including microscopy. Diseases of the urinary system and other parts of the body may be diagnosed with this valuable clinical tool. For example, albumin is a protein normally present in the bloodstream. If it appears in the urine, it is a physical sign of abnormal renal filtration. The condition is called _____. This constructed term contains two word parts and is written albumin/uria.

anuresis
an yoo REE siss

anuria
an YOO ree ah

11.9 The inability to pass urine is a sign of a blockage of the urinary tract or kidney failure. It is called _____, which is a constructed term written as an/uresis. It literally means "without urination." Alternatively, the suffix -uria may be substituted to form the term _____ and is written an/uria. It means "pertaining to without urine." Clinically, anuria is the production of less than 100 mL of urine per day.

azotemia
az oh TEE mee ah

11.10 The sign of abnormally high levels of urea and other nitrogen-containing compounds in the blood is called **azotemia.** _____ is a constructed term and is written azot/emia.

bacteriuria
bak ter ee YOO ree ah
bacteri/uria

11.11 The abnormal presence of bacteria in the urine is a sign of a urinary tract infection and is called _____. This constructed term includes two word parts, which are revealed when the term is written as _____/_____.

diuresis
DYE yoo REE siss

11.12 The excessive discharge of urine is a sign of the endocrine disorders known as diabetes insipidus and diabetes mellitus. This is known as **diuresis,** which literally means "urination through." The constructed form of _____ is written di/uresis. Note that the *a* in the prefix *dia-* is not used in order to make the term easier to pronounce. It may also be called **polyuria** (Frame 11.19).

dysuria
diss YOO ree ah

11.13 Recall that the prefix *dys-* means "bad, abnormal, painful, or difficult." When *dys-* is combined with the suffix for "pertaining to urine, urination," the resulting term refers to difficulty or pain experienced during urination. It is a symptom of a urinary tract disease often caused by a bacterial infection. The symptom is called _____. It is a constructed term written dys/uria.

glycosuria
glye kohs YOO ree ah

11.14 The combining form *glycos/o* means "sweet, sugar." The abnormal presence of glucose (sugar) in the urine is a sign of an endocrine disease, such as diabetes mellitus, or a kidney disorder, or perhaps both. The sign is called _____, which is a constructed term written glycos/uria.

hematuria
HEE mah TOO ree ah

11.15 The abnormal presence of blood in the urine is a sign of urinary disease. It is called _____, which means "pertaining to bloody urine or urination" (Figure 11.4■). The constructed form of this term is written hemat/uria.

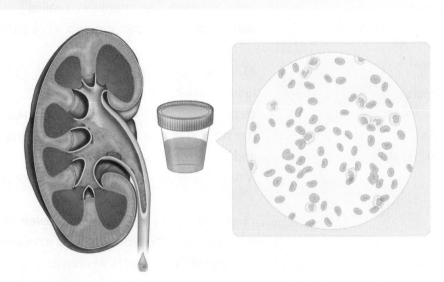

Figure 11.4 ■
Hematuria. An analysis of urine is performed to evaluate kidney function. In this illustration, the beaker contains urine that is red, indicating the sign of blood within the urine, which is confirmed by microscopic analysis.

ketonuria
kee tohn YOO ree ah

11.16 The abnormal presence of ketone bodies in the urine is called **ketonuria.** The constructed form of _____ uses the combining form for ketone bodies (*keton/o*) and is written keton/uria. It is a common sign of a metabolic disorder, a high-protein/low-carbohydrate diet, starvation, or diabetes mellitus.

WORDS TO WATCH OUT FOR

▶▶▶▶▶ **Terms with No Combining Vowels**

Most of the terms related to the signs and symptoms of the urinary system contain no combining vowel. For example, terms such as *ketonuria* and *hematuria* only contain a word root and suffix. This is because the suffixes in this section (*-emia, -urea, -uresis, -uria*) all begin with a vowel, so no combining vowel is needed to make the terms easier to pronounce.

nocturia nok TOO ree ah	**11.17** The need to urinate frequently at night is a possible symptom of diabetes mellitus or benign prostate hyperplasia (BPH). It is called **nocturia.** As a constructed term, _____ includes two word parts and is written noct/uria.
oliguria all ig YOO ree ah	**11.18** Reduced urination becomes a clinical problem when the volume of urine declines to less than 500 mL within a 24-hour period. It is known as **oliguria** and is a possible sign of a kidney disorder. _____ may also be a sign of congestive heart failure, dehydration, or a blockage in the urinary tract. This constructed term is written olig/uria.
polyuria pall ee YOO ree ah	**11.19** Chronic excessive urination is a common sign of an endocrine disease, usually diabetes insipidus or diabetes mellitus. The sign is called _____, which is a constructed term written poly/uria. It is also known as diuresis (Frame 11.12).
proteinuria proh tee NYOO ree ah	**11.20** In Frame 11.8 you learned that albuminuria is the presence of the protein albumin in the urine. The presence of any protein in the urine is called _____. This constructed term is written protein/uria.
pyuria pye YOO re ah	**11.21** Pus is a mixture of white blood cells, bacteria, and cell debris that forms during an infection. Its appearance in the urine indicates a urinary tract infection. The presence of pus in urine is called _____, which is a constructed term written py/uria. The combining form that means "pus" is *py/o.*

PRACTICE: Signs and Symptoms of the Urinary System

The Right Match

Match the term on the left with the correct definition on the right.

_____ 1. albuminuria
_____ 2. bacteriuria
_____ 3. diuresis
_____ 4. glycosuria
_____ 5. hematuria
_____ 6. ketonuria
_____ 7. nocturia
_____ 8. oliguria
_____ 9. polyuria

a. urination at night
b. presence of blood in the urine
c. presence of bacteria in the urine
d. chronic excessive urination
e. ketone bodies in the urine
f. presence of sugar in the urine
g. presence of albumin in the urine
h. reduced urination
i. literally "urination through"

Break the Chain

Analyze these medical terms:

   a) Separate each term into its word parts; each word part is labeled for you (**p** = prefix, **r** = root, **cf** = combining form, and **s** = suffix).

   b) For the Bonus Question, write the requested definition in the blank that follows.

The first set has been completed as an example.

1. a) proteinuria   _protein/uria_
                                            r   s

   b) *Bonus Question:* What is the definition of the suffix? _pertaining to urine or urination_

2. a) azotemia   _____/_____
                                             r   s

   b) *Bonus Question:* What is the definition of the word root? _____

3. a) dysuria   _____/_____
                                             p   s

   b) *Bonus Question:* What is the definition of the suffix? _____

4. a) anuresis   _____/_____
                                             p   s

   b) *Bonus Question:* What is the definition of the prefix? _____

5. a) pyuria   _____/_____
                                             r   s

   b) *Bonus Question:* What is the definition of the word root? _____

Diseases and Disorders of the Urinary System

Review some of the word parts that specifically apply to the diseases and disorders of the urinary system that are covered in the following section. Note that the word parts are color-coded to help you identify them: prefixes are green, combining forms are red, and suffixes are blue.

Prefix	Definition
an-	without, absence of
dia-	through
dys-	bad, abnormal, painful, difficult
en-	within, upon, on, over
epi-	upon, over, above, on top
hypo-	deficient, abnormally low, below
poly-	excessive, over, many

Combining Form	Definition
albumin/o	albumin (a protein)
azot/o	urea, nitrogen
bacteri/o	bacteria
blast/o	germ, bud, developing cell
cyst/o	bladder, sac
glomerul/o	little ball, glomerulus
hemat/o	blood
hydr/o	water
ket/o, keton/o	ketone
lith/o	stone
nephr/o	kidney
olig/o	few in number
py/o	pus
pyel/o	renal pelvis
ren/o	kidney
spadias/o	rip, tear
sten/o	narrow
ur/o	urine
ureter/o	ureter
urethr/o	urethra

Suffix	Definition
-al	pertaining to
-cele	hernia, swelling, protrusion
-emia	condition of blood
-ia	condition of
-iasis	condition of
-ic	pertaining to
-itis	inflammation
-megaly	abnormally large
-oma	tumor
-osis	condition of
-pathy	disease
-ptosis	drooping
-sis	state of
-urea	urine
-uresis	urination

KEY TERMS A–Z

cystitis
siss TYE tiss

11.22 The combining form for bladder is cyst/o. An inflammation of the urinary bladder is called _____. This constructed term is written cyst/itis. It is usually caused by a bacterial infection that travels up the urethra. An infection of the urinary bladder and the urethra is called **urethrocystitis** (yoo REE throh siss TYE tiss), which is written urethr/o/cyst/itis.

cystocele
SISS toh seel

11.23 A herniation of the urinary bladder is called a **cystocele.** In females, the protrusion pushes into the adjacent vagina. The term _____ is a constructed term with three word parts, written cyst/o/cele.

cystolith
SISS toh lith

11.24 A _____ is a stone, or calculus, in the urinary bladder. If it is too large to pass through the urethra, medical intervention is required to eliminate it. This constructed term is written cyst/o/lith.

enuresis
ehn yoo REE siss

11.25 An involuntary release of urine, which usually occurs due to a lack of bladder control among children or the elderly, is known as **enuresis.** When this occurs during sleep, it is known as **nocturnal** _____, or bedwetting. This constructed term is written en/uresis.

epispadias
EP ih SPAY dee ass

11.26 A congenital defect resulting in the abnormal positioning of the urinary meatus is known as **epispadias** (Figure 11.5■). In males, the meatus opens on the dorsal (upper) surface of the penis, and in females the meatus opens dorsal to the clitoris. _____ is a constructed term written epi/spadias, which literally means "a rip or tear upon."

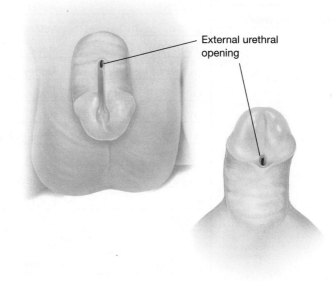

External urethral opening

Figure 11.5 ■
Epispadias and hypospadias. In the male, epispadias is an abnormally placed opening of the urethra on the dorsal side of the penis (left), and in hypospadias, the opening is on the underside (ventral) of the penis (right).

glomerulonephritis
gloh MAIR yoo loh neh FRYE tiss

11.27 A glomerulus is a ball of specialized capillaries within a kidney nephron (the term *glomerulus* means "little ball"). Any disease of the glomeruli is called a **glomerulonephropathy** (gloh MAIR yoo loh neh FROH path ee), which is a constructed term written glomerul/o/nephr/o/pathy. An example is inflammation of the glomeruli, which is known as _____. It is either an autoimmune disease resulting from an attack on glomeruli by the body's own white blood cells, or it may be caused by a bacterial infection. The constructed term is written glomerul/o/nephr/itis.

11.28 The production of urine by the kidneys is a physiological process that is continual throughout your lifetime. If the exit of urine out of the kidneys becomes blocked by an obstruction in a ureter, the urine will back up to cause distension of the renal pelvis. This condition is known as **hydronephrosis** and is illustrated in Figure 11.6■. The term _____ is written hydr/o/nephr/osis. Recall that *hydr/o* means "water," which refers to the fluid (urine) blockage that occurs in this condition.

hydronephrosis
HIGH droh neh FROH siss

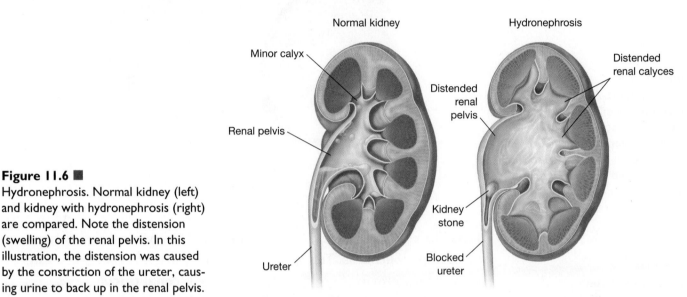

Normal kidney   Hydronephrosis

Minor calyx

Distended renal calyces

Distended renal pelvis

Renal pelvis

Kidney stone

Ureter

Blocked ureter

Figure 11.6 ■
Hydronephrosis. Normal kidney (left) and kidney with hydronephrosis (right) are compared. Note the distension (swelling) of the renal pelvis. In this illustration, the distension was caused by the constriction of the ureter, causing urine to back up in the renal pelvis.

11.29 You learned in Frame 11.26 that epispadias is a congenital defect in which the urinary meatus has shifted dorsally. In **hypospadias,** the change in location of the urinary meatus is ventral (see Figure 11.5). In males, it opens on the underside of the penis, and in females the meatus is within the vagina. _____ is a constructed term written hypo/spadias, which literally means "a rip or tear below."

hypospadias
HIGH poh SPAY dee ass

11.30 The inability to control urination is called **urinary** _____. In **stress incontinence,** an involuntary discharge of urine occurs during a cough, sneeze, or strained movement.

incontinence
in KON tih nens

11.31 One word root for kidney is *nephr*, and it is found in many terms describing a kidney disease or procedure. For example, inflammation of a kidney is known as **nephritis.** Its usual cause is a bacterial infection, and if left untreated it can lead to the more serious condition of glomerulonephritis (Frame 11.27). _____ is a constructed term written nephr/itis.

nephritis
neh FRYE tiss

nephroblastoma
NEFF roh blass TOH mah

11.32 A **nephroblastoma** is a tumor originating from kidney tissue that includes developing embryonic cells (Figure 11.7■). It is also called **Wilms' tumor** after the 19th-century German physician who published the first description of the disease. _____ is a constructed term written nephr/o/blast/oma.

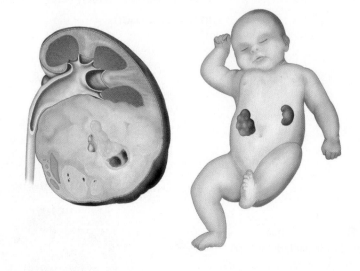

Figure 11.7 ■
Nephroblastoma. A sectioned kidney reveals the presence of a very large tumor, which arose from fetal cells during development. A newborn with nephroblastoma is illustrated to show the location and relative size of the tumor.

nephrolithiasis
NEFF roh lith EYE ah siss

11.33 The presence of one or more stones, or calculi, within a kidney is called **nephrolithiasis.** This constructed term is written nephr/o/lith/iasis. An alternate term for _____ is **renal calculi** (REE nal * KAL kyoo lye) and is further described in Figure 11.8■.

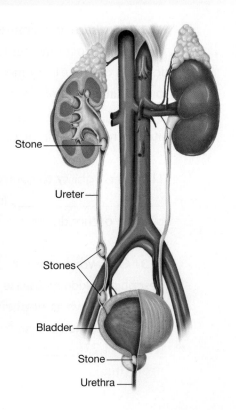

Stone

Ureter

Stones

Bladder

Stone

Urethra

Figure 11.8 ■
Nephrolithiasis. Stones, or calculi, may form in several areas within the urinary tract. When they form in the kidney, they usually arise within the renal pelvis to form the condition nephrolithiasis. Kidney stones may dislocate to form obstructions in the ureter, urinary bladder, or urethra, usually at their junctions.

nephroma
neff ROH mah

11.34 A general term for a tumor arising from kidney tissue is _____. This constructed term is written nephr/oma.

nephromegaly
neff roh MEG ah lee

11.35 The suffix -*megaly* means "abnormally large." An abnormal enlargement of one or both kidneys is called _____. The word parts of this term can be shown as nephr/o/megaly.

nephroptosis
neff ropp TOH siss

11.36 The condition of a downward displacement ("drooping") of a kidney is known as **nephroptosis.** The constructed form of this term is nephr/o/ptosis. It occurs when the kidney is no longer held in its proper position against the posterior abdominal wall. _____ is commonly called **floating kidney.**

polycystic
PALL ee SISS tik

11.37 A kidney condition characterized by the presence of numerous cysts (fluid-filled capsules) occupying much of the kidney tissue is called **polycystic kidney disease.** The cysts replace normal tissue, resulting in a loss of kidney function (Figure 11.9■). The term _____ is a constructed term composed of three word parts, poly/cyst/ic, and literally means "pertaining to many bladders."

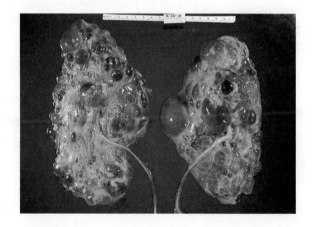

Figure 11.9 ■
Polycystic kidney disease. Notice the presence of numerous fluid-filled sacs, or cysts, in these kidneys, which were removed from a patient who died of renal failure.
Source: Courtesy of Dr. Edwin P. Ewing, Centers for Disease Control, Public Health Image Library, Atlanta, GA.

pyelitis
PYE eh LYE tiss

11.38 The combining form for renal pelvis is pyel/o. Inflammation of the renal pelvis is called _____. It is usually caused by a bacterial infection. The constructed form of this term is pyel/itis.

pyelonephritis
PYE eh loh neh FRYE tiss

11.39 An inflammatory condition of the renal pelvis and nephrons is called **pyelonephritis.** The constructed form of _____ is written pyel/o/nephr/itis.

strictures
STRIK cherz

11.40 A condition of abnormal narrowing is known as a **stricture.** Examples of urinary _____ include **ureteral stricture,** in which the ureter is narrowed; **urethral stricture,** in which the urethra is narrowed; and **ureterovesical stricture,** in which the junction of the ureter and bladder is narrowed. Because the medical term **stenosis** also refers to an abnormal narrowing, it may be used as an alternative term to _stricture_ in each of these terms. An example term is **ureterostenosis** (yoo REE ter oh steh NOH siss), which is a ureteral stricture, or narrowing. The constructed form of this term is ureter/o/sten/osis.

uremia
yoo REE mee ah

11.41 In the condition **uremia,** an excess of urea and other nitrogenous wastes are present in the blood. The constructed form of this term is ur/emia. _____ is caused by failure of the kidneys to remove urea and is associated with renal insufficiency or renal failure (Frame 11.46).

WORDS
TO
WATCH
OUT
FOR

▶▶▶▶▶ **Hematuria versus Uremia**

Here is a pair of opposites. The term _hematuria_ is a sign of any condition in which urine contains blood or red blood cells. On the other hand, the term _uremia_ refers to a condition in which the blood contains urine (actually, an excess of urea and other nitrogenous wastes). Uremia is often the result of advanced kidney disease and is also known as _azotemia._

---

ureteritis
yoo REE ter EYE tiss

11.42 The ureters are the paired narrow tubes that transport urine from the kidneys to the urinary bladder. Inflammation of a ureter is called _____ and is often the result of a bacterial infection. This constructed term is written ureter/itis.

ureterocele
yoo REE ter oh seel

11.43 A herniated ureter is called a **ureterocele.** The constructed form of _____ is ureter/o/cele.

ureterolithiasis
yoo REE ter oh lith EYE ah siss

11.44 The presence of one or more stones, or calculi, within a ureter is called **ureterolithiasis.** The constructed form of _____ includes a combining form _and_ a word root and is written ureter/o/lith/iasis.

urinary retention
YOO rih nair ee * ree TEN shun

11.45 The abnormal accumulation of urine within the urinary bladder is called **urinary retention.** The condition of _____ _____ results from an inability to void, or urinate.

urinary suppression
 YOO rih nair ee * suh PREH shun

11.46 An acute stoppage of urine formation by the kidneys is known as **urinary suppression.** The condition of _____ _____ is a consequence of **acute renal failure,** in which kidney function ceases.

urinary tract infection
 YOO rih nair ee * trakt * in FEK shun

11.47 Commonly called by its abbreviation of **UTI,** a _____ _____ _____ is an infection of urinary organs, usually the urethra and urinary bladder. The symptoms are illustrated in Figure 11.10■ and include fever, dysuria (Frame 11.13), and lumbar or abdominal pain. It is more common in females and is usually caused by *Staphylococci* or *E. coli* bacteria.

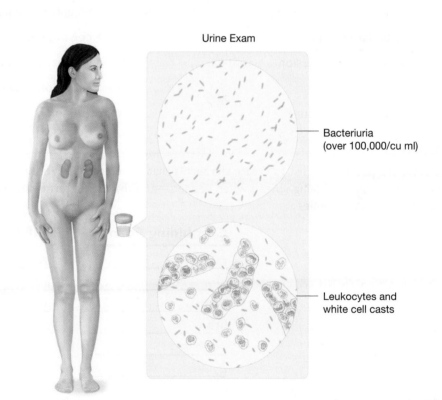

Urine Exam

Bacteriuria
(over 100,000/cu ml)

Leukocytes and
white cell casts

Figure 11.10 ■
Urinary tract infection. A UTI is characterized by fever, lumbar or abdominal pain, and pain or burning during urination. A diagnosis may be confirmed in a urine exam that reveals the presence of bacteria (bacteriuria) and white blood cells (pyuria).

PRACTICE: Diseases and Disorders of the Urinary System

The Right Match

Match the term on the left with the correct definition on the right.

_____ 1. cystocele   a.   condition of excess urea in the blood

_____ 2. cystolith   b.   protrusion of the urinary bladder

_____ 3. nephritis   c.   stone(s) in the urinary bladder

_____ 4. nephromegaly   d.   urinary meatus opens on the penis underside

_____ 5. uremia   e.   inflammation of a kidney

_____ 6. hypospadias   f.   enlargement of a kidney

_____ 7. polycystic kidney disease   g.   a condition of stones in the kidneys

_____ 8. renal calculi   h.   an acute stoppage of urine formation

_____ 9. urinary incontinence   i.   involuntary discharge of urine

_____ 10. urinary retention   j.   a condition of many cysts within a kidney

_____ 11. urinary suppression   k.   abnormal accumulation of urine in the bladder

_____ 12. stricture   l.   a condition in which kidney function ceases

_____ 13. acute renal failure   m.   condition of abnormal narrowing

Linkup

Link the word parts in the list to create the terms that match the definitions. You may use word parts more than once. Remember to add combining vowels when needed—and that some terms do not use any combining vowel. The first one is completed as an example.

Combining Form	Suffix
cyst/o	-ia
glomerul/o	-itis
hydr/o	-oma
lith/o	-osis
nephr/o	
pyel/o	

Definition		Term
1.	inflammation of the urinary bladder	*cystitis*
2.	inflammation of the glomeruli	_____
3.	inflammation of the renal pelvis and the nephrons	_____
4.	presence of one or more stones within a kidney	_____
5.	condition of blockage of urine (water) in the kidney	_____
6.	tumor that arises from kidney tissue	_____
7.	inflammation of the renal pelvis	_____

Treatments, Procedures, and Devices of the Urinary System

Review some of the word parts that specifically apply to the treatments, procedures, and devices of the urinary system that are covered in the following section. Note that the word parts are color-coded to help you identify them: prefixes are green, combining forms are red, and suffixes are blue.

Prefix	Definition
a-	without, absence of
dia-	through

Combining Form	Definition
cyst/o	bladder, sac
hemat/o, hem/o	blood
lith/o	stone
meat/o	opening, passage
nephr/o	kidney
peritone/o	to stretch over, peritoneum
pyel/o	renal pelvis
ren/o	kidney
son/o	sound
tom/o	to cut
ureter/o	ureter
urethr/o	urethra
ur/o, urin/o	urine
vesic/o	bladder

Suffix	Definition
-al	pertaining to
-ectomy	surgical excision, removal
-gram	a record or image
-graphy	recording process
-logy	study or science of
-lysis	loosen, dissolve
-meter	measure, measuring instrument
-pexy	surgical fixation, suspension
-plasty	surgical repair
-rrhaphy	suturing
-scopy	process of viewing
-stomy	surgical creation of an opening
-tomy	incision, to cut
-tripsy	surgical crushing

KEY TERMS A–Z

blood urea nitrogen
blud * YOO ree ah

11.48 A clinical lab test that measures urea concentration in a sample of blood as an indicator of kidney function is **blood urea nitrogen.** Abbreviated **BUN,** elevated values of _____ _____ _____ indicate kidney disease.

creatinine
kree ATT ih neen

11.49 The protein **creatinine** is a normal component of urine and is a by-product of muscle metabolism. It may be measured in a urine sample. Elevated levels of _____ indicate a problem during kidney filtration, suggesting kidney disease.

cystectomy
siss TEK toh mee

11.50 Because the combining form cyst/o means "bladder, sac" and the suffix -ectomy means "surgical excision, removal," the surgical removal of the urinary bladder is called _____. This constructed term is written cyst/ectomy.

cystogram
SISS toh gram

11.51 An X-ray procedure producing an image of the urinary bladder with injection of a contrast medium or dye is called **cystography** (siss TOG rah fee). This constructed term is written cyst/o/graphy. The X-ray image is called a _____. If the procedure includes the ureters, it is called a **cystoureterography** (SISS toh yoo REE ter OG rah fee), and the image obtained is a **cystoureterogram** (SISS toh yoo REE ter oh gram). The constructed form of the term *cystoureterography* is cyst/o/ureter/o/graphy. If the procedure includes the urethra, it is a **cystourethrography** (SISS toh yoo reeth ROG rah fee), and the image is a **cystourethrogram.** The constructed form of the term is written cyst/o/urethr/o/gram. In a **voiding** _____ (**VCUG**), X-rays are taken before, during, and after urination to observe bladder function.

cystourethrogram
SISS toh you REE throh gram

WORDS TO WATCH OUT FOR ▶▶▶▶▶ *-graphy* **or** *-gram*?

Remember that the suffix *-graphy* means "a recording process," whereas the suffix *-gram* means "a record or image." In each of these procedures, switching the suffix from *-graphy* to *-gram* creates the term that refers to the *record* that is a result of the *recording process*.

---

cystolithotomy
siss toh lith OTT oh mee
cyst/o/lith/o/tomy

11.52 A procedure in which an incision is made through the urinary bladder wall to remove a stone is called _____. The constructed form of this term includes five word parts and is written _____/__/_____/__/_____.

cystoplasty
SISS toh plass tee

11.53 Surgical repair of the urinary bladder is a procedure called _____. The constructed form of this term is cyst/o/plasty, which reveals three word parts.

cystorrhaphy
sist OR ah fee

11.54 Suturing the urinary bladder wall is a procedure called _____. The constructed form of the term is cyst/o/rrhaphy, which literally means "suturing bladder."

cystoscopy
siss TOSS koh pee

11.55 A procedure using a modified endoscope to view the interior of the urinary bladder is known as _____. The instrument is inserted through the urinary meatus and urethra to enter the bladder cavity (Figure 11.11■). The constructed form of this term is cyst/o/scopy. The **cystoscope** may also be used as a surgical instrument.

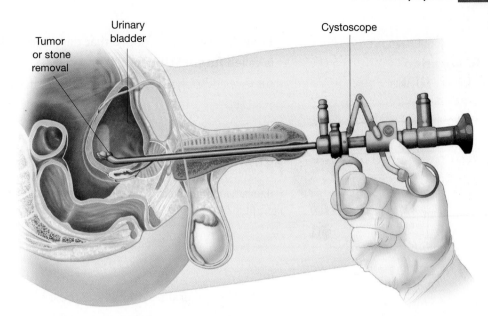

Tumor
or stone
removal

Urinary
bladder

Cystoscope

Figure 11.11 ■
Cystoscopy. In this procedure, a specialized endoscope with a rigid tube, known as a cystoscope, is used to view the internal environment of the urinary bladder. As shown, the cystoscope may be outfitted to include surgical devices to remove tumors or stones.

cystostomy

siss TOSS toh mee

11.56 Recall that the suffix -*stomy* means "surgical creation of an opening." The surgical creation of an artificial opening into the urinary bladder is a procedure called _____. It is performed to provide an alternate exit pathway for urine if the normal passageway through the urethra is blocked or the urethra is surgically removed (Figure 11.12■). *Cystostomy* is a constructed term written cyst/o/stomy.

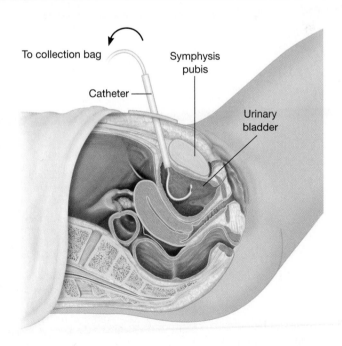

To collection bag

Catheter

Symphysis
pubis

Urinary
bladder

Figure 11.12 ■
Cystostomy. An artificial opening is made through the urinary bladder wall during this procedure. As the illustration suggests, it is often performed to enable a patient to bypass obstructions for voiding.

cystotomy

siss TOTT oh mee

11.57 The suffix -*tomy* means "incision" or "to cut." Therefore, the term _____ refers to an incision through the urinary bladder wall. It is also called **vesicotomy** (VESS ih KOTT oh mee) because both *cyst* and *vesic* are word roots meaning "bladder."

fulguration
full guh RAY shun

11.58 A surgical procedure that destroys living tissue with an electric current is called **fulguration**. _____ is commonly used to remove tumors and polyps from the interior wall of the urinary bladder.

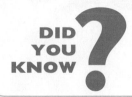

DID YOU KNOW?

▶▶▶▶▶ **Fulguration**

Fulguration is derived from the Latin word *fulguratio,* which means "flash of lightning."

hemodialysis
HEE moh dye AL ih siss

11.59 The general term dia/lysis means "dissolving through" and refers to the movement of substances across a permeable membrane during the process of filtration. Also, *hem/o* is the combining form that means "blood." Combining these word parts forms the term _____, which is a procedure that pushes a patient's blood through permeable membranes within an instrument (Figure 11.13■). It is performed to artificially remove nitrogenous wastes and excess ions that accumulate during normal body metabolism, temporarily replacing the function of kidney filtration for patients with kidney disease or kidney failure. *Hemodialysis* is a constructed term, written hem/o/dia/lysis.

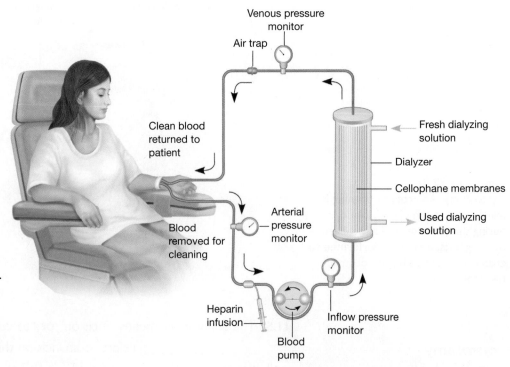

Figure 11.13 ■
Hemodialysis. The process of hemodialysis replaces the kidney function of blood filtration by forcing blood from the patient through cellophane membranes, as shown in this schematic.

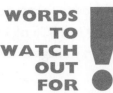

A Misplaced Prefix?

Most prefixes appear in the very beginning of a term, but in the term *hemodialysis*, note that the prefix (*dia-*) appears as the second word part (just after the combining form *hem/o*).

lithotripsy
LITH oh trip see

11.60 The suffix *-tripsy* means "surgical crushing." A surgical technique that applies concentrated sound waves to pulverize or dissolve stones into smaller pieces that may then pass with urine through the urethra is called _____. This constructed term is written lith/o/tripsy. In the procedure **extracorporeal shock wave lithotripsy (ESWL)**, ultrasonic energy from a source outside of the body is used on stones that are too large to pass through the urethra. It is a noninvasive technique and therefore avoids the risks of surgery. Both procedures are shown in Figure 11.14■.

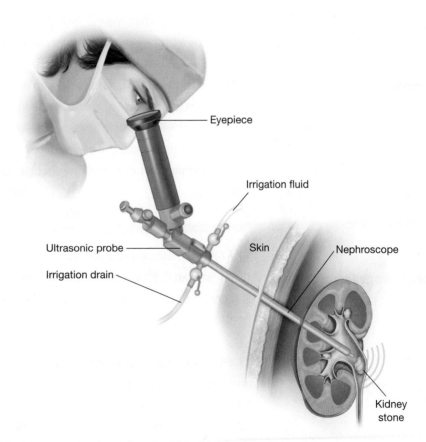

Figure 11.14 ■
Lithotripsy. The direction of a sound pulse crushes the stones into smaller fragments that can be passed with urine.

nephrectomy
neh FREK toh mee

11.61 Recall that one of the combining forms for kidney is *nephr/o*. A surgical procedure that removes a kidney is called _____. This constructed term is written nephr/ectomy.

nephrogram
NEFF roh gram

11.62 An X-ray technique producing an image of a kidney after injection of a contrast medium or dye is called **nephrography** (neh FROG rah fee). It is a constructed term written nephr/o/graphy. The X-ray image of the kidney obtained in this procedure is called a _____.

nephrology
neff ROL oh jee

11.63 The medical field that studies and treats disorders associated with the kidneys is called _____. This constructed term is written nephr/o/logy. A physician specializing in this field is a **nephrologist** (neff ROL oh jist).

nephrolysis
neh FRALL ih siss

11.64 The suffix -lysis means "loosen, dissolve." Combining it with the combining form for kidney, nephr/o, forms the constructed term _____. It is a surgical procedure during which abnormal adhesions are removed from a kidney, loosening the organ. This constructed term is written nephr/o/lysis.

nephropexy
NEFF roh pek see

11.65 The suffix that means "surgical fixation, suspension" is -pexy. Surgical fixation of a kidney is sometimes necessary if the kidney is abnormally loose within the abdominal cavity, such as in the condition nephroptosis or floating kidney (Frame 11.36). The procedure is called _____, and the constructed form of this term is written nephr/o/pexy.

nephroscopy
neh FROSS koh pee

11.66 Remember that the suffix -scopy means "process of viewing." Therefore, visual examination of kidney nephrons may be performed in the procedure known as _____, during which a modified fiber-optic endoscope called a **nephroscope** (NEFF roh skope) is used.

nephrosonography
neff roh son OG rah fee

11.67 An ultrasound procedure that provides an image of a kidney for diagnostic analysis is known as **nephrosonography**. _____ is a constructed term that contains five word parts and is written nephr/o/son/o/graphy.

nephrostomy
neff ROSS toh mee

nephr/o/**stomy**

11.68 A procedure that surgically creates an opening through the body wall and into a kidney is called a _____. It is usually established to allow a catheter to be inserted from the exterior to a renal pelvis for urine drainage and is also called a **pyelostomy** (PYE ell OSS toh mee). The constructed form of **nephrostomy** is written _____/__/_____, and the term pyelostomy is pyel/o/stomy.

nephrotomogram
NEH froh toh moh gram

11.69 A diagnostic procedure that images the kidney with sectional X-rays to observe internal details of kidney structure is known as **nephrotomography** (NEH froh toh MOG rah fee). The suffix that means "a record or image" is *-gram*, so the image obtained from this procedure is a _____. *Nephrotomography* is a constructed term that is written nephr/o/tom/o/graphy, which literally means "recording process of cut kidney."

peritoneal dialysis
pair ih TOH nee al * dye AL ih siss

11.70 You learned about hemodialysis in Frame 11.59. A similar procedure is **peritoneal dialysis,** which also processes fluids and electrolytes by artificial filtration as a cleansing treatment to compensate for kidney failure. Thus, _____ _____ removes toxins and other wastes as a replacement for kidney function. In contrast to hemodialysis, peritoneal dialysis processes fluids from the peritoneal cavity rather than directly from the bloodstream. The constructed form of this term is written peritone/al dia/lysis.

pyelogram
PYE ell oh gram

11.71 An X-ray image of the renal pelvis (a **pyelogram**) is a useful diagnostic tool that is often used to examine kidney-related disorders. In obtaining an image called a **retrograde** _____, the procedure involves injection of contrast medium into the ureter using a cystoscope. As the X-ray is taken, it moves in a direction opposite from the norm (retrograde means "opposite of normal"). It is abbreviated **RP,** and an example is shown in Figure 11.15■. In an **intravenous pyelogram,** iodine is used as the contrast medium and is injected into the bloodstream. It is abbreviated **IVP.**

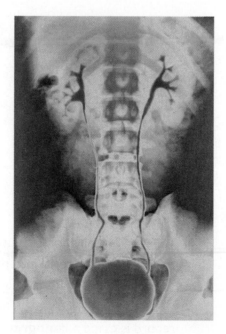

Figure 11.15
Retrograde pyelogram. A contrast medium is injected into the ureter using a cystoscope, and the X-ray moves in a direction opposite from the norm, producing the image that is shown. It serves to highlight the internal features of the renal pelvis and ureters.
Source: CNRI/Photo Researchers, Inc.

pyelolithotomy
pye ell oh lith OTT oh mee

11.72 A kidney stone may sometimes form within the renal pelvis. A surgery performed to remove the stone from the renal pelvis involves an incision into the kidney and is called a **pyelolithotomy.** The constructed form of the term _____ is written pyel/o/lith/o/tomy, which literally means "to cut stone from renal pelvis."

pyeloplasty
PYE ell oh PLASS tee

11.73 The suffix that means "surgical repair" is -*plasty*. Surgical repair of the renal pelvis is a procedure called _____. This constructed term is written pyel/o/plasty.

renal transplant

11.74 The replacement of a dysfunctioning kidney with a donor kidney is a surgery called _____ _____ (Figure 11.16■). The donated kidney is often provided by a close relative with a similar genetic makeup. Alternatively, a donor kidney can be implanted with the use of cytological drugs that suppress the immune response, reducing the chance of rejection.

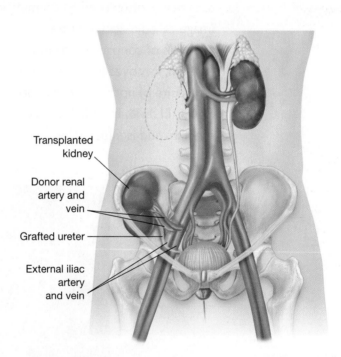

Transplanted kidney

Donor renal artery and vein

Grafted ureter

External iliac artery and vein

Figure 11.16 ■
Renal transplant. A transplanted kidney is placed within the pelvic cavity below the location of the kidney requiring replacement.

renography
ree NOG rah fee

11.75 An examination that uses nuclear medicine by IV (intravenous) injection of radioactive material into the patient's kidneys is called **renography.** The radioactive materials highlight internal details of the kidney during the _____. This constructed term is written ren/o/graphy. The record is called a **renogram** (REE noh gram).

specific gravity	**11.76** The measurement of the density of substances in a liquid compared to water is called **specific gravity** (**SG**). The _____ _____ of a urine sample is often measured with an instrument called a urinometer (Frame 11.85). The specific gravity of a urine sample helps to reveal the efficiency of renal filtration and the reabsorption of water.
ureterectomy yoo REE ter EK toh mee	**11.77** The suffix that means "surgical excision, removal" is *-ectomy*. The surgical removal of a ureter is called _____. The constructed form of this term is written ureter/ectomy.
ureterostomy yoo REE ter OSS toh mee **ureterotomy** yoo ree ter OTT oh mee	**11.78** The surgical creation of an external opening from the ureter to the body surface is called _____. It is performed to provide an alternate exit route for urine that bypasses the urethra. The procedure includes an incision into the wall of the ureter, called _____. Both terms are constructed of word parts: *ureterostomy* is written ureter/o/stomy, and *ureterotomy* is written ureter/o/tomy.

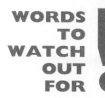 **WORDS TO WATCH OUT FOR**

 ▶▶▶▶▶ *-stomy* **or** *-tomy*?

The suffix *-stomy* means "surgical creation of an opening," whereas *-tomy* means "incision, to cut." The two suffixes represent two different surgical techniques. In general, an incision is a cut through tissue, whereas the surgical creation of an opening establishes an artificial window into the body, usually for the drainage of fluids or waste. Can you see how the small addition of an *s* makes a big difference in meaning?

urethropexy yoo REE throh pek see	**11.79** Surgical fixation of the urethra is a procedure called **urethropexy**. A _____ is often performed to correct stress incontinence (Frame 11.30). It is a constructed term written urethr/o/pexy.
urethroplasty yoo REE throh plass tee	**11.80** Surgical repair of the urethra is a procedure called _____. This constructed term is written urethr/o/plasty.
urethrostomy yoo REE THROSS toh mee **urethrotomy** yoo ree THROTT oh mee	**11.81** The surgical creation of an opening through the urethra is called _____. It is performed to provide an alternate exit route for urine. The procedure includes an incision into the wall of the urethra, called _____. Both terms are constructed of word parts: *urethrostomy* is written urethr/o/stomy, and *urethrotomy* is written urethr/o/tomy.

urinalysis
YOO rin AL ih siss

11.82 A combination of clinical lab tests that are performed on a urine specimen is called **urinalysis** (Figure 11.17■). The term _____ is a constructed term written urin/alysis, in which *alysis* is a shortened form of the word *analysis* to make the term easier to pronounce. It literally means "analysis of urine." Abbreviated **UA,** it provides information on the quality and composition of urine, including specific gravity, creatinine levels, glucose levels, protein levels, and the abnormal presence of red blood cells, white blood cells, and pus for diagnostic purposes.

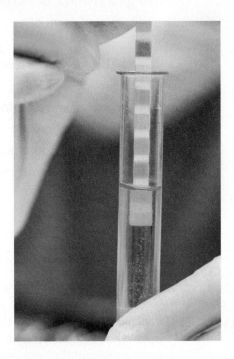

Figure 11.17 ■
Urinalysis. During a simple urinalysis, a stick with colored blocks is dipped into a urine specimen. Color changes in the blocks are noted and compared to a known standard.
Source: © Max Tactic/Fotolia.

urinary catheterization
YOO rih nair ee *
KATH eh ter ih ZAY shun

11.83 A **catheter** is a flexible tube that is inserted into an opening of the body to transport fluids in or out. A **urinary catheter** is usually inserted through the urethra to enter the urinary bladder and is often used to drain urine from a patient who is immobile. The process of inserting the urinary catheter is called _____ _____. It is illustrated in Figure 11.18■.

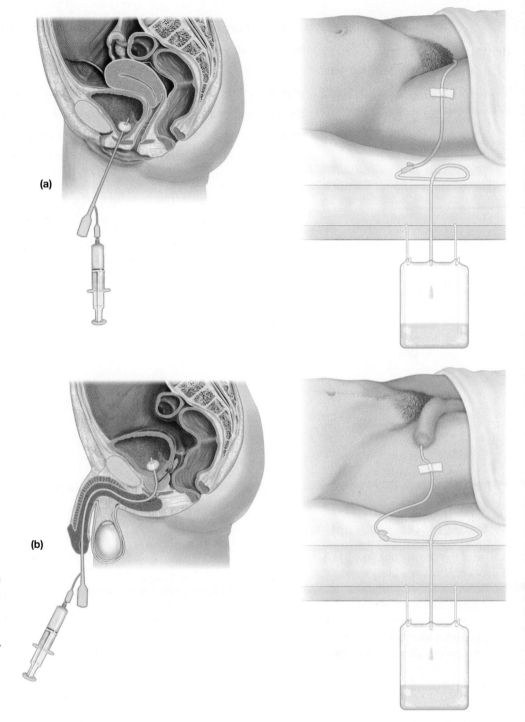

Figure 11.18 ■
Urinary catheterization. The procedure involves the insertion of a flexible tube, or catheter, through the urethra and into the urinary bladder. Voiding occurs through the catheter and is collected in a plastic bag adjacent to the patient.
(a) Catheterization of a female patient.
(b) Catheterization of a male patient.

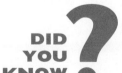

DID YOU KNOW ?

▶▶▶▶▶ **Catheter**

The term *catheter* is from the Greek word *katheter,* which means "to send down," so named because it is a flexible tube that lets urine down from the urinary bladder.

urinary endoscopy
YOO rih nair ee * ehn DOSS koh pee

11.84 The procedural use of an endoscope to observe internal structures of the urinary system is generally known as _____ _____. A specialized endoscope is associated with each urinary organ, including a **meatoscope** (mee AT oh skope) for inserting into the urinary meatus, a **nephroscope** (NEFF roh skope) for viewing a kidney, a **urethroscope** (yoo REE throh skope) for viewing the urethra, and a **cystoscope** (SISS toh skope) for observing the interior of the urinary bladder.

urinometer
yoo rih NOM eh ter

11.85 An instrument that measures the specific gravity (density of substances in water) in a sample of urine is known as a **urinometer.** This constructed term is composed of three word parts and is written urin/o/meter. A _____ is illustrated in Figure 11.19■.

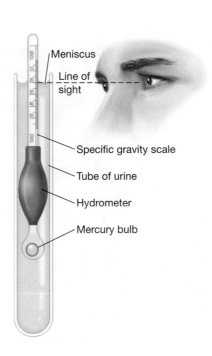

Figure 11.19 ■
Urinometer. Specific gravity is a measure of the density of a liquid. In this procedure, a urine sample and urinometer are placed within a tube, and the liquid level is compared to the scale on the urinometer. The procedure provides information on the concentration of solids within a urine sample.

urologist
yoo RAHL oh jist

11.86 The medical field specializing in disorders of the urinary system is called **urology** (yoo RAHL oh jee). A physician who treats patients in this discipline is called a _____.

vesicourethral
vess ih koh yoo REE thral

11.87 A surgery that is performed to stabilize the position of the urinary bladder is called **vesicourethral suspension.** The term _____ contains four word parts and is written vesic/o/urethr/al. It is performed to treat stress incontinence (Frame 11.30).

PRACTICE: Treatments, Procedures, and Devices of the Urinary System

Break the Chain

Analyze these medical terms:

    a) Separate each term into its word parts; each word part is labeled for you (**p** = prefix, **r** = root, **cf** = combining form, and **s** = suffix).

    b) For the Bonus Question, write the requested definition in the blank that follows.

---

1. a) cystography   _____/___/_____
                                          cf   s

    b) *Bonus Question:* What is the definition of the suffix? _____

---

2. a) cystolithotomy   _____/___/_____/___/_____
                                       cf   cf   s

    b) *Bonus Question:* What is the definition of the suffix? _____

---

3. a) lithotripsy   _____/___/_____
                              cf   s

    b) *Bonus Question:* What is the definition of the combining form? _____

---

4. a) hemodialysis   _____/___/_____/_____
                            cf   p   s

    b) *Bonus Question:* What is the definition of the prefix? _____

---

5. a) cystorrhaphy   _____/___/_____
                          cf   s

    b) *Bonus Question:* Does this term contain a prefix? _____

---

6. a) nephrolysis   _____/___/_____
                          cf   s

    b) *Bonus Question:* What is the definition of the suffix? _____

---

7. a) nephrogram   _____/___/_____
                          cf   s

    b) *Bonus Question:* What is the meaning of the suffix? _____

---

8. a) nephrotomography   _____/___/_____/___/_____
                                cf   cf   s

    b) *Bonus Question:* What is the definition of the *first* combining form? _____

---

9. a) ureterostomy   _____/___/_____
                          cf   s

    b) *Bonus Question:* What is the definition of the suffix? _____

The Right Match

Match the term on the left with the correct definition on the right.

_____ 1. cystorrhaphy
_____ 2. extracorporeal shock wave lithotripsy
_____ 3. nephrectomy
_____ 4. nephrostomy
_____ 5. vesicourethral suspension
_____ 6. fulguration
_____ 7. renal transplant
_____ 8. blood urea nitrogen
_____ 9. peritoneal dialysis
_____ 10. creatinine
_____ 11. specific gravity
_____ 12. urinary catheter

a. removal of a kidney
b. creates a new opening through the renal pelvis to the outside
c. stabilizes the position of the urinary bladder
d. suture of the urinary bladder
e. technique that uses ultrasonic energy to crush stones
f. test for protein levels in a urine sample
g. test for water concentration in urine
h. electric current that kills unwanted tissue
i. test for urea in the blood
j. insertion of a tube to drain urine
k. surgical procedure replacing a diseased kidney
l. blood filtration using the peritoneal cavity

Abbreviations of the Urinary System

The abbreviations that are associated with the urinary system are summarized here. Study these abbreviations, and review them in the exercise that follows.

Abbreviation	Definition
BUN	blood urea nitrogen
cath	catheter, catheterization
ESWL	extracorporeal shock wave lithotripsy
HD	hemodialysis
IVP	intravenous pyelogram

Abbreviation	Definition
RP	retrograde pyelogram
SG	specific gravity
UA	urinalysis
UTI	urinary tract infection
VCUG	voiding cystourethrogram

PRACTICE: Abbreviations

Fill in the blanks with the abbreviation or the complete medical term.

Abbreviation	Medical Term
1. UA	_____
2. _____	retrograde pyelogram
3. cath	_____
4. _____	voiding cystourethrogram
5. IVP	_____
6. _____	urinary tract infection
7. HD	_____

Chapter Review

Word Building

Construct medical terms from the following meanings. (Some are built from word parts, some are not.) The first question has been completed as an example.

1. inability to pass urine   *an*uresis

2. absence of urine   an_____

3. presence of bacteria in the urine   bacteri_____

4. presence of a stone in the bladder   _____lith

5. inflammation of a kidney   nephr_____

6. presence of blood in the urine   _____uria

7. protrusion of a ureter   uretero_____

8. involuntary release of urine   _____uresis

9. presence of stones in the kidney   nephro_____

10. fixation of an abnormally mobile kidney   nephro_____

11. surgical creation of an opening into the renal pelvis   _____stomy

12. surgical repair of the urethra   urethro_____

13. incision into the ureter wall   uretero_____

14. X-ray image of the urinary bladder   cysto_____

15. X-ray technique imaging a kidney   nephro_____

16. X-ray image of the renal pelvis with iodine   intravenous _____gram

17. an endoscope modified to view a kidney   _____scope

18. lab test measuring urea in the blood   blood urea _____ (BUN)

19. instrument measuring water concentration in urine   urino_____

20. urine test that includes multiple parameters   urin_____

▶▶▶▶ Medical Report Exercises

Read the following medical report, then answer the questions that follow.

PEARSON GENERAL HOSPITAL

PGH

5500 University Avenue Metropolis, NE
Phone: (211) 594-4000 • Fax: (211) 594-4001

Medical Consultation: Urology

Date: 6/25/2011

Patient: Sylvia Hernandez-Brown

Patient Complaint: Pain in the lower lumbar region (right and left sides). The patient also complains of feeling tired, shortness of breath, general body aches with mild fever, and loss of appetite, all within the past month.

History: 60-year-old Hispanic female, 40 pounds overweight with Type 2 diabetes without drug assist, history of periodic UTIs.

Family History: Father deceased at 72 years old with COPD and CHF. Mother alive at 77 years with Type 2 diabetes under care; lost one kidney at age 70 due to polycystic disease.

Allergies: None

Physical Examination: Vital signs: moderate fever of 99.9 °F, pulse rate 82/min., bp 129/90. Blood test reveals uremia. Urinalysis reveals albumin high, and blood in the urine.

Diagnosis: Renal failure of left kidney apparent with increasing insufficiency of right kidney due to PD evident by nephrotomography and confirmed by nephroscopy.

Treatment: Immediate dialysis, to repeat every other day until surgery. Admit patient for radical nephrectomy. Schedule dialysis treatments postoperative and include patient to renal transplant database.

Joshua Ryan, M.D.
‾‾‾‾‾‾‾‾‾‾‾‾‾‾‾‾‾‾‾‾‾‾‾‾‾‾‾‾
Joshua Ryan, M.D.

Photo Source: Gravicapa/Shutterstock

Comprehension Questions

1. What patient complaints point to the kidneys as the source of the disease? _____

_____

_____

2. Describe the meaning of the terms *nephrotomography* and *nephrectomy*. _____

_____

_____

3. Why does the urologist order dialysis for the patient prior to surgery? _____

_____

_____

Case Study Questions

The following Case Study provides further discussion regarding the patient in the medical report. Fill in the blanks with the correct terms. Choose your answers from the following list of terms. (Note that some terms may be used more than once.)

albuminuria	nephroscopy	renal transplant
hematuria	nephrotomography	urinalysis
hemodialysis	polycystic kidney disease	
nephromegaly	pyelonephritis	

A 60-year-old female, Sylvia Hernandez-Brown, was admitted to urology by her general practitioner following a physical exam that included blood tests revealing abnormally high levels of urea in the blood. A generalized test of urine composition, or (a) _____, revealed elevated levels of albumin, a symptom known as (b) _____, and the presence of red blood cells in the urine, or (c) _____. Following diagnostic exams that included an X-ray technique imaging the kidney by sections called (d) _____, and an endoscopic evaluation of the kidney known as (e) _____, the attending physician concluded a diagnosis of enlargement of both kidneys, or (f) _____, caused by multiple cysts, or (g) _____ _____ _____, which had resulted in inflammation of the renal pelvis and nephrons, or (h) _____ and renal failure. Artificial filtration of the blood, or (i) _____, was ordered, due to a growing insufficiency to reduce blood metabolites (metabolic wastes). Surgical removal of both diseased kidneys was scheduled immediately, and the patient was placed on a waiting list for a replacement kidney as a (j) _____ _____.

Del Hamilton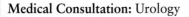

For a greater challenge, read the following medical report and answer the critical thinking questions that follow from the information in the chapter.

PGH

PEARSON GENERAL HOSPITAL

5500 University Avenue Metropolis, PA
Phone: (211) 594-4000 • Fax: (211) 594-4001

Medical Consultation: Urology

Date: 08/22/2011

Patient: Del Hamilton

Patient Complaint: Intermittent pain in the left lumbar region radiating to the left flank; dysuria; nocturia.

History: 45-year-old male with Type 2 DM diagnosed 2 years ago at 270 pounds of weight; present weight is 190 pounds under doctor-supervised diet management program; no additional complications.

Family History: Father diagnosed with renal calculi and treated successfully with lithotripsy at age 62 years; mother died of breast cancer at age 58 years.

Allergies: None

Physical Examination: Vital signs normal. RP positive for pelvic calculi, confirmed by nephroscopy.

Diagnosis: Renal calculi with pelvis of right kidney and pyelonephritis as complicating factor.

Treatment: Extracorporeal lithotripsy.

Karl Moss, M.D.

Karl Moss. M.D.

Photo Source: Monkey Business Images

Comprehension Questions

1. What conditions other than the one diagnosed might caused the reported symptoms? _____

   _____

   _____

2. Do you think the prediagnosed condition of Type 2 DM contributed to the condition of renal calculi? _____

   _____

   _____

3. Describe the meaning of the terms *renal calculi* and *pyelonephritis*. _____

   _____

   _____

Case Study Questions

The following case study provides further discussion regarding the patient in the medical report. Fill in the blanks with the correct terms, using information in this chapter.

Del Hamilton, a 45-year-old male, was admitted to the hospital after presenting himself to the emergency department in acute distress. He complained of intermittent pain in the left lumbar region, radiating to the left flank. He also complained of pain and difficulty voiding, a symptom called (k) _____, with the sensation of the need to void at night, known as (l) _____, which interrupted his sleep. A generalized lab test of his urine sample, called a (m) _____, revealed no abnormalities. A review of his family history revealed stones in the renal pelvis, called (n) _____. The attending physician referred the patient to a (o) _____. The specialist in treating urinary disorders, called a (p) _____, immediately prepared the patient for diagnostics that included an X-ray technique that images the renal pelvis with an injected contrast medium, known as a (q) _____ _____, followed with an endoscopic evaluation of the kidney called a (r) _____. Both exams revealed the presence of stones in the renal pelvis, or renal calculi. The stones were pulverized successfully using the (s) _____ procedure and passed the next day.

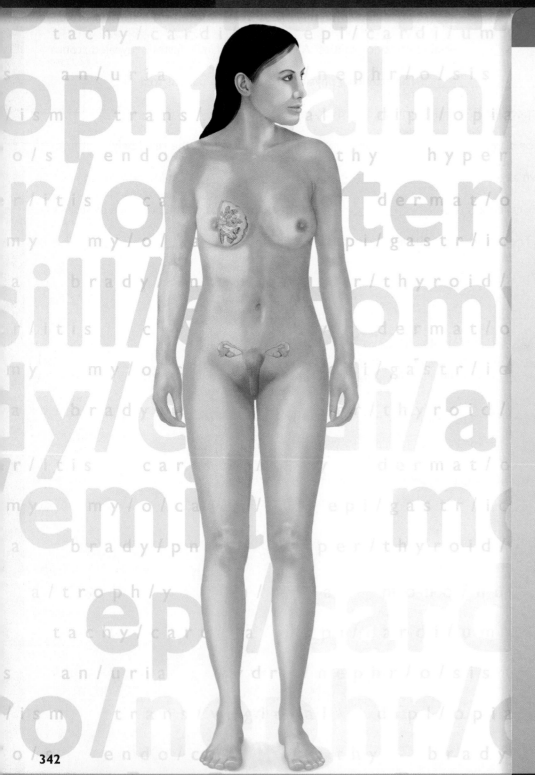

CHAPTER

12

Reproductive System and Obstetrics

LEARNING OBJECTIVES

After completing this chapter, you will be able to:

1. Define and spell the word parts used to create terms for the reproductive system and obstetrics.

2. Break down and define common medical terms used for symptoms, diseases, disorders, procedures, treatments, and devices associated with the reproductive system and obstetrics.

3. Build medical terms from the word parts associated with the reproductive system and obstetrics.

4. Pronounce and spell common medical terms associated with the reproductive system and obstetrics.

342

Anatomy and Physiology Terms ▶▶▶▶▶

The following table provides the combining forms that specifically apply to the anatomy and physiology of the reproductive system and obstetrics. Note that the combining forms are colored red to help you identify them when you see them again later in the chapter.

Combining Form	Definition	Combining Form	Definition
amni/o, amnion/o	amnion	mast/o	breast
andr/o	male	men/o, menstru/o	month, menstruation
balan/o	glans penis	orchi/o, orchid/o	testis
cervic/o	neck, cervix	pen/o	penis
chori/o	membrane, chorion	prostat/o	prostate gland
cyes/o, cyesi/o	pregnancy	semin/o	seed, sperm
embry/o	embryo	sperm/o, spermat/o	seed, sperm
epididym/o	epididymis	test/o	testis, testicle
episi/o	vulva	testicul/o	little testis, testicle
fet/o	fetus	urethr/o	urethra
gravid/o, gravidar/o	pregnancy	vas/o	vessel
mamm/o	breast		

reproductive

testes

ovaries

obstetrics
ob STET riks

12.1 The reproductive systems are separated in this chapter to reflect the differences between the male and female. In both sexes, the _____ system performs the role of producing sex cells, or gametes (GAH meets), in preparation for fertilization and the development of new offspring. The male gametes are called spermatozoa, or sperm cells, and are produced by the male gonads, the testes. Other male organs include the scrotum that houses the testes, the penis, the tubes that convey sperm (epididymis, vas deferens, and urethra), and the glands that contribute to semen (seminal vesicles, prostate gland, and bulbourethral glands). The male sex hormone, testosterone, is also produced by the _____. The female gametes are called ova and are produced by the female gonads, the ovaries. Other female organs include the fallopian tubes, uterus, vagina, and vulva. The female hormones, estrogen and progesterone, are produced by cells within the _____.

Once a new life has been conceived, the developing embryo enters into the segment of life called **prenatal** (pree NAY tal) **development,** which includes the changes in body form that occur through the mother's pregnancy until birth. The clinical field of **obstetrics** is focused on this period of life. _____ is often referred to by its abbreviation, **OB.** It supports the mother during childbirth and during the first month or so following childbirth.

gamete
GAMM eet

12.2 The general function of the reproductive system is the creation of offspring, which occurs when the male gamete (sperm) unites successfully with a female _____ (ovum). The resulting fertilized egg is the origin of a new human life.

12.3 Use the anatomy terms that appear in the left column to fill in the corresponding blanks in Figures 12.1■ through 12.3■.

1. **vas**
2. **prostate**
3. **testis**
4. **epididymis**

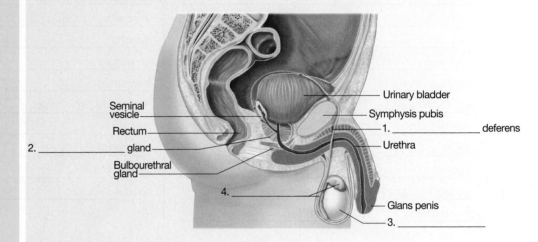

Seminal vesicle

Rectum

2. _____ gland

Bulbourethral gland

4. _____

Urinary bladder

Symphysis pubis

1. _____ deferens

Urethra

Glans penis

3. _____

Figure 12.1 ■
The male reproductive system.

5. **vagina**
6. **ovary**
7. **minora**

8. **cervix**
9. **vagina**

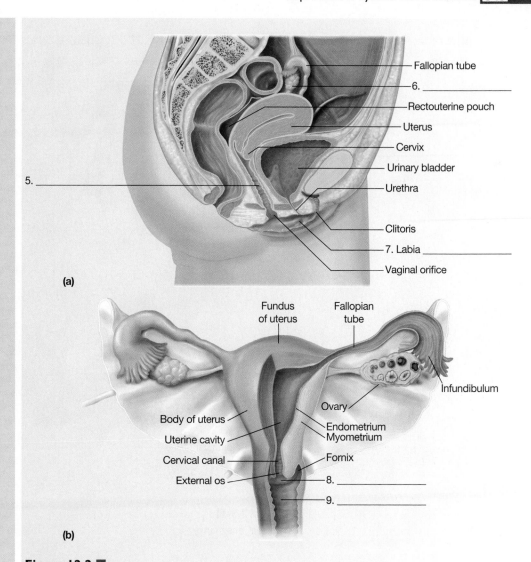

(a)

Fallopian tube

6. _____

Rectouterine pouch

Uterus

Cervix

Urinary bladder

Urethra

Clitoris

7. Labia _____

Vaginal orifice

5. _____

Fundus of uterus

Fallopian tube

Infundibulum

Body of uterus

Uterine cavity

Cervical canal

External os

Ovary

Endometrium

Myometrium

Fornix

8. _____

9. _____

(b)

Figure 12.2 ■
The female reproductive system. (a) Sagittal section through the pelvis. (b) Top view of pelvic organs.

10. placenta
11. uterus

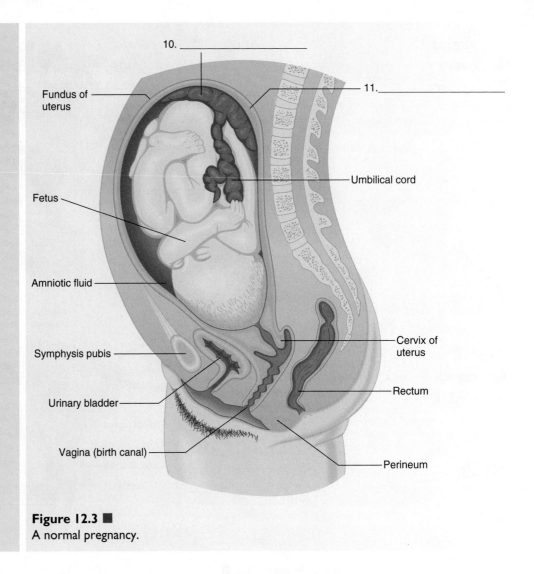

10. _____

11. _____

Fundus of uterus

Umbilical cord

Fetus

Amniotic fluid

Cervix of uterus

Symphysis pubis

Rectum

Urinary bladder

Vagina (birth canal)

Perineum

Figure 12.3 ■
A normal pregnancy.

Medical Terms for the Reproductive System and Obstetrics ▶▶▶▶

reproductive

urologist
yoo RAHL oh jist

gynecology
GYE neh KALL oh jee

12.4 The medical field of **reproductive medicine** manages the health care of both the male and female _____ systems. Because the male urethra is responsible for transporting both urine and semen, diseases of the male reproductive system are usually treated within the field of **urology** (yoo RAHL oh jee) by a _____. Diseases of the female reproductive system are generally treated by a physician called a **gynecologist** (gye neh KAHL oh jist), who specializes within the field of _____. In both sexes, reproductive diseases are often diagnosed initially during a physical examination. The diseases that require confirmation or an internal evaluation may be further analyzed using the noninvasive procedures of MRI, CT scan, or ultrasound imaging.

pathogens

12.5 The reproductive systems of the male and female are subject to infections, tumors, injury, endocrine disorders, and inherited diseases. For many people, the most common threat to health is the exposure to _____ during sexual contact. Although the reproductive tract is lined with a protective mucous membrane, certain bacteria, viruses, fungi, and protozoa are able to gain entry into the bloodstream directly or by way of breaks in the mucosal lining. Once established, these pathogens may spread throughout the body. Most **sexually** _____ **infections (STIs)**, also called **sexually transmitted diseases (STDs)** or venereal diseases, infect the body in this manner. Thus, STIs are infections acquired during intimate physical contact that occurs during sexual intercourse or other sexual activities. The most common forms of STIs are described in this chapter.

transmitted

12.6 In the following sections, you will study the prefixes, combining forms, and suffixes that combine to build the medical terms of the reproductive system and obstetrics.

Signs and Symptoms of the Male Reproductive System

Here are the word parts that specifically apply to the signs and symptoms of the male reproductive system that are covered in the following section. Note that the word parts are color-coded to help you identify them: prefixes are green, combining forms are red, and suffixes are blue.

Prefix	Definition	Combining Form	Definition	Suffix	Definition
a-	without, absence of	balan/o	glans penis	-algia	condition of pain
		olig/o	few in number	-ia	condition of
		orchi/o, orchid/o	testis	-itis	inflammation
		prostat/o	prostate gland	-rrhea	discharge
		sperm/o	seed, sperm		
		test/o	testis		
		urethr/o	urethra		
		zo/o	animal, living		

KEY TERMS A–Z

aspermia
ah SPER mee ah

12.7 As you know, the prefix *a-* means "without, absence of." Therefore, the inability to produce or ejaculate sperm is a sign of male infertility known as _____. The constructed form of this term is a/sperm/ia, which literally means "condition of without seed."

azoospermia AY zoh oh SPER mee ah a/zo/o/sperm/ia	**12.8** The absence of living sperm in semen is called **azoospermia** and is another sign of infertility. The term _____ literally means "condition of without living seed." This constructed term has five word parts and is written as __/____/__/_____/____.
balanorrhea BAL ah noh REE ah	**12.9** The combining form for the distal end of the penis, known as the glans penis, is *balan/o*. Recall that the suffix *-rrhea* means "discharge." Therefore, an abnormal condition of discharge from the glans is called _____, which is a symptom of the sexually transmitted infection called gonorrhea (Frame 12.134). Balanorrhea is a constructed term that can be written balan/o/rrhea.
chancres SHANG kerz	**12.10** The sexually transmitted infection syphilis (Frame 12.137) may be diagnosed by the presence of small ulcers on the skin of the penis, which are called **chancres**. The term _____ is a French word meaning "cancer."
oligospermia all ih goh SPER mee ah	**12.11** An abnormally low sperm count is the most common sign of male infertility. Combining the word part that means "few in number," *olig/o*, with the word parts meaning "condition of sperm," the term that results is the condition _____. It is a constructed term that can be represented as olig/o/sperm/ia.
papilloma pap ih LOH mah	**12.12** **Papillomas** are wartlike lesions on the skin and mucous membranes. A _____ is a sign of infection by the sexually transmitted human papillomaviruses (Frame 12.136), and they are commonly called **genital warts**.
prostatitis pross tah TYE tiss	**12.13** Inflammation of the prostate gland is called _____. It is usually a sign of either BPH (Frame 12.20) or prostate cancer (Frame 12.28). This constructed term is written prostat/itis.
prostatorrhea PROSS tah toh REE ah	**12.14** An abnormal discharge from the prostate gland is known as _____. This is a constructed term that is written prostat/o/rrhea.
testalgia test AHL jee ah	**12.15** A suffix that means "condition of pain" is *-algia*. The condition of testicular pain is known as _____, which is written test/algia. It is also known as **orchialgia** (OR kee ALL jee ah) and **orchidalgia** (OR kid ALL jee ah) because *test/o*, *orchi/o*, and *orchid/o* are each combining forms that mean "testis."

urethritis	12.16 Inflammation of the urethra is called _____. It is
yoo ree THRYE tiss	a symptom of an irritation of the urethra, usually resulting from a sexually transmitted infection. This constructed term is written urethr/itis.

PRACTICE: Signs and Symptoms of the Male Reproductive System

The Right Match

Match the term on the left with the correct definition on the right.

_____ 1. chancres

_____ 2. balanorrhea

_____ 3. prostatitis

_____ 4. papillomas

_____ 5. azoospermia

a. excessive discharge from the glans penis

b. inflammation of the prostate gland

c. absence of living sperm in semen

d. small ulcers on the skin of the penis, sign of syphilis

e. wartlike lesions

Break the Chain

Analyze these medical terms:

   a) Separate each term into its word parts; each word part is labeled for you (**p** = prefix, **r** = root, **cf** = combining form, and **s** = suffix).

   b) For the Bonus Question, write the requested definition in the blank that follows.

The first set has been completed as an example.

1. a) prostatorrhea   _prostat/o/rrhea_
                                          cf   s

   b) *Bonus Question:* What is the definition of the suffix? _excessive discharge_____

2. a) oligospermia   _____/___/_____/_____
                                          cf   r   s

   b) *Bonus Question:* What is the definition of the prefix? _____

3. a) testalgia   _____/_____
                                          r   s

   b) *Bonus Question:* What is the definition of the word root? _____

4. a) urethritis   _____/_____
                                          r   s

   b) *Bonus Question:* What is the definition of the suffix? _____

5. a) aspermia   _____/_____/_____
                                          p   r   s

   b) *Bonus Question:* What is the definition of the prefix? _____

Diseases and Disorders of the Male Reproductive System

Here are the word parts that specifically apply to the diseases and disorders of the male reproductive system that are covered in the following section. Note that the word parts are color-coded to help you identify them: prefixes are green, combining forms are red, and suffixes are blue.

Prefix	Definition
an-	without, absence of
hyper-	excessive, abnormally high, above
para-	alongside, abnormal

Combining Form	Definition
andr/o	male
balan/o	glans penis
crypt/o	hidden
epididym/o	epididymis
hydr/o	water
orchi/o, orchid/o	testis
prostat/o	prostate gland
varic/o	dilated vein

Suffix	Definition
-cele	hernia, swelling, or protrusion
-ism	condition or disease
-itis	inflammation
-pathy	disease
-plasia	formation, growth

KEY TERMS A–Z

andropathy
an DROPP ah thee

12.17 A combining form that means "male" and the suffix meaning "disease" may be combined to form a general term for a disease afflicting only males, _____. This constructed term includes three word parts, which can be represented as andr/o/pathy.

anorchism
an OR kizm
an/orch/ism

12.18 A word root that means "testis" is orchi or orchid. When the prefix meaning "without, absence of" is added along with the suffix -ism, the constructed term _____ is created. It means "condition of without testis" and refers to the absence of one or both testes. The constructed form of the term is written _____/_____/_____. The term **anorchidism** may also be used with the same meaning.

balanitis
bal ah NYE tiss

12.19 Inflammation of the glans penis is a disorder called _____. It is a constructed term with two word parts, written balan/itis.

benign prostatic hyperplasia
bee NINE * pross TAT ik * HIGH per PLAY zee ah

12.20 Among many men older than 50 years, the prostate gland enlarges to constrict the urethra passing through it. Known as **benign prostatic hyperplasia,** symptoms include nocturia (nighttime urination) and a frequent need to void (Figure 12.4■). It is not a form of cancer and does not spread to other tissues, but its symptoms are uncomfortable. _____ _____ _____ is also called **benign prostatic hypertrophy;** both are abbreviated **BPH.**

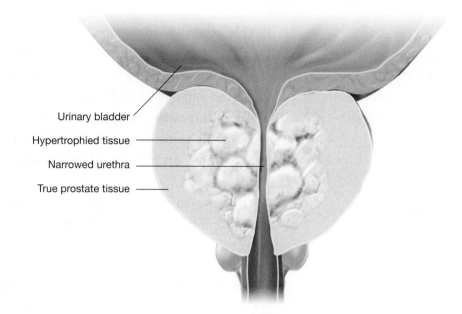

Urinary bladder

Hypertrophied tissue

Narrowed urethra

True prostate tissue

Figure 12.4 ■
Benign prostatic hyperplasia. The condition results when an inner capsule of nonfunctional prostate tissue swells, pushing against the walls of the urethra to cause a restriction of urine flow.

cryptorchidism
kript OR kid izm

12.21 The condition of an undescended testis is called **cryptorchidism.** Note that the combining form *crypt/o* means "hidden" and is used in this term to describe the hidden location of an undescended testis within the abdomen or pelvic cavity (Figure 12.5■). The constructed form of _____ is crypt/orchid/ism. An alternate name for this condition is **cryptorchism** (KRIPT or kizm).

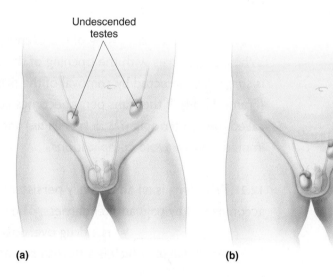

Undescended testes

Partially descended testis

(a)   **(b)**

Figure 12.5 ■
Cryptorchidism. (a) In complete cryptorchidism, the testes of a newborn have failed to descend into the scrotum and remain within the pelvic cavity where they originally developed. (b) A partial cryptorchidism of the left testis.

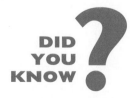

DID YOU KNOW ▶▶▶▶ **Cryptorchidism**

Cryptorchidism is derived from the Greek word *kruptorkhos,* which literally means "a condition of a hidden testis." It is named this way because an undescended testis is in a location that is hidden from view.

epididymitis ep ih did ih MY tiss	**12.22** Inflammation of the epididymis is a condition called _____. The constructed form of this term is written epididym/itis. Recall that *orchi* means "testis." Therefore, when the epididymis and one or both testes are inflamed, the condition is known as **orchiepididymitis** (OR kee ep ih did ih MY tiss), which may be written orchi/epididym/itis. If the inflammation is limited to one or more testes, the term becomes **orchitis** (or KYE tiss), written orch/itis.
erectile dysfunction ee REK tile * diss FUNK shun	**12.23** Many men experience **erectile dysfunction** at some time in their life, which is the inability to achieve an erection sufficient to perform sexual intercourse. The term _____ _____ is abbreviated **ED** and is also known as **impotence** (IM poh tens). Failing health, certain drugs, fatigue, circulatory disorders, and diabetes mellitus can cause ED.
hydrocele HIGH droh seel	**12.24** Injury is the most frequent cause of **hydrocele**, which is the swelling of the scrotum caused by fluid accumulation. _____ is a constructed term containing three word parts and is written hydr/o/cele.
Peyronie disease pay ROHN eez	**12.25** A hardness, or induration, of the erectile tissue within the penis is a condition known as **Peyronie disease.** _____ _____ can cause erectile dysfunction (Frame 12.23), especially if the induration is greater on one side to cause a curvature of the penis.
phimosis figh MOH siss	**12.26** A congenital narrowing of the prepuce opening is known as **phimosis.** When it interferes with the opening of the urethra, _____ is surgically corrected by removal of the prepuce in a circumcision (Frame 12.34). If the glans penis becomes strangulated, the condition is called **paraphimosis** (PAR ah figh MOH siss) and must be surgically corrected immediately to avoid complications.
priapism PRY ah pizm	**12.27 Priapism** is an abnormally persistent erection of the penis, often accompanied by pain and tenderness. The most common cause of _____ is a drug overdose. The term is derived from the Latin word *priapus,* which is a Roman scarecrow figure with an erect penis.

prostate cancer
PROSS tayt * KANN ser

12.28 The prostate gland is subject to an aggressive form of cancer, commonly known as _____ _____. Also called **prostatic carcinoma** (pro STAT ik * kar sih NOH mah), it increases the size of the prostate before it spreads into the pelvic region and beyond and can often be felt as a hard nodule on the prostate during a digital rectal exam (Frame 12.35). It is illustrated in Figure 12.6■.

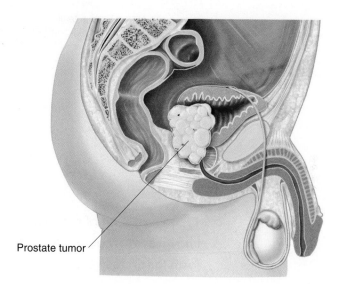

Prostate tumor

Figure 12.6 ■
Prostate cancer. In this example, a large mass has grown into the urinary bladder. Prostate cancer is highly metastatic, sending tumor cells to the pelvic area and beyond, where they may form secondary tumor sites.

testicular carcinoma
tess TIK yoo ler * kar sih NOH mah

12.29 A cancer originating from the testis is known as _____ _____. Its occurrence and mortality rate is highest among the 20- to 40-year-old age group. The most common form is called **seminoma** (sem ih NOH mah), which arises from sperm-forming cells and metastasizes to nearby lymph nodes. It is the most common cancer diagnosis among American young men, with 8,290 new cases reported in 2011 and 350 deaths, according to the American Cancer Society.

testicular torsion
tess TIK yoo ler * TOR shun

12.30 A **testicular torsion** occurs when the spermatic cord becomes twisted, causing a reduced blood flow to the testis (Figure 12.7■). If _____ _____ is not corrected within a few hours by surgery, the affected testicular tissue can die.

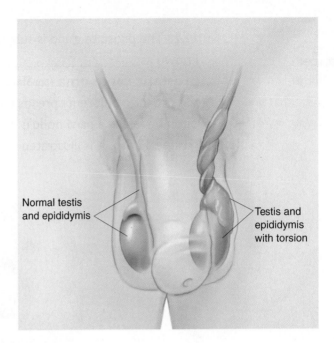

Figure 12.7 ■
Testicular torsion.

Normal testis
and epididymis

Testis and
epididymis
with torsion

---

varic/o/cele
varicocele
VAIR ih koh seel

12.31 Herniation of the veins within the spermatic cord is a condition known as **varicocele.** It is a constructed term that uses the combining form for dilated vein, *varic/o*, and can be written _____/__/_____. A _____ is caused by failure of the valves within the veins, allowing blood to pool and dilate the veins.

PRACTICE: Diseases and Disorders of the Male Reproductive System

The Right Match

Match the term on the left with the correct definition on the right.

_____ 1. benign prostatic hyperplasia

_____ 2. erectile dysfunction

_____ 3. Peyronie disease

_____ 4. priapism

_____ 5. phimosis

_____ 6. testicular torsion

a. the inability to achieve an erection sufficient to perform sexual intercourse

b. an abnormally persistent erection of the penis

c. reduced blood flow to the testis due to a twisted spermatic cord

d. enlargement of the prostate gland that constricts the urethra

e. a hardness of the erectile tissue within the penis

f. a congenital narrowing of the prepuce

Linkup

Link the word parts in the list to create the terms that match the definitions. You may use word parts more than once. Remember to add combining vowels when needed—and that some terms do not use any combining vowel. The first one is completed as an example.

Combining Form	Suffix
andr/o	-pathy
balan/o	-itis
epididym/o	-cele
hydr/o	
varic/o	

	Definition	Term
1.	a disease that afflicts only males	*andropathy*
2.	inflammation of the glans penis	
3.	inflammation of the epididymis	
4.	fluid accumulation in the scrotum	
5.	herniation of the veins within the spermatic cord	

Treatments, Procedures, and Devices of the Male Reproductive System

Here are the word parts that specifically apply to the treatments, procedures, and devices of the male reproductive system that are covered in the following section. Note that the word parts are color-coded to help you identify them: prefixes are green, combining forms are red, and suffixes are blue.

Prefix	Definition	Combining Form	Definition	Suffix	Definition
anti-	against, opposite of	balan/o	glans penis	-al	pertaining to
		cyst/o	bladder, sac	-cele	hernia, swelling, protrusion
poly-	excessive, over, many	hydr/o	water	-ectomy	surgical excision, removal
		orchi/o, orchid/o	testis	-logy	study or science of
trans-	through, across, beyond	prostat/o	prostate gland	-pexy	surgical fixation, suspension
		urethr/o	urethra	-plasty	surgical repair
		ur/o	urine	-stomy	surgical creation of an opening
		vas/o	vessel		
		vesicul/o	small bag	-tomy	incision, to cut

KEY TERMS A–Z

anti-impotence therapy
an tye IM poh tens * THAIR ah pee

12.32 A collection of therapies that address erectile dysfunction (Frame 12.23) is called **anti-impotence therapy.** _____ _____ includes drugs such as sildenafil (Viagra) or implantation of a penile implant (Frame 12.40).

balanoplasty
BAL ah noh plass tee

12.33 The suffix that means "surgical repair" is -*plasty*. The surgical repair of the glans penis is therefore called _____. The constructed form of this term is balan/o/plasty.

circumcision
ser kum SIH zhun

12.34 A common, routine procedure in many parts of the world is the removal of the prepuce. Known as **circumcision** after the circular cut that is made around the base of the glans penis, it is usually performed within hours after birth. Alternate procedures of _____ are illustrated in Figure 12.8■.

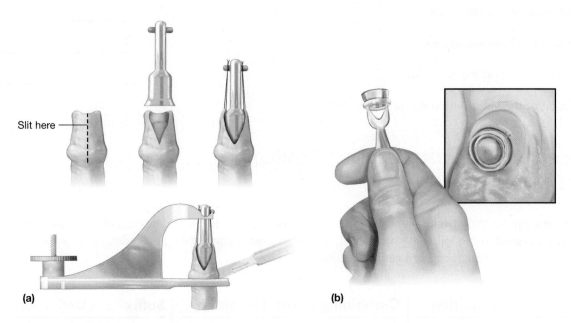

Slit here

(a)

(b)

Figure 12.8 ■
Circumcision. Alternate procedures may be used with the common goal of removing the prepuce from the penis. (a) Use of the Yellen clamp, in which a cone is inserted over the glans and clamped in place, followed by the excision of the prepuce. (b) Use of the PlastiBell, which is inserted over the glans and the prepuce cut away. The plastic rim remains in place for three to four days until healing occurs, then falls away.

digital rectal examination

12.35 A **digital rectal examination** is a physical exam that involves the insertion of a finger into the rectum to feel the size and shape of the prostate gland through the wall of the rectum (Figure 12.9■). A _____ _____ _____ is used to screen the patient for BPH (Frame 12.20) and prostate cancer (Frame 12.28), and is abbreviated **DRE.**

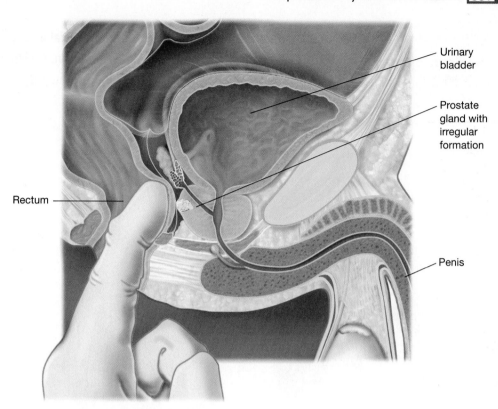

Urinary bladder

Prostate gland with irregular formation

Rectum

Penis

Figure 12.9 ■
Digital rectal exam (DRE). The physician's index finger is inserted into the rectum and pressed against the prostate gland as a test for BPH and prostate cancer.

hydrocelectomy HIGH droh see LEK toh mee	**12.36** Recall that the suffix -*ectomy* means "surgical excision, removal." The surgical removal of a hydrocele (Frame 12.24) is a procedure called _____. The constructed form of this term is written hydr/o/cel/ectomy.
orchidectomy OR kid EK toh mee	**12.37** The surgical removal of a testis is called _____, or **orchiectomy**. A bilateral **orchidectomy** is commonly called **castration** (kass TRAY shun).
orchidopexy or KID oh pek see	**12.38** Surgical fixation of a testis is sometimes required to draw an undescended testis into the scrotum. The procedure is called _____, or **orchiopexy**, because the suffix -*pexy* means "surgical fixation, suspension." The constructed form of **orchidopexy** reveals three word parts and is written orchid/o/pexy.
orchidoplasty OR kid oh PLASS tee orchid/o/tomy	**12.39** A general term for a surgical repair of a testis is _____, or **orchidoplasty**. An incision into the testis is a form of **orchidoplasty** and is called **orchidotomy** (OR kid OTT oh mee). The constructed form of the term *orchidotomy* is written _____/__/_____. Similar to other terms of the testis, an alternate term for orchidotomy is **orchiotomy** (OR kee OTT oh mee).

penile implants
PEE nile * IM plants

12.40 A **penile implant** is the surgical insertion of a prosthesis, or artificial device, to correct erectile dysfunction. Optional _____ _____ include semirigid rods and inflatable balloonlike cylinders (Figure 12.10■).

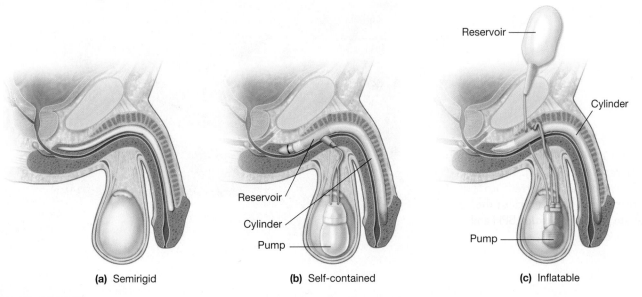

(a) Semirigid   (b) Self-contained   (c) Inflatable

Figure 12.10 ■

Penile implants. (a) Semirigid rods may be surgically implanted into the penis, which provides a partial erection that is persistent. (b) Inflatable cylinders implanted into the penis may be self-contained, producing an erection when the pump is activated by physical contact. (c) Inflatable cylinders may alternatively include a pump that requires a more directed hand pumping action to activate.

prostatectomy
pross tah TEK toh mee

12.41 The surgical removal of the prostate gland is a procedure called _____. This constructed term is written prostat/ectomy. It is a treatment for BPH (Frame 12.20) and prostate cancer (Frame 12.28). During a suprapubic prostatectomy, the prostate gland is removed through an abdominal incision made above the pubic bone and a second incision through the urinary bladder wall. The second incision is called a **prostatocystotomy** (pross TAH toh siss TOTT oh mee).

prostate-specific antigen
PROSS tayt * speh SIH fik * AN tih jenn

12.42 A **prostate-specific antigen** is a clinical test that measures levels of the protein, prostate-specific antigen, in the blood. _____-_____ _____ is commonly called **PSA.** Elevated levels suggest a possible presence of prostate cancer and indicate a need for additional tests before a diagnosis can be made.

transurethral resection of the prostate gland

trans you REE thrall

12.43 Transurethral resection of the prostate gland is a procedure that treats BPH (Frame 12.20) through the noninvasive removal of prostate tissue (Figure 12.11■). It involves the scraping of the urethral section of prostate tissue using a specialized endoscope, called a resectoscope. The resectoscope is inserted through the urethra to the prostate wall, where it scrapes the capsule (outer covering) of the prostate while as much inner tissue is left intact as possible. _____ _____ _____ _____ _____ _____

is abbreviated **TURP.** *Transurethral* is a constructed term that can be written as trans/urethr/al.

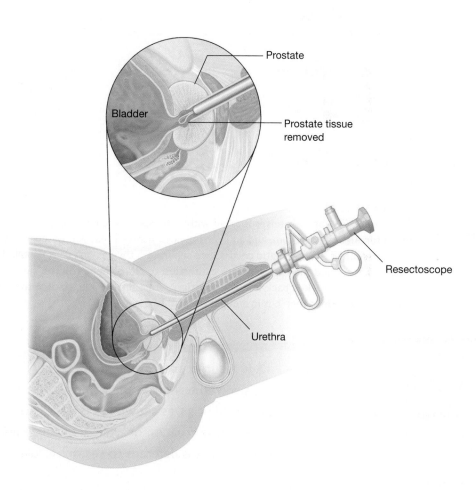

Figure 12.11 ■
Transurethral resection of the prostate (TURP). As a treatment for BPH, part of the prostate gland is removed in this procedure to reduce the pressure against the urethra, allowing for a less restricted flow of urine.

urology

yoo RAHL oh jee

12.44 The department within a hospital or clinic that treats urinary tract problems (in both sexes) is called **urology.** The constructed form of _____ is written ur/o/logy. A specialist in this field is a **urologist** (yoo RAHL oh jist). Male reproductive conditions are also treated by a urologist.

vasectomy

vas EK toh mee

12.45 A male can elect to become **sterile,** or unable to produce and ejaculate sperm, by undergoing a **vasectomy.** This constructed term literally means "surgical removal of vessel," where the "vessel" is the vas deferens. It is a simple, quick procedure in which the vas deferens is severed to block the flow of sperm during ejaculation (Figure 12.12■). A _____ does not affect a man's ability to ejaculate (the fluid is a spermless semen) or his experience of sexual pleasure. *Vasectomy* is a constructed term with two word parts, written vas/ectomy.

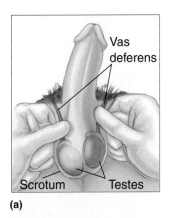
(a)

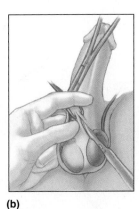
(b)

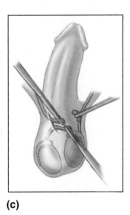
(c)

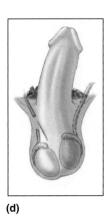
(d)

Figure 12.12 ■
Vasectomy. (a) Vas deferens is located within the spermatic cord on both sides. (b) A small incision is made through the scrotum, and an instrument is inserted that gently separates the vas deferens from other tissues of the spermatic cord. Once separated, the vas deferens is pulled out gently. (c) The vas deferens is cut and the exposed ends cauterized to close them. (d) The vas deferens is returned to the spermatic cord, tucked back into the scrotum, and a single suture closes the incision. The vas deferens on the other side is then cut in a duplicate procedure.

vasovasostomy

VAS oh vah SOSS toh mee

12.46 A surgery to reverse a vasectomy is known as a **vasovasostomy.** This constructed term uses the combining form for "vessel" twice and contains five word parts, as shown in vas/o/vas/o/stomy. A _____ involves the creation of artificial openings and reconnection of the severed ends of the vas deferens to restore fertility.

vesiculectomy

veh SIK yoo LEK toh mee

12.47 A procedure to remove the seminal vesicles is called a _____. The constructed form of this term is vesicul/ectomy.

PRACTICE: Treatments, Procedures, and Devices of the Male Reproductive System

The Right Match

Match the term on the left with the correct definition on the right.

_____ 1. anti-impotence therapy

_____ 2. circumcision

_____ 3. penile implant

_____ 4. prostate-specific antigen

_____ 5. urology

a. the removal of the prepuce

b. blood protein that is measured in the PSA test

c. a collection of therapies that address erectile dysfunction

d. department that treats urinary tract problems

e. surgical insertion of a prosthesis to correct erectile dysfunction

Break the Chain

Analyze these medical terms:

    a) Separate each term into its word parts; each word part is labeled for you (**p** = prefix, **r** = root, **cf** = combining form, and **s** = suffix).

    b) For the Bonus Question, write the requested definition in the blank that follows.

1. a) vasectomy   _____/_____
                                     r   s

    b) *Bonus Question:* Which vessel does the word root refer to in this procedural term? _____

2. a) hydrocelectomy   _____/___/_____/_____
                                       cf   s   s

    b) *Bonus Question:* What is the definition of the first suffix? _____

3. a) orchidopexy   _____/___/_____
                                       cf   s

    b) *Bonus Question:* What is the definition of the combining form? _____

4. a) prostatectomy   _____/_____
                                     r   s

    b) *Bonus Question:* What is the definition of the suffix? _____

5. a) vasovasostomy   _____/___/_____/___/_____
                                     cf   cf   s

    b) *Bonus Question:* What is the definition of the suffix? _____

Signs and Symptoms of the Female Reproductive System

Here are the word parts that specifically apply to the signs and symptoms of the female reproductive system that are covered in the following section. Note that the word parts are color-coded to help you identify them: prefixes are green, combining forms are red, and suffixes are blue.

Prefix	Definition
a-	without, absence of
dys-	bad, abnormal, painful, difficult
poly-	excessive, over, many

Combining Form	Definition
colp/o	vagina
hemat/o	blood
hydr/o	water
leuk/o	white
mamm/o	breast
mast/o	breast
men/o	month, menstruation
metr/o	uterus
olig/o	few in number
py/o	pus
salping/o	trumpet

Suffix	Definition
-algia	condition of pain
-dynia	condition of pain
-rrhagia	abnormal discharge
-rrhea	discharge
-salpinx	trumpet

KEY TERMS A–Z

amenorrhea
ay MEN oh REE ah

12.48 The absence of a menstrual discharge in a woman of childbearing age is a symptom of reproductive disease. It is called **amenorrhea.** Its constructed form is written a/men/o/rrhea. _____ literally means "without menstrual discharge." The term **menorrhea** (MEN oh REE ah) is used to describe a normal discharge.

colpodynia
KOL poh DIN ee ah

colp/o/**rrhagia**

12.49 The combining form *colp/o* means "vagina." Attaching the suffix meaning "condition of pain" creates the term _____, which is the symptom of vaginal pain. Similarly, adding the suffix meaning "abnormal discharge" produces the term **colporrhagia** (KOL poh RAJ ee ah), which is the symptom of profuse vaginal bleeding. Colporrhagia is a constructed term that is represented as _____/__/_____.

dysmenorrhea
DISS men oh REE ah

12.50 Dysmenorrhea is the symptom of abnormal pain during menstruation. The constructed form of this term is dys/men/o/rrhea. Because the prefix *dys-* means "bad, abnormal, painful, difficult," the term _____ literally means "bad, abnormal, painful, or difficult menstruation discharge."

hematosalpinx
HEE mah toh SAL pinks

12.51 The Greek word *salpinx* means "trumpet" and is used to form terms associated with the fallopian tubes due to their trumpetlike appearance. In the term _____, the combining form for blood, *hemat/o*, is added for the condition of retained menstrual blood in a fallopian tube. The constructed form of the term is written hemat/o/salpinx.

hydrosalpinx
HIGH droh SAL pinks

12.52 Fluid accumulation is another symptom of a disease associated with a fallopian tube. Called _____, it is usually a symptom of an inflammation within the fallopian tube, called salpingitis (Frame 12.80). The constructed form of this term is hydr/o/salpinx.

WORDS TO WATCH OUT FOR

▶▶▶▶▶ *salping* or *-salpinx*?

The term for fallopian tube is the word root *salping*, which is derived from the Greek word that means "trumpet" because of the resemblance of its shape to that of the musical instrument. The combining form of the term is *salping/o*. When it is used as a suffix, the ending is changed to form *-salpinx*.

leukorrhea
LOO koh REE ah

12.53 The term **leukorrhea** literally means "white discharge." It is a white or yellow discharge from the vagina, which is a sign of infection. The constructed form of _____ is written leuk/o/rrhea.

mastalgia
mass TAL jee ah

12.54 A combining form for breast is mast/o, which is derived from the Greek word for breast, *mastos*. A condition of pain in the breast is called _____. The constructed form is mast/algia.

menorrhagia
men oh RAY jee ah

men/o/metr/o/rrhagia

12.55 Recall that the suffix *-rrhagia* means "abnormal discharge." The sign of profuse bleeding during menstruation is called _____. The constructed form is written men/o/rrhagia, which uses the combining form that means "month, menstruation," *men/o*. If the combining form for uterus is used instead, the meaning changes. Thus, **metrorrhagia** (METT roh RAY jee ah) is "abnormal discharge from the uterus." When both combining forms are used, as in **menometrorrhagia** (MEN oh METT roh RAY jee ah), the meaning becomes "abnormal discharge from the uterus during and between menstrual periods." The constructed form of *menometrorrhagia* reveals five word parts and is written _____/__/_____/__/_____.

mittelschmerz
MIT ehl shmerts

12.56 The term for the symptom of abdominal pain occurring during ovulation is a German word, **mittelschmerz**. _____ occurs when bleeding from ovulation irritates the peritoneum.

oligomenorrhea ALL ih goh men oh REE ah	**12.57** An abnormally reduced discharge during menstruation may also be a sign of reproductive disease. It is called _____. The constructed form is written olig/o/men/o/rrhea.
pyosalpinx pye oh SAL pinks	**12.58** The combining form that means "pus" is *py/o*, and the combining form for fallopian tube is *salping/o*. Therefore, the discharge of pus from a fallopian tube is called _____. It is a sign of an infection. The constructed form is written py/o/salpinx and literally means "trumpet pus."

PRACTICE: Signs and Symptoms of the Female Reproductive System

Linkup

Link the word parts in the list to create the terms that match the definitions. You may use word parts more than once. Remember to add combining vowels when needed—and that some terms do not use any combining vowel.

Prefix	Combining Form	Suffix
a-	colp/o	-algia
	hemat/o	-dynia
	mast/o	-rrhagia
	men/o	-rrhea
	olig/o	
	salping/o	

Definition | **Term**

1. absence of menstrual discharge in a woman of childbearing age _____

2. vaginal pain _____

3. condition of pain in the breast _____

4. profuse discharge during menstruation _____

5. blood in a fallopian tube _____

6. abnormally reduced menstrual discharge _____

Diseases and Disorders of the Female Reproductive System

Review some of the word parts that specifically apply to the diseases and disorders of the female reproductive system that are covered in the following section. Note that the word parts are color-coded to help you identify them: prefixes are green, combining forms are red, and suffixes are blue.

Prefix	Definition
a-	without, absence of
endo-	within
ex-	outside, away from
poly-	excessive, over, many
pre-	to come before

Combining Form	Definition
cervic/o	neck, cervix
colp/o	vagina
cyst/o	bladder, sac
fibr/o	fiber
hyster/o	uterus
lei/o	smooth
mamm/o	breast
mast/o	breast
metr/i, metr/o	uterus
my/o	muscle
oophor/o	ovary
ovar/o	ovary
rect/o	rectum
salping/o	trumpet
vagin/o	sheath, vagina
vesic/o	bladder
vulv/o	vulva

Suffix	Definition
-al	pertaining to
-atresia	closure or absence of a normal body opening
-cele	hernia, swelling, protrusion
-ia	condition of
-ic	pertaining to
-itis	inflammation
-oma	tumor
-osis	condition of
-pathy	disease
-ptosis	drooping
-s	plural

KEY TERMS A–Z

amastia
ay MASS tee ah

poly/mast/ia

12.59 Recall that a combining form for breast is *mast/o*. The term that means "condition of without breast" is _____. Although the areola and nipple are present, the lack of breast tissue results in this condition. In the condition **polymastia** (pahl ee MASS tee ah), the individual has more than two elevated areas on the chest or abdomen with areola and nipple. The constructed form of this term is _____/_____/___.

breast cancer

12.60 A malignant tumor arising from breast tissue is known as
_____ _____. The most common form
is called **infiltrating ductal carcinoma,** abbreviated **IDC** (Figure 12.13■).

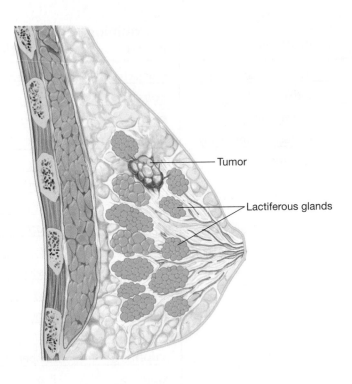

Tumor

Lactiferous glands

Figure 12.13 ■
Breast cancer. Notice the tumor growing within a lactiferous gland, which occurs in infiltrating ductal carcinoma.

carcinoma in situ
  kar sih NOH mah * in * SIGH tyoo

12.61 A form of cervical cancer arises from cells of the cervix, which change in appearance before developing into a spreading malignancy. It is called **carcinoma in situ (CIS) of the cervix** (Figure 12.14■). The change in cells is a process called **dysplasia.** There is evidence that exposure to HPV (Frame 12.136) may increase the risk of developing _____ _____ _____.

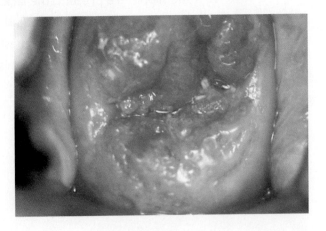

Figure 12.14 ■
Carcinoma in situ (CIS) of the cervix. Photograph of the cervix as seen during a gynecological exam. The reddish tissue is inflamed and indicative of carcinoma in situ of the cervix.
Source: Courtesy of the Centers for Disease Control.

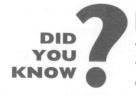

▶▶▶▶▶ **in situ**

The term *in situ* (pronounced in * SIGH tyoo) is a Latin phrase that literally means "in site." Its use in modern medicine refers to confinement to a site of origin. Carcinoma in situ describes a tumor that is confined to its organ of origin, rather than a metastatic tumor in a secondary site.

cervical cancer
SER vih kal * KANN ser

12.62 A malignant tumor of the cervix is known as _____ _____ (Figure 12.15■). The most common form is a squamous cell carcinoma, arising from the epithelial cells lining the opening into the uterus. It is called **cervical intraepithelial neoplasia** (SER vih kal * in trah ep ih THEE lee al * nee oh PLAY zee ah), or **CIN.** A smaller percentage, about 20%, are adenocarcinomas, arising from the underlying glandular tissue. In 2011, an estimated 11,200 women were diagnosed in the United States, and roughly 3,400 died of the disease. It is hoped that the vaccine against HPV may reduce the incidences of cervical cancer.

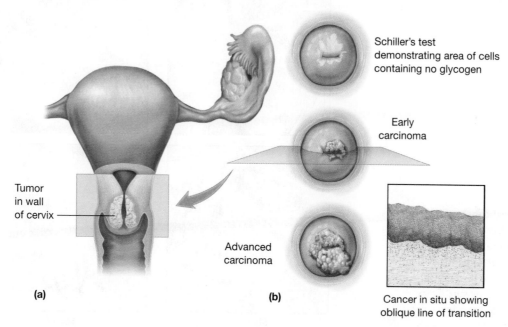

Schiller's test demonstrating area of cells containing no glycogen

Early carcinoma

Advanced carcinoma

Tumor in wall of cervix

Cancer in situ showing oblique line of transition

(a)   (b)

Figure 12.15 ■
Cervical cancer (a) Top view of the uterus showing the presence of a tumor in the wall of the cervix. (b) Three successive stages in the development of cervical cancer, as seen through a gynecological exam. The insert shows a histological exam revealing the tumor and how it differs from normal tissue that borders it.

cervicitis
SER vih SIGH tiss

endo/cervic/itis

12.63 Inflammation of the cervix is a condition known as _____. The constructed form of this term is written cervic/itis. The most common form of cervicitis occurs when the inner lining of the cervix becomes inflamed. It is called **endocervicitis** (EHN doh ser vih SIGH tiss). The constructed form is written _____/_____/_____.

cystocele
SISS toh seel

endometrial cancer
ehn doh MEE tree al * KANN ser

12.64 A protrusion of the urinary bladder against the wall of the vagina may occur if the attachments between the two organs weaken. It is called a **cystocele,** which is a constructed term written cyst/o/cele. A large _____ may affect urinary bladder function. Similarly, a **rectocele** (REK toh seel) is a protrusion of the rectum against the wall of the vagina. This constructed term is written rect/o/cele.

12.65 A malignant tumor arising from the endometrial tissue lining the uterus is called _____ _____. The four stages of endometrial cancer are illustrated in Figure 12.16■. Most endometrial cancers arise from the glandular cells of the endometrium and are therefore called adenocarcinomas. Nearly 40,000 new cases occurred in 2011 with roughly 7,000 deaths.

Stage I
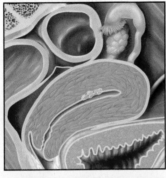

Stage II
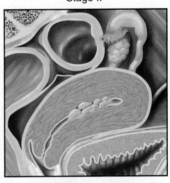

Stage III
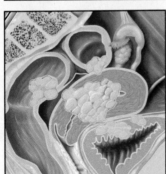

Stage IV
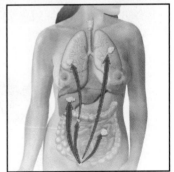

Figure 12.16 ■
Stages of endometrial cancer. Stage I: Mutated cells arise from glandular epithelium of the endometrium to form a tumor. Stage II: Tumor expands within the uterine cavity. Stage III: Tumor metastasizes to nearby organs. Stage IV: Metastasis progresses to form secondary tumors throughout the body.

endometriosis
EHN doh mee tree OH siss

12.66 The abnormal growth of endometrial tissue may occur throughout areas of the pelvic cavity, including the external walls of the uterus, fallopian tubes, urinary bladder, and even on the peritoneum. The condition is called **endometriosis.** This constructed term is written endo/metr/i/osis, which literally means "condition of within the uterus." Because endometrial tissue responds to hormonal changes by undergoing the cyclic bleeding and proliferation of menstruation, the unwanted tissue located outside the uterus that forms in _____ performs in the same manner, resulting in scarring, adhesions, and pelvic pain.

endometritis
EHN doh meh TRY tiss

12.67 Inflammation of the endometrium is a condition called _____. It is usually caused by bacterial infection. The constructed form of this term is written endo/metr/itis.

fibrocystic breast disease
figh broh SISS tik

12.68 In the condition **fibrocystic breast disease,** one or more benign, fibrous cysts develop within the breast. _____ _____ _____ is an inherited condition that has no known association with breast cancer. The term *fibrocystic* is a constructed term that can be written as fibr/o/cyst/ic.

fistulas
FISS tyoo lahs

12.69 A **fistula** is an abnormal passage from one organ or cavity to another (Figure 12.17■). Two major types of vaginal _____ may occur. A **rectovaginal** (rek toh VAJ ih nal) **fistula** occurs between the vagina and rectum, and a **vesicovaginal** (vess ih koh VAJ ih nal) **fistula** is located between the urinary bladder and the vagina.

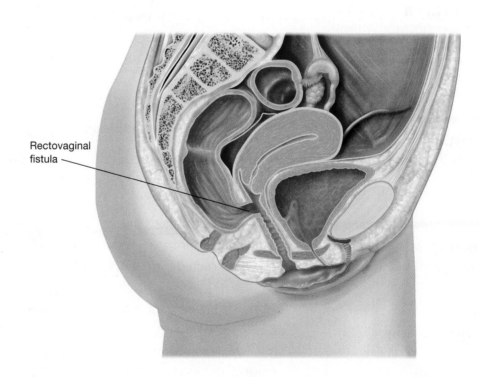

Rectovaginal fistula

Figure 12.17 ■
Rectovaginal fistula. It is an abnormal passageway between the rectum and vagina.

hysteratresia
hiss ter ah TREE zee ah

12.70 The suffix *-atresia* means "closure or absence of a normal body opening." Adding this suffix to the word root for uterus forms the term _____, which means a closure of the uterus. The closure results in an abnormal obstruction within the uterine canal that may interfere with childbirth. The constructed form of this term is written hyster/atresia.

leiomyoma
lye oh my OH mah

12.71 The muscular wall of the uterus is the origin of benign tumors known as **leiomyomas**. Also known as **fibroid tumors** because of their tough, fibrous structure, their presence can produce abnormal pain during menstruation (Figure 12.18■). _____ is a constructed term written as lei/o/my/oma, which literally means "tumor of smooth muscle."

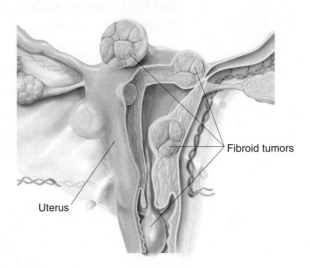

Fibroid tumors

Uterus

Figure 12.18 ■
Fibroid tumors, or leiomyomas. Fibroids develop from the uterus to form a variety of hard, round benign structures.

mastitis
mass TYE tiss

12.72 Inflammation of the breast is a condition known as _____. It is often caused by bacterial infection of the lactiferous ducts within breast tissue. The constructed form of this term is written mast/itis.

mastoptosis
mass top TOH siss

12.73 The suffix -ptosis means "drooping." A breast that is abnormally pendulous or drooping is the condition known as _____. The constructed form of this term is mast/o/ptosis.

oophoropathy
oh OFF or OPP ah thee

oophoritis
oh OFF or EYE tiss

12.74 A combining form that means "ovary" is oophor/o. Any disease of an ovary is known as _____. An example of an oophoropathy is inflammation of an ovary, which is called _____. This constructed term is written oophor/itis. Inflammation of an ovary and fallopian tube is called **oophorosalpingitis** (oh OFF or oh sal pinj EYE tiss). This term is also constructed of word parts and can be written as oophor/o/salping/itis.

ovarian cancer
oh VAIR ee an * KANN ser

12.75 Aside from breast cancer (Frame 12.60), the most lethal form of reproductive cancer in women is **ovarian cancer.** Older women and women who have not given birth are at higher risk, and there is some evidence for a genetic link. The incidences of _____ _____ in 2011 were about 22,000 new diagnoses and roughly 15,000 deaths.

ovarian cyst
oh VAIR ee an * sist

12.76 A cyst is a fluid-filled sac that forms within the body from mutated cells. An _____ _____ is a cyst on an ovary that is usually benign and asymptomatic, although in some cases it may cause pelvic pain and dysmenorrhea (Frame 12.50). The term **polycystic ovary syndrome** is quite different. It is a hormonal disturbance characterized by lack of ovulation (called anovulation), amenorrhea (Frame 12.48), and infertility. Numerous ovarian cysts may develop, sometimes increasing the size of the ovary dramatically. If cyst development spreads into the fallopian tube, the condition is called **parovarian cyst** (par oh VAIR ee an * sist).

pelvic inflammatory disease

12.77 An inflammation involving some or all of the female organs within the pelvic cavity is called **pelvic inflammatory disease,** abbreviated **PID.** It is usually caused by bacterial infection that spreads from organ to organ. Complications of _____ _____ _____ include obstruction of the fallopian tubes and infertility.

premenstrual syndrome
pre MEN stroo al * SIN drohm

12.78 Premenstrual syndrome is a collection of symptoms, including nervous tension, irritability, breast pain (mastalgia, Frame 12.54), edema, and headache, which usually occur during the ten days preceding menstruation. _____ _____ is abbreviated **PMS.**

prolapsed uterus

12.79 The uterus is suspended in the pelvic cavity by ligaments. If these ligaments weaken, often due to a congenital deformity or trauma, the uterus may become displaced to droop downward into the vagina. The condition is called **prolapsed uterus,** and in some cases it may even fall completely within the vagina (Figure 12.19■). Another term for _____ _____ is **hysteroptosis** (HISS ter op TOH siss), which is a constructed term that is written hyster/o/ptosis.

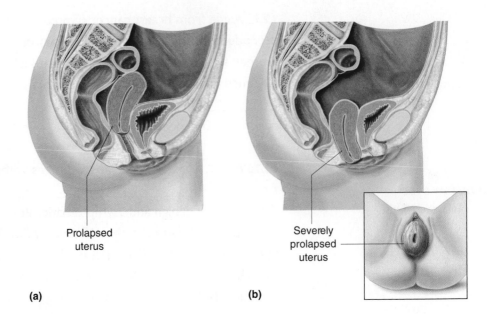

Figure 12.19 ■
Prolapsed uterus. (a) A prolapse is the abnormal drop of the uterus into the vagina, representing the most common type of uterine displacement. It is usually caused by weakened uterine ligaments.
(b) A severely prolapsed uterus may extend through the vaginal orifice, as shown.

Prolapsed uterus

Severely prolapsed uterus

(a) (b)

salpingitis sal pin JYE tiss	12.80 Inflammation of a fallopian tube is called _____. The constructed form of this term is salping/itis. It is usually caused by bacterial infection and is often associated with **PID** (Frame 12.77).
salpingocele sal PING goh seel	12.81 A protrusion, or herniation, of a fallopian tube wall is known as _____. The constructed form is salping/o/cele.
toxic shock syndrome	12.82 **Toxic shock syndrome,** or **TSS,** is a severe bacterial infection characterized by a sudden high fever, skin rash, mental confusion, acute renal failure, and abnormal liver function. _____ _____ _____ is caused by a type of *Staphylococcus* and is most common in menstruating women using noncotton tampons.
vaginitis vaj ih NYE tiss	12.83 Inflammation of the vagina is known as _____. Because *colp/o* is an alternate combining form for vagina, it is also called **colpitis** (kol PYE tiss). In a common form known as **atrophic vaginitis** (ay TROH fik * vaj ih NYE tiss), the usual symptoms of redness and swelling are accompanied by thinning of the vaginal wall and loss of moisture, usually due to a depletion of estrogen.
vulvitis vul VYE tiss **vulv/o/vagin/itis**	12.84 Inflammation of the external genitals, or vulva, is called _____. When the vagina is also inflamed, the condition is known as **vulvovaginitis** (VUL voh vaj ih NYE tiss). The constructed form of this term is written _____/__/_____/____.

PRACTICE: Diseases and Disorders of the Female Reproductive System

The Right Match

Match the term on the left with the correct definition on the right.

_____ 1. breast cancer

_____ 2. carcinoma in situ

_____ 3. cervical cancer

_____ 4. fibrocystic breast disease

_____ 5. fistula

_____ 6. ovarian cancer

_____ 7. ovarian cyst

_____ 8. pelvic inflammatory disease

_____ 9. premenstrual syndrome

_____ 10. prolapsed uterus

_____ 11. toxic shock syndrome

a. a malignant tumor of the cervix

b. the most common form is infiltrating ductal carcinoma

c. a form of cervical cancer

d. a common form of reproductive cancer in women

e. a condition in which one or more benign, fibrous cysts develop within the breast

f. an abnormal passage from one hollow organ to another

g. inflammation that involves some or all of the female organs within the pelvic cavity

h. a severe bacterial infection

i. a fluid-filled sac on an ovary

j. collection of symptoms that occur during the ten days preceding menstruation

k. displacement of the uterus into the vagina

Break the Chain

Analyze these medical terms:
   a) Separate each term into its word parts; each word part is labeled for you (**p** = prefix, **r** = root, **cf** = combining form, and **s** = suffix).
   b) For the Bonus Question, write the requested words or definition in the blank that follows.

1. a) vulvitis   _____/_____
                              r   s

   b) *Bonus Question:* What is the definition of the word root? _____

2. a) salpingocele   _____/___/_____
                                   cf   s

   b) *Bonus Question:* What anatomical part does the combining form refer to? _____

3. a) amastia   _____/_____/_____
                              p   r   s

   b) *Bonus Question:* What is the definition of the word root? _____

4. a) endometriosis   _____/_____/___/_____
                              p   cf   s

   b) *Bonus Question:* What is the definition of the prefix? _____

5. a) leiomyoma   _____/___/_____/_____
                              cf   r   s

   b) *Bonus Question:* What is the definition of the combining form? _____

Treatments, Procedures, and Devices of the Female Reproductive System

Here are the word parts that specifically apply to the treatments, procedures, and devices of the female reproductive system that are covered in the following section. Note that the word parts are color-coded to help you identify them: prefixes are green, combining forms are red, and suffixes are blue.

Prefix	Definition
endo-	within
trans-	through, across, beyond

Combining Form	Definition
cervic/o	neck, cervix
colp/o	vagina
episi/o	vulva
gyn/o, gynec/o	woman
hyster/o	uterus
lapar/o	abdomen
mamm/o	breast
mast/o	breast
metr/i	uterus
oophor/o	ovary
path/o	disease
salping/o	trumpet
son/o	sound
vagin/o	sheath, vagina
vulv/o	vulva

Suffix	Definition
-al	pertaining to
-ectomy	surgical excision, removal
-gram	a record or image
-graphy	recording process
-ic	pertaining to
-logist	one who studies
-logy	study or science of
-pexy	surgical fixation, suspension
-plasty	surgical repair
-rrhaphy	suturing
-scopy	process of viewing
-stomy	surgical creation of an opening
-tomy	incision, to cut

KEY TERMS A–Z

biopsy
BYE op see

12.85 A minor surgical procedure that involves the surgical extraction of tissue for microscopic analysis is called a _____. Abbreviated **bx** or **Bx,** the sample may be removed from the cervix, endometrium, or breast. Any one of several procedures may be used, including excision, aspiration, or needle biopsy (Figure 12.20■).

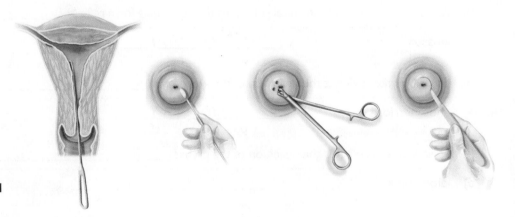

Figure 12.20 ■
Biopsy. Various forms of gynecological biopsy are shown.

cervicectomy
SER vih SEK toh mee

12.86 To remove precancerous or cancerous tissue from the cervix, the anterior part of the cervix can be removed in a **cervical conization** (SER vih kal * koh nih ZAY shun). In this procedure, a cone-shaped section of the cervix is removed. If the cancer is developed, the cervix may be removed in a _____. The constructed form of this term is written cervic/ectomy.

colpectomy
kol PEK toh mee

12.87 Recall that a word root for vagina is colp. Removal of the vagina is a surgery called a _____, or alternatively called **vaginectomy** (VAJ ih NEK toh mee).

colpoplasty
KOL poh plass tee

colporrhaphy
kol POR ah fee

colp/o/**scopy**

12.88 Surgical repair of the vagina is a procedure called _____. This constructed term may be written as colp/o/plasty. A colpoplasty often includes suturing the wall of the vagina in a procedure called _____. Also a constructed term, it is written colp/o/rrhaphy. Both procedures often follow an endoscopic evaluation of the vagina, called a **colposcopy.** This constructed term is written _____/__/_____.

dilation and curettage
dye LAY shun * and * koo reh TAZH

12.89 A common procedure that is used for both diagnostic and treatment purposes is called **dilation and curettage,** abbreviated **D&C.** During a _____ _____ _____, the cervix is dilated to permit the insertion of a spoon-shaped instrument called a **curette,** which is used to scrape the lining of the endometrium. It is often performed to control bleeding, obtain a tissue sample for biopsy, or remove polyps.

endometrial ablation
ehn doh MEE tree al * ahb LAY shun

12.90 If the endometrium requires more treatment than can be provided by a D&C, an **endometrial ablation** may be applied. In an _____ _____, lasers, electricity, or heat may be used to destroy the endometrium. The procedure is effective in treating dysmenorrhea (Frame 12.50).

gynecology
GYE neh KOL oh jee

gynopathology
GYE no path ALL oh jee

12.91 Two combining forms that mean "woman" are *gynec/o* and *gyn/o*. The branch of medicine focusing on women is known as _____, abbreviated **GYN**. The constructed form of this term is *gynec/o/logy*. Frequently, a physician known as an **obstetrician-gynecologist** combines these two areas of expertise; this is abbreviated **OB/GYN**. Also, the study of diseases that afflict women is known as _____. As a constructed term, it is written *gyn/o/path/o/logy*. A physician specializing in this field of medicine is called a **gynopathologist** (GYE no path ALL oh jist).

hormone replacement therapy

12.92 As a common therapy for hormonal management, **hormone replacement therapy**, abbreviated **HRT,** can be very effective in correcting disrupted menstrual and ovarian cycles. In _____ _____ _____, the hormones estrogen and progesterone are frequently prescribed in pill form. It is also the most effective means of **female contraception** for the prevention of unwanted pregnancy.

hysterectomy
HISS teh REK toh mee

12.93 The surgical removal of the uterus is commonly called _____. The surgery may involve surrounding structures, as shown in Figure 12.21■.

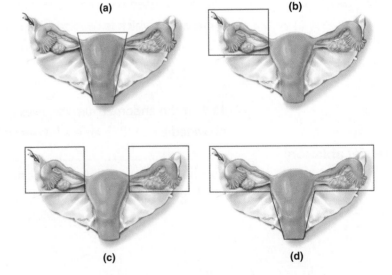

(a) (b) (c) (d)

Figure 12.21 ■
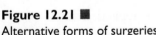
Alternative forms of surgeries involving the uterus, ovaries, and fallopian tubes. The solid lines indicate excision.
(a) Hysterectomy.
(b) Right salpingo-oophorectomy.
(c) Bilateral salpingo-oophorectomy.
(d) Bilateral hysterosalpingo-oophorectomy, or panhysterectomy.

hysteropexy
HISS ter oh PEK see

12.94 The surgical procedure that may be used to correct a prolapsed uterus (Frame 12.79) by strengthening its connections to the abdominal wall to correct its position is called _____. This constructed term is written *hyster/o/pexy* and means "surgical fixation of the uterus."

WORDS TO WATCH OUT FOR ❗

▶▶▶▶▶ *-pexy* **or** *-plasty*?

The meanings of these two suffixes both relate to surgery—but they are very different forms of surgery. Remember that *-pexy* means "surgical *fixation, suspension*," and *-plasty* means "surgical *repair*." One way to remember the meaning of *-pexy* is that it uses an *x*, as does the word *fixation* in its definition. Similarly, a way to remember the meaning of *-plasty* is that it uses a *p*, as does the word *repair* in its definition.

hysteroscopy
HISS ter OSS koh pee

laparoscopy
lap ahr OSS koh pee

12.95 A noninvasive diagnostic technique that uses a modified endoscope, called a **hysteroscope** (HISS ter oh skope), to evaluate the uterine cavity is called _____. The constructed form is hyster/o/scopy. To evaluate the external appearance of the uterus and other organs of the pelvic cavity, a **laparoscope** (LAP ahr oh skope) is inserted through a small incision through the lower abdominal wall during a _____. The procedure is shown in Figure 12.22■. This is also a constructed term, written as lapar/o/scopy (the word root *lapar* means "abdomen").

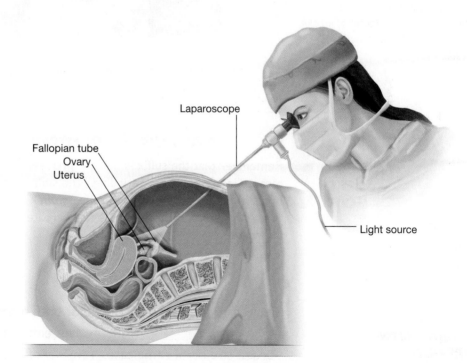

Figure 12.22 ■
Laparoscopy. A lighted endoscope specialized for insertion into the abdomen, called a laparoscope, is used to view reproductive organs. The laparoscope may also be outfitted with surgical devices for excision of structures.

mammography

mam OG rah fee

12.96 An X-ray procedure that produces an X-ray image of a breast, called a **mammogram,** is called _____. The procedure and a mammogram are shown in Figure 12.23■. The procedure is an early screening for breast cancer. The term **mammography** is a constructed word, written as mamm/o/graphy.

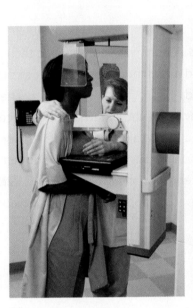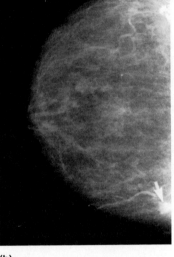

(a)   (b)

Figure 12.23 ■
Mammography. (a) A health-care professional assists the patient to ensure the breast is placed ideally for the X-ray.
Source: Keith Brofsky/Photodisc/ Thinkstock.com
(b) A mammogram. A tumor is visible in this mammogram, indicated by the arrow in the lower right corner.
Source: Courtesy of Dr. Dwight Kaufman, National Institutes of Health, National Cancer Institute Visuals Online, Bethesda, MD.

WORDS TO WATCH OUT FOR !

▶▶▶▶▶ *-graph, -graphy,* or *-gram*?

Remember that the suffix *-y* means "process of." Thus, because the suffix *-graph* means "instrument for recording," the suffix *-graphy* means "recording process." In a slightly different twist, the suffix *-gram* means "a record or image." In each of these suffixes, switching the ending creates the term used for recording information.

mammoplasty

MAM moh PLASS tee

12.97 The surgical repair of one or both breasts is called a _____. It involves either the enlargement or reduction of breast size or, in some cases, removal of a tumor. Mammoplasty is also an important reconstructive procedure for women who have had a mastectomy (Frame 12.98).

12.98 In addition to the combining form *mamm/o*, the combining form *mast/o* also means "breast." Thus, a procedure involving the removal of breast tissue is a _____ (Figure 12.24■). In a **simple mastectomy**, one entire breast is removed while leaving underlying muscles and lymph nodes intact. In a **radical mastectomy** (or Halsted mastectomy), the entire affected breast is removed along with muscles and lymph nodes of the chest. In a **modified radical mastectomy,** the affected breast and lymph nodes are removed but the muscles are left intact. Finally, a **lumpectomy** is the removal of the cancerous lesions only, which conserves the breast.

mastectomy

mass TEK toh mee

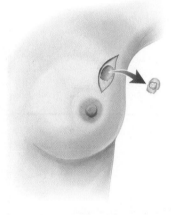
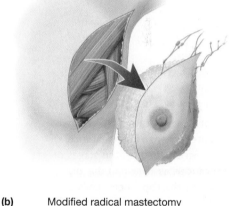

Figure 12.24 ■
Breast surgery. Surgical removal of all or part of the breast is a treatment against the spread of breast cancer.

(a)   Lumpectomy

(b)   Modified radical mastectomy

oophorectomy

oh OFF oh REK toh mee

12.99 Surgical removal of an ovary is performed in an _____. This constructed term is written oophor/ectomy.

Pap smear

12.100 A common diagnostic procedure that screens for precancerous cervical dysplasia and cervical cancer is known as the **Papanicolaou smear** (pap an IK oh law * smeer), commonly called a _____ _____. It involves the gentle scraping of cells from the cervix and vagina followed by their microscopic examination (Figure 12.25■).

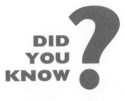

Figure 12.25 ■
Pap smear. Cells of the cervix (shown in the center) change in appearance as they progress through the stages of cervical cancer, as shown in this diagram. During the Pap smear, cells are obtained from the cervix and studied under the microscope for changes. Based on the appearance of cells, a diagnosis can be made.

DID YOU KNOW?

▶▶▶▶▶ **Papanicolaou Smear**

Named after Dr. George Papanicolaou, an anatomist and cytologist, the Pap smear is a screening test for cervical cancer that has made early detection possible. The American Cancer Society recommends annual tests at ages 20 and 21, followed by tests at two-year or three-year intervals throughout later years.

salpingectomy
SAL pin JEK toh mee

12.101 The surgical removal of a fallopian tube is performed in the procedure called a _____. This constructed term is written salping/ectomy. If an ovary is also removed, the procedure is called a **salpingo-oophorectomy** (sal ping goh oh OFF oh REK toh mee). Also a constructed term, it includes four word parts and is written _____/__-_____/_____.

salping/o-oophor/ectomy

WORDS
TO
WATCH
OUT
FOR

▶▶▶▶▶ **The Os in Salpingo-oophorectomy**

When two combining forms are joined together to form a term, the first combining form keeps its combining vowel, even if the second begins with a vowel. Thus, in the term *salpingo-oophorectomy,* the combining form *salping/o* retains its combining vowel. In this long term, the hyphen is included to distinguish between the two adjacent combining forms and to make pronunciation easier. This makes for a lot of o's, so be careful when you spell this term.

---

salpingopexy
sal PING oh PEK see

salping/o/stomy

12.102 Surgical fixation of a fallopian tube may become necessary if the ligaments that support the tube within the pelvic cavity weaken. The procedure is called _____. This constructed term is written salping/o/pexy. Often, a **salpingopexy** is accompanied by a procedure to open a blocked fallopian tube or to drain fluid from an inflamed tube. This procedure is called a **salpingostomy** (SAL ping GOSS toh mee), which can be written as _____/__/_____.

---

sonohysterography
son oh HIST er OG rah fee

12.103 A noninvasive diagnostic procedure that uses ultrasound waves to visualize the uterus within the pelvic cavity is called **sonohysterography.** The constructed term _____ contains five word parts, represented as son/o/hyster/o/graphy. In the diagnostic procedure known as **transvaginal sonography** (trans VAJ ih nal * son OG rah fee), an ultrasound probe is inserted through the vagina to record images of the uterine cavity and fallopian tubes. The constructed form of these terms is trans/vagin/al son/o/graphy. In addition to its use for observing tumors or cysts, it is used to monitor pregnancy.

tubal ligation
TOO bal * lye GAY shun

12.104 The most common form of female sterilization as a contraceptive measure is called **tubal ligation,** during which the fallopian tubes are severed and closed to prevent the migration of sperm upward into the tubes (Figure 12.26■). The term _____ _____ includes the word that means "to tie up," _ligate._

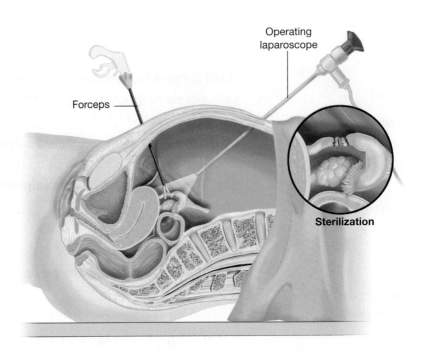

Figure 12.26 ■
Tubal ligation. To minimize the size of the incisions necessary, laparoscopic surgery may be used to enter the abdominal cavity through a small incision, cut the fallopian tubes, and ligate (tie off).

vaginal speculum
VAJ ih nal * SPEK yoo lum

12.105 A **vaginal speculum** is an instrument used during a gynecological exam. A _____ _____ is used to open the vaginal orifice wide enough to permit visual examination of the vagina and cervix.

vulvectomy
vuhl VEK toh mee

12.106 The surgical removal of the vulva is called a _____. The constructed form of this term is written vulv/ectomy.

PRACTICE: Treatments, Procedures, and Devices of the Female Reproductive System

The Right Match

Match the term on the left with the correct definition on the right.

_____ 1. biopsy

_____ 2. dilation and curettage

_____ 3. cervical conization

_____ 4. Papanicolaou smear

_____ 5. hormone replacement therapy

_____ 6. transvaginal sonography

_____ 7. endometrial ablation

_____ 8. tubal ligation

_____ 9. vaginal speculum

a. removal of the cervix

b. severs and closes the fallopian tubes to prevent migration of sperm

c. common therapy for hormone imbalances

d. destroys the endometrium with a laser

e. a procedure in which the cervix is dilated, and a curette is inserted to scrape the endometrium

f. instrument that opens the vaginal orifice to permit visual examination

g. records images of the uterine cavity and fallopian tubes

h. microscopic examination of cells scraped from the cervix and vagina

i. surgical extraction of tissue for microscopic analysis

Linkup

Link the word parts in the list to create the terms that match the definitions. You may use word parts more than once. Remember to add combining vowels when needed—and that some terms do not use any combining vowel.

Combining Form	Suffix
colp/o	-ectomy
gynec/o	-gram
hyster/o	-logy
mamm/o	-pexy
oophor/o	-plasty
salping/o	-rrhaphy
vulv/o	

Definition	Term
1. surgical removal of the vulva	_____
2. surgical repair of the vagina	_____
3. branch of medicine that focuses on women	_____
4. surgical removal of the uterus	_____
5. suturing the wall of the vagina	_____
6. surgical fixation of the uterus	_____
7. X-ray image of a breast	_____
8. surgical removal of an ovary	_____
9. surgical removal of a fallopian tube	_____

Signs and Symptoms of Obstetrics

Here are the word parts that specifically apply to the signs and symptoms of obstetrics that are covered in the following section. Note that the word parts are color-coded to help you identify them: prefixes are green, combining forms are red, and suffixes are blue.

Prefix	Definition
dys-	bad, abnormal, painful, difficult
hyper-	excessive, abnormally high, above
poly-	excessive, over, many

Combining Form	Definition
amni/o	amnion
cyes/o	pregnancy
gravid/o	pregnancy
hydr/o	water
lact/o	milk
pseud/o	false
toc/o	birth

Suffix	Definition
-cyesis	pregnancy
-emesis	vomiting
-ia	condition of
-rrhea	discharge
-s	plural

KEY TERMS A–Z

amniorrhea
AM nee oh REE ah

12.107 Recall that the suffix -rrhea means "discharge." The abnormal discharge of amniotic fluid is a sign of a ruptured amniotic sac. The sign is called _____. This constructed term is written amni/o/rrhea.

dystocia
diss TOH see ah

12.108 The combining form for birth is toc/o. When the prefix dys- and the suffix -ia are added, the new term is _____ and means "condition of difficult labor." The constructed form is written dys/toc/ia.

hyperemesis gravidarum
HIGH per EM eh siss *
grav ih DAR um

12.109 The symptom of severe nausea and emesis (vomiting) during pregnancy is called **hyperemesis gravidarum.** The term literally means "excessive vomiting when pregnant." _____ _____ can cause severe dehydration in the mother and fetus if left untreated.

lactorrhea
LAK toh REE ah

12.110 A normal, spontaneous discharge of milk is known as _____. This constructed term contains three word parts, shown as lact/o/rrhea.

polyhydramnios
PALL ee high DRAM nee ohs

12.111 An excessive production of amniotic fluid during fetal development is called **polyhydramnios.** If left untreated, _____ can cause unwanted pressure on the fetus that can disturb development. The term is a constructed term, written as poly/hydr/amni/o/s.

pseudocyesis
SOO doh sigh EE siss

12.112 A sensation of being pregnant when a true pregnancy does not exist is called **pseudocyesis,** which literally means "false pregnancy." The constructed form of _____ is written pseud/o/cyesis.

PRACTICE: Signs and Symptoms of Obstetrics

Break the Chain

Analyze these medical terms:

    a) Separate each term into its word parts; each word part is labeled for you (**p** = prefix, **r** = root, **cf** = combining form, and **s** = suffix).

    b) For the Bonus Question, write the requested definition in the blank that follows.

1. a) dystocia   _____ / _____ / _____
                                       p   r   s

    b) *Bonus Question:* What is the definition of the suffix? _____

2. a) hyperemesis   _____ / _____
                                        p   s

    b) *Bonus Question:* What is the definition of the prefix? _____

3. a) pseudocyesis   _____ / __ / _____
                                        cf   s

    b) *Bonus Question:* What is the definition of the combining form? _____

4. a) polyhydramnios   _____ / _____ / _____ / __ / _____
                                        p   r   cf   s

    b) *Bonus Question:* What is the definition of the combining form? _____

Diseases and Disorders of Obstetrics

Here are the word parts that specifically apply to the diseases and disorders of obstetrics that are covered in the following section. Note that the word parts are color-coded to help you identify them: prefixes are green, combining forms are red, and suffixes are blue.

Combining Form	Definition	Suffix	Definition
blast/o	germ, bud, developing cell	-al	pertaining to
chori/o	membrane, chorion	-osis	condition of
erythr/o	red	-sis	state of
fet/o	fetus		
plasm/o	form		
tox/o	poison		

KEY TERMS A–Z

abruptio placentae
ah BRUP shee oh * plah SEN tee

12.113 The premature separation of the placenta from the uterine wall is called **abruptio placentae.** This Latin word means "abrupt (loss) of placenta." _____ _____ results in either a miscarriage, stillbirth, or premature birth and is illustrated in Figure 12.27■.

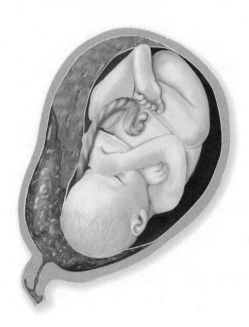

Figure 12.27 ■
Abruptio placentae. The placenta becomes prematurely detached from the uterine wall.

breech presentation

12.114 An abnormal childbirth in which the buttocks, feet, or knees appear through the birth canal first is commonly called a **breech presentation.** A _____ _____ is relatively common and places the child at risk due to an increased risk of complications during birth.

congenital anomaly
kon JENN ih tal * ah NOM ah lee

12.115 A **congenital anomaly** is an abnormality present at birth. As an example, **cleft palate** is a failure of the roof of the mouth to close during prenatal development. Another _____ _____ is **esophageal atresia** (eh sof ah GEE al * ah TREE zhe ah) in which the child is born with an absence of part of the esophagus. This constructed term literally means "closure of the esophagus." A severe, relatively common congenital anomaly is **Down syndrome.** Also called trisomy 21 to identify the chromosome number that contains the defective genes, it is an abnormality present at birth and characterized by mental retardation, glossomegaly (enlarged tongue), stubby fingers, and a fold over the eyelids.

eclampsia

eh KLAMP see ah

12.116 A condition that places a pregnant woman and her child at risk is a circulatory disorder called **pregnancy-induced hypertension** (**PIH**), or **preeclampsia** (pree eh KLAMP see ah). It is characterized by high blood pressure, proteinuria (protein in the urine), and edema, all due to toxemia (toxins in the bloodstream) during pregnancy. In some women, it may progress to the more dangerous condition known as _____, in which the high blood pressure worsens to cause convulsions and possibly coma and death.

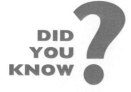

▶▶▶▶▶ **Eclampsia**

The term *eclampsia* is derived from the Greek word *eclampsis,* which means "to shine forth rapidly or flash." It refers to a sudden development and was chosen to be used for this condition in modern times because of the sudden onset of convulsions that often marks the disease.

ectopic pregnancy

ek TOP ik * PREG nan see

12.117 Normally, about eight days after fertilization the zygote will implant into the inner lining of the uterus. However, in some cases the zygote may implant in other tissues, such as the fallopian tube lining or even the peritoneum, and from there proceed through embryonic and fetal development (Figure 12.28■). The term *ectopic* means "out of place." Therefore, a pregnancy occurring outside the uterus is called _____ _____.

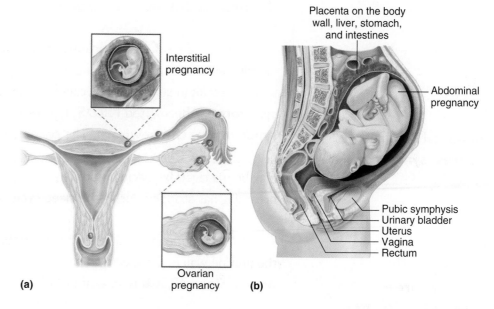

Figure 12.28 ■
Ectopic pregnancies. (a) An ectopic pregnancy may occur in any of the locations shown. Interstitial pregnancy is the most common, with implantation occurring near the union of a fallopian tube and uterus. An ovarian pregnancy has the unfortunate result of destroying the ovary.
(b) An abdominal pregnancy is shown at full term. Note that the fetus is surrounded by the amnion, but outside the uterus.

(a)

(b)

erythroblastosis fetalis
eh RITH roh blass TOH siss *
fee TAL iss

12.118 A condition of neonates, or newborns, in which red blood cells are destroyed due to an incompatibility between the mother's blood and baby's blood is called **erythroblastosis fetalis.** It occurs when the mother has RH− blood and has previously had an RH+ child (Figure 12.29■). The term _____ _____ is constructed as erythr/o/blast/osis fetalis and means "condition of fetal development of red (cells)." It is also called **hemolytic disease of the newborn.**

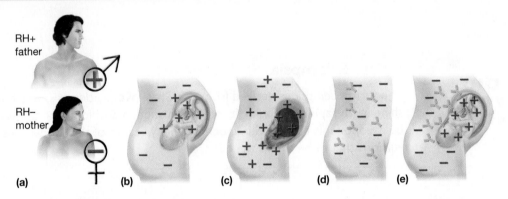

RH+ father

RH− mother

(a) (b) (c) (d) (e)

Figure 12.29 ■
Erythroblastosis fetalis. (a) The condition occurs with an RH+ father and RH− mother. (b) First pregnancy with an RH+ fetus stimulates the mother's blood to form antibodies against the fetal blood. (c) As the placenta separates during birth, the mother is further exposed to the RH+ blood, increasing her blood's reaction against it. (d) The mother carries antibodies against the RH+ blood. (e) In a subsequent pregnancy with an RH+ fetus, the mother's antibodies attack the RH+ blood of the fetus, causing hemolysis of the fetal red blood cells resulting in the disease that can kill the child.

fetal alcohol syndrome

12.119 A neonatal condition caused by excessive alcohol consumption by the mother during pregnancy is known as **fetal alcohol syndrome, or FAS.** The _____ _____ _____ often causes brain dysfunction and growth abnormalities that usually afflict the child throughout life.

neonatal respiratory distress syndrome

12.120 A lung disorder of neonates, particularly premature infants, in which certain cells of the lungs fail to mature at birth to cause lung collapse that can result in suffocation, is called **neonatal respiratory distress syndrome.** Abbreviated **NRDS,** it is also called **respiratory distress syndrome of the newborn.** The condition of _____ _____ _____ _____ may be managed by placing monitors around the baby that trigger when breathing has stopped during the sleep cycle.

placenta previa
plah SEN tah * PREH vee ah

12.121 A condition in which the placenta is abnormally attached to the uterine wall in the lower portion of the uterus is called **placenta previa.** Figure 12.30■ is an example of _____ _____.

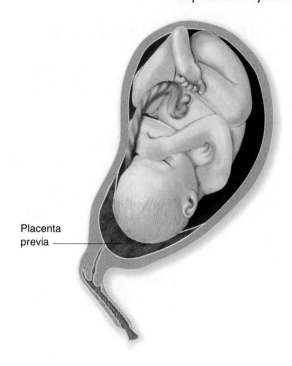

Placenta previa

Figure 12.30 ■
Placenta previa. The condition is caused by the development of the placenta over the cervical canal, creating an occlusion.

toxoplasmosis TAHK soh plaz MOH siss	**12.122** Caused by the protozoan *Toxoplasma gondii,* the disease _____ may be contracted by exposure to animal feces, most commonly from household cats. This constructed term is written tox/o/plasm/osis and means "condition of toxic form." It is a danger to pregnant women because the protozoa are capable of crossing the placental barrier to infect the fetus and cause birth defects.

PRACTICE: Diseases and Disorders of Obstetrics

The Right Match

Match the term on the left with the correct definition on the right.

_____ 1. congenital anomaly

_____ 2. breech presentation

_____ 3. eclampsia

_____ 4. abruptio placentae

_____ 5. ectopic pregnancy

_____ 6. fetal alcohol syndrome

_____ 7. neonatal respiratory distress syndrome

_____ 8. placenta previa

a. severely high blood pressure in the pregnant woman

b. brain dysfunction and growth abnormalities caused by excessive alcohol consumption by the mother during pregnancy

c. abnormality present at birth

d. placenta is abnormally located

e. lung disorder of neonates

f. abnormal birth position in which the buttocks, feet, or knees appear through the birth canal first

g. pregnancy that occurs outside the uterus

h. premature separation of the placenta from the uterine wall

Treatments, Procedures, and Devices of Obstetrics

Here are the word parts that specifically apply to the treatments, procedures, and devices of obstetrics that are covered in the following section. Note that the word parts are color-coded to help you identify them: combining forms are red, and suffixes are blue.

Prefix	Definition
epi-	upon, over, above, on top

Combining Form	Definition
abort/o	miscarry
amni/o	amnion
dur/o	hard
episi/o	vulva
fet/o	fetus
obstetr/o	midwife

Suffix	Definition
-al	pertaining to
-centesis	surgical puncture
-ic	pertaining to
-ician	one who practices
-metry	measurement, process of measuring
-tomy	incision, to cut

KEY TERMS A–Z

abortion
ah BOR shun

12.123 A term derived from the Latin word, *aborto*, which means "miscarry," is **abortion**. It is the termination of pregnancy by expulsion of the embryo or fetus from the uterus. A natural expulsion is called a **miscarriage** or **spontaneous abortion (SAB)**. An _____ induced by surgery or drugs is called a **therapeutic abortion (TAB)**. A drug that induces TAB is called an **abortifacient** (ah BOR tih FAY shent).

amniocentesis
AM nee oh sehn TEE siss

12.124 A procedure that involves penetration of the amnion with a syringe and aspiration of a small amount of amniotic fluid for analysis is known as **amniocentesis**. This constructed term is written amni/o/centesis. _____ literally means "surgical puncture of amnion." It is shown in Figure 12.31■.

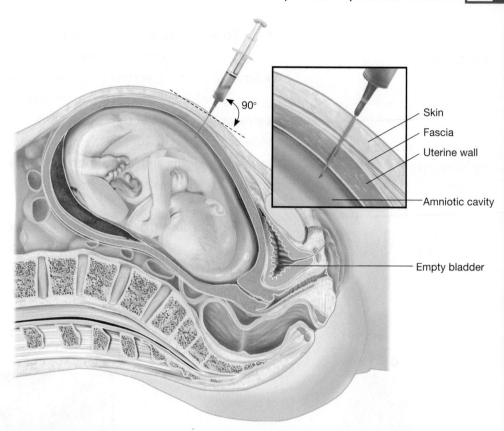

90°

Skin
Fascia
Uterine wall
Amniotic cavity
Empty bladder

Figure 12.31 ■
Amniocentesis. In this examination procedure, amniotic fluid is aspirated with a syringe that is inserted through the abdominal wall, uterine wall, and amnion.

cesarean section
seh ZAIR ee an * SEK shun

12.125 An alternative to the nonsurgical birth of a child through the birth canal, birthing can be accomplished surgically by making an incision through the abdomen and uterus. This procedure is called _____ _____; it is abbreviated **C-section.**

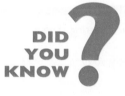

DID YOU KNOW ?

▶▶▶▶ **Cesarean section**

The term *cesarean section* was first used to describe this surgical alternative to vaginal birth during Roman times because it was thought that Julius Caesar was born in this way. However, his family name, Caesar, had its origin from such a birth, which literally means "to cut," centuries before the birth of Julius.

contraception
kon trah SEP shun

12.126 The term **contraception** literally means "against conception," or prevention of birth. It is the use of devices and drugs to prevent fertilization, implantation of a fertilized egg, or both. The most effective _____ is surgical sterilization, including the vasectomy in males (Frame 12.45) and tubal ligation in females (Frame 12.104). The most popular method is the birth control pill, taken orally by females to block ovulation. Other methods include condoms, diaphragms, and intrauterine devices (IUDs).

epidural

episiotomy
eh peez ee OTT oh mee

12.127 To reduce pain during childbirth, a patient may request an
_____ **block,** during which an anesthetic is injected into the epidural space of the vertebral column to block sensation from the pelvic region. _Epidural_ is a constructed term, written epi/dur/al. Another elective treatment may be made to prevent tearing of the vulva and perineum during childbirth. This procedure involves an incision through these tissues to widen the vaginal opening and is called **episiotomy.** _____ is a constructed term, written episi/o/tomy.

fetometry
fee TOM eh tree

12.128 A procedure that measures the size of a fetus is called
_____. This constructed term is written fet/o/metry and means "fetal measurement." It is performed using ultrasound technology on the pregnant mother in the technique known as **obstetrical sonography** (ob STET rih kal * son OG rah fee), which is shown in Figure 12.32■.

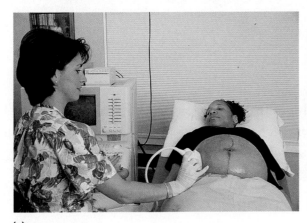
(a)

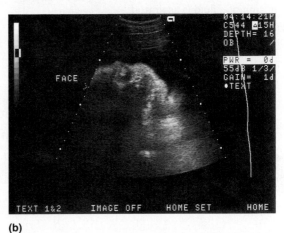
(b)

Figure 12.32 ■
Obstetrical sonography and fetometry. (a) The procedure is performed in a clinical setting. The instrumentation includes a monitor, control panel, and ultrasound probe.
Source: Courtesy of Jim Gathany, Centers for Disease Control Public Health Image Library, Atlanta, GA.
(b) An ultrasound image reveals the fetus within the uterus.
Source: Christophe Testi/Shutterstock.

obstetrics
ob STET riks

obstetrician

12.129 The combining form _obstetr/o_ is derived from the Latin word _obstetrix_, which means "midwife." The medical field of _____ is a discipline concerned with prenatal development, pregnancy, childbirth, and the postpartum period. It is abbreviated **OB.** A physician practicing in this field is called an _____ (OB steh TRISH an).

PRACTICE: Treatments, Procedures, and Devices of Obstetrics

The Right Match

Match the term on the left with the correct definition on the right.

_____ 1. cesarean section

_____ 2. miscarriage

_____ 3. abortifacient

_____ 4. therapeutic abortion

_____ 5. contraception

_____ 6. obstetrics

a. termination of pregnancy by a natural expulsion of the embryo or fetus; also called *spontaneous abortion*

b. the use of devices and drugs to prevent fertilization, implantation of a fertilized egg, or both

c. an abortion induced by surgery or drugs

d. an assisted birth procedure using a surgical incision through the abdomen and uterus

e. medical field concerned with fetal development, pregnancy, childbirth, and the postpartum period

f. a drug that induces therapeutic abortion

Linkup

Link the word parts in the list to create the terms that match the definitions. You may use word parts more than once. Remember to add combining vowels when needed—and that some terms do not use any combining vowel.

Combining Form	Suffix
amni/o	-centesis
episi/o	-metry
fet/o	-tomy

Definition   **Term**

1. aspiration of amniotic fluid for analysis   _____

2. an incision made through the vulva and perineum during childbirth   _____

3. procedure that measures the size of a fetus   _____

Sexually Transmitted Infections (STIs)

acquired immunodeficiency syndrome
ah KWIE erd *
ih MYOO noh deh FISH en see *
SIN drom

12.130 The disease that results from infection with the human immunodeficiency virus, or **HIV,** is called **acquired immunodeficiency syndrome,** abbreviated **AIDS.** It is acquired mainly through the exchange of body fluids during sex, such as semen, blood, and vaginal secretions. It can also be acquired by the use of contaminated instruments, such as intravenous needles. The onset of _____ _____

_____ is characterized by the development of opportunistic infections, which arise as the white blood cell count (mainly helper T cells) declines.

candidiasis
KAN dih DYE ah siss

12.131 Infection by the yeastlike fungus *Candida albicans* is often sexually transmitted to cause the infection known as _____. It is characterized by skin and mucuous membrane irritation and can lead to fatal systemic disease such as endocarditis and septicemia. Candidiasis may also be caused by an interference with normal flora, such as antibiotic therapy, and occurs most frequently in women.

chlamydia
klah MID ee ah

12.132 The most common bacterial STI in North America is **chlamydia.** Its symptoms include urethral or vaginal discharge and pelvic pain among women, urethritis and proctitis in men, and inflammation of the eye's conjunctiva in newborns that can lead to blindness. The term _____ is derived from the Greek word *chlamydos,* which means "cloak."

genital herpes
JENN ih tal * HER peez

12.133 **Genital herpes** is the most common viral STI in North America. _____ _____ is caused by the herpes simplex virus Type 2, or **HSV-2.** It is characterized by periodic outbreaks of ulcer-like sores on the genital and anorectal skin and mucous membranes.

gonorrhea
gahn oh REE ah

12.134 An STI that is caused by the bacterium *Neisseria gonorrhoeae* is called _____. It produces ulcerlike lesions on the mucous membranes and skin of the genital region and is characterized by urethral discharge. The term means "a flow of seed."

hepatitis B

12.135 Hepatitis is an inflammatory disease of the liver that has many different forms that are categorized as type A through E. In _____, commonly called **hep B,** the cause is a virus that is primarily transmitted via blood exchange, often through blood transfusions or sharing IV needles. It may also be acquired through sexual exchange of body fluids. Hep B causes liver damage that can lead to liver failure and death. (Recall from Chapter 10 that hepatitis is a constructed term, hepat/itis: *hepat/o* means "liver," and *-itis* means "inflammation.")

human papillomavirus

12.136 The **human papillomavirus,** or **HPV,** is a virus that is extremely common in the human population and is transmitted during intercourse. In some people, _____ _____ forms the symptom of papillomas or genital warts, which are transient vesicles on the penis or within the vagina. There is evidence that HPV creates an increased risk of cervical cancer (Frame 12.62). A recently developed vaccine is believed to provide protection from HPV infection.

syphilis
SIFF ih liss

12.137 An STI that is caused by a bacterium called a spirochete (*Treponema pallidum*) is known as **syphilis.** It is transmitted by sexual contact and usually first appears as red, painless pustules on the skin that erode to form small ulcers known as **chancres** (SHANG kerz) (Frame 12.10). If left untreated, _____ can result in mental confusion, organ destruction, and death.

trichomoniasis
TRIK oh moh NYE ah siss

12.138 An STI caused by the protozoan *Trichomonas*, which is an amoebalike single-celled organism, is called _____. It is spread by sexual contact and infects both women and men. In women, the sexually transmitted form is called *Trichomonas vaginalis* and causes vaginal swelling and pain. In men, the urethra and prostate gland become infected, causing inflammation and pelvic pain.

PRACTICE: Sexually Transmitted Infections (STIs)

The Right Match

Match the term on the left with the correct definition on the right.

_____ 1. chlamydia

_____ 2. genital herpes

_____ 3. acquired immunodeficiency syndrome

_____ 4. hepatitis B

_____ 5. human papillomavirus

_____ 6. syphilis

_____ 7. gonorrhea

_____ 8. trichomoniasis

_____ 9. candidiasis

a. extremely common STI that causes genital warts in some people and may also increase risk of cervical cancer

b. caused by a bacterium called a spirochete

c. the most common bacterial STI in North America; symptoms include urethritis and inflammation of the conjunctiva

d. characterized by skin and mucous membrane irritation; can lead to endocarditis and septicemia

e. a bacterial infection that produces ulcerlike lesions on the mucous membranes and skin of the genital region and urethral discharge

f. results from infection with the human immunodeficiency virus (HIV)

g. infection caused by a protozoan that causes inflammation of the urethra and prostate, and pelvic pain

h. a form of an inflammatory disease of the liver caused by a virus that is sexually transmitted

i. characterized by periodic outbreaks of ulcer-like sores on the genital and anorectal skin and mucous membranes

Abbreviations of the Reproductive System and Obstetrics

The abbreviations associated with the reproductive system and obstetrics are summarized here. Study these abbreviations, and review them in the exercise that follows.

Abbreviation	Definition
AIDS	acquired immunodeficiency syndrome
BPH	benign prostatic hyperplasia
Bx, bx	biopsy
CIN	cervical intraepithelial neoplasia
CIS	carcinoma in situ
C-section	cesarean section
D&C	dilation and curettage
DRE	digital rectal exam
ED	erectile dysfunction
FAS	fetal alcohol syndrome
FBD	fibrocystic breast disease
GYN	gynecology
HBV	hepatitis B virus
HIV	human immunodeficiency virus
HPV	human papillomavirus
HRT	hormone replacement therapy

Abbreviation	Definition
HSV-2	herpes simplex virus type 2
IDC	infiltrating ductal carcinoma
NRDS	neonatal respiratory distress syndrome
OB	obstetrics
OB/GYN	obstetrics/gynecology
Pap smear (test)	Papanicolaou smear (or test)
PID	pelvic inflammatory disease
PIH	pregnancy-induced hypertension
PMS	premenstrual syndrome
PSA	prostate-specific antigen
SAB	spontaneous abortion
STI	sexually transmitted infection
TAB	therapeutic abortion
TSS	toxic shock syndrome
TURP	transurethral resection of the prostate
TVS	transvaginal sonography

PRACTICE: Abbreviations

Fill in the blanks with the abbreviation or the complete medical term.

Abbreviation	Medical Term
1. PSA	_____
2. _____	sexually transmitted infection
3. HIV	_____
4. _____	transurethral resection of the prostate
5. BPH	_____
6. _____	acquired immunodeficiency syndrome
7. _____	hepatitis B virus
8. HSV-2	_____
9. _____	digital rectal exam
10. HPV	_____
11. _____	cervical intraepithelial neoplasia
12. D&C	_____
13. _____	carcinoma in situ
14. HRT	_____
15. _____	neonatal respiratory distress syndrome
16. PMS	_____
17. _____	therapeutic abortion
18. TSS	_____
19. _____	pelvic inflammatory disease
20. TVS	_____
21. _____	gynecology
22. Bx	_____
23. _____	Papanicolaou smear
24. ED	_____
25. _____	fibrocystic breast disease
26. OB	_____
27. _____	cesarean section
28. OB/GYN	_____
29. _____	spontaneous abortion
30. PIH	_____
31. _____	fetal alcohol syndrome
32. IDC	_____

▶▶▶▶ Chapter Review

Word Building _____

Construct medical terms from the following meanings. (Some are built from word parts, some are not.) The first question has been completed as an example.

1. absence of one or both testes   _____*an*orchism

2. cancer originating from a testis   testicular carcin_____

3. abnormally persistent erection   _____ism

4. constriction of the prepuce   _____mosis

5. excision of the prepuce   circum_____

6. an STI that causes liver inflammation   _____itis

7. incision into a testis   _____tomy

8. condition of an undescended testis   _____orchidism

9. condition of abnormally few sperm   _____spermia

10. inflammation of a testis   orch_____

11. herniation of veins in the spermatic cord   _____cele

12. absence of menstrual discharge   _____menorrhea

13. white or yellow discharge from the uterus   _____rrhea

14. condition of pain in the breast   _____algia

15. profuse bleeding during menstruation   meno_____

16. abnormally reduced bleeding during menstruation   _____menorrhea

17. spread of endometrial tissue into the myometrium   endometri_____

18. inflammation of the cervix   _____itis

19. closure of the uterus   _____atresia

20. condition of a sagging breast   masto_____

21. inflammation of the vulva and vagina   _____vaginitis

22. displacement of the uterus downward   _____ uterus (2 words)

23. excision of a fallopian tube and ovary   salpingo-_____ (hyphenated term)

24. incision to prevent tearing of the vulva and perineum during childbirth   _____tomy

25. endoscopic examination of the uterus   hystero_____

26. breast X-ray procedure   mammo_____

27. a false pregnancy   pseudo_____

28. termination of pregnancy by expulsion of the fetus   _____ (do this one on your own)

29. separation of the placenta from the uterine wall   _____ placentae (2 words)

▶▶▶▶ Medical Report Exercises

Marsha Williams _____

Read the following medical report, then answer the questions that follow.

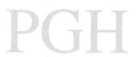

PEARSON GENERAL HOSPITAL

5500 University Avenue Metropolis, MN
Phone: (211) 594-4000 • Fax: (211) 594-4001

Medical Consultation: Gynecology

Date: 7/10/2011

Patient: Marsha Williams

Patient Complaint: Dysmenorrhea accompanied by menorrhagia with possible leukorrhea between menstrual periods.

History: 45-year-old female, nulligravida, with history of occasional dysmenorrhea since puberty. No record of STI or other reproductive pathology. D&C performed on 3/1/07 but failed to correct symptoms.

Family History: Father 79-year-old with hepatic cancer in remission; mother 82-year-old with total hysterectomy at age 44 as a treatment for dysmenorrhea and menorrhagia.

Allergies: None

Physical Examination: Vital signs normal. Pap smear positive for anaplasia. HPV confirmed with culture. Colposcopy positive for CIS and confirmed with blood test.

Diagnosis: Carcinoma in situ of the cervix.

Treatment: Perform cervical conization to confirm CIS; if confirmed, perform cervicectomy and follow with lab tests.

Jennifer Holland, M.D.
_____
Jennifer Holland, M.D.

Photo Source: Peter Baxter/Shutterstock

Comprehension Questions

1. Which patient complaints are consistent with the evidence? _____

_____

_____

2. Why was a Pap smear performed? _____

_____

_____

3. What is the meaning of the terms *dysmenorrhea* and *menorrhagia*? _____

_____

_____

Case Study Questions

The following Case Study provides further discussion regarding the patient in the medical report. Fill in the blanks with the correct terms. Choose your answers from the following list of terms. (Note that some terms may be used more than once.)

carcinoma in situ of the cervix	dilation and curettage	leukorrhea
cervical conization	dysmenorrhea	menorrhagia
colposcopy	HPV (human papillomavirus)	Papanicolaou (Pap) smear

A 45-year-old woman, Marsha Williams, was admitted after complaining of excessive pain during menstruation,

or (a)_____, that was often accompanied by profuse bleeding, or (b)_____.

A white discharge, or (c)_____, was also mentioned by the patient, usually between periods.

A prior treatment in which the cervix was dilated and the endometrium scraped, called a (d)_____

_____ _____, did not eliminate the symptoms. The woman had no prior history

of reproductive disease, STI, or cancer. A scraping of the vagina and cervix for microscopic evaluation of cells, or

(e)_____ _____, showed abnormalities of cells. Culturing the cells indicated a type

of virus that produces vaginal warts, called (f)_____, was present and may have been the source of

the abnormalities. Further evaluation of the cervix, in which a tissue sample is removed with the aid of endoscopy and

known as (g)_____, indicated a premetastatic population of mutated cells that were cancerous, a

condition called (h)_____ _____ _____ _____

_____. This finding was confirmed by a negative blood test for ovarian cancer cells. To eliminate

the possibility of metastasis, the location of the anaplastic cell population, at the end of the cervix, was confirmed by

(i)_____ before it was surgically removed in a cervicectomy procedure.

Richard Miller

For a greater challenge, read the following medical report, then answer the critical thinking questions that follow.

PEARSON GENERAL HOSPITAL

PGH

5500 University Avenue Metropolis, OR
Phone: (211) 594-4000 • Fax: (211) 594-4001

Medical Consultation: Urology

Date: 10/15/2011

Patient: Richard Miller

Patient Complaint: Pain in the sacral and genital areas; discomfort during urination; balanorrhea.

History: 22-year-old male. Urology history negative; patient reported sexually active with frequent unprotected sex in the past year.

Family History: Mother and father with urology negative.

Allergies: None

Physical Examination: Vital signs are normal. Physical exam confirmed balanorrhea, culture positive for gonorrhea; sensitivity in scrotal and genital region; palpable lump on lateral aspect of right testis; bx positive for non-seminoma testicular cancer in both testes.

Diagnosis: Gonorrhea, testicular cancer of right testis with mets to left testis.

Treatment: Antibiotic therapy to defeat STI. Bilateral orchidectomy to remove testicular cancer with lymph node dissection and exploratory into pelvic region, followed with 6 months of chemotherapy and radiation therapy.

Samantha M. Ramapurthy, M.D.

Samantha M. Ramapurthy, M.D.

Photo Source: vgstudio/Shutterstock

Comprehension Questions

1. What evidences support the diagnosis of testicular cancer? _____
   _____
   _____

2. How was the gonorrhea infection obtained? _____
   _____
   _____

3. What is a bilateral orchidectomy? _____
   _____
   _____

Case Study Questions

The following case study provides further discussion regarding the patient in the medical report. Recall the terms from this chapter to fill in the blanks with the correct terms.

A 22-year-old male presented with symptoms that included abnormally few sperm in a semen sample, called

(j) _____, pain in the scrotal and perineal regions, inflammation of the right testis and epididymis,

known as (k) _____, and a palpable lump on his right testis. An evaluation of his medical history

revealed excessive discharge from the glans, called (l) _____, caused by a concurrent infection

resulting in the STI known as (m) _____. The STI was treated with antibiotics and reported cleared.

A biopsy taken from the right testis was positive for (n) _____ cancer. The left testis also showed

evidence of early metastasis, so both testes were removed during a bilateral (o) _____ that included

lymph node dissection from the pelvic region, followed with chemotherapy and radiation therapy. Intervention proved

successful: the patient survived and is recovering from the treatment with no late stage metastasis evident. However, the

patient is now (p) _____, or incapable of producing viable gametes.

The Nervous System and Mental Health

13

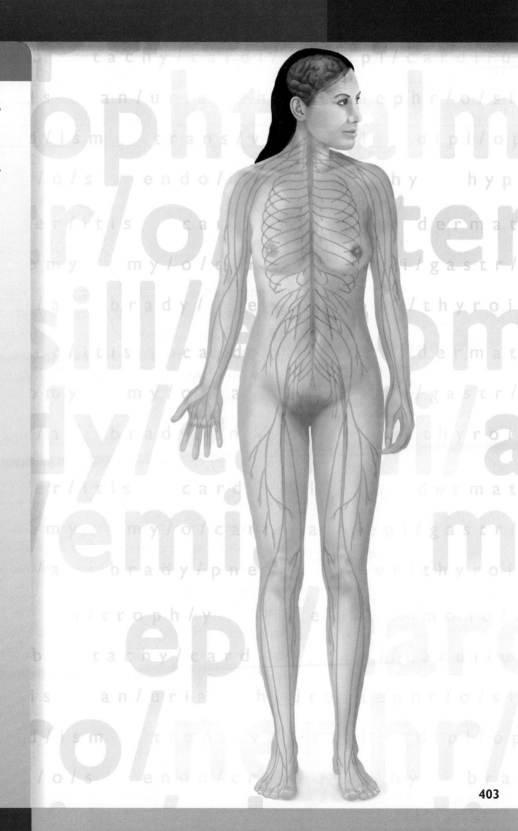

LEARNING OBJECTIVES

After completing this chapter, you will be able to:

1. Define and spell the word parts used to create terms for the nervous system.

2. Identify the major organs of the nervous system.

3. Break down and define common medical terms used for symptoms, diseases, disorders, procedures, treatments, and devices associated with the nervous system and mental health.

4. Build medical terms from the word parts associated with the nervous system and mental health.

5. Pronounce and spell common medical terms associated with the nervous system and mental health.

Anatomy and Physiology Terms ▶▶▶▶▶

The following table provides the combining forms that specifically apply to the anatomy and physiology of the nervous system. Note that the combining forms are colored red to help you identify them when you see them again later in the chapter.

Combining Form	Definition
cephal/o	head
cerebell/o	little brain, cerebellum
cerebr/o	brain, cerebrum
crani/o	skull, cranium
encephal/o	brain
gangli/o	swelling, knot
mening/i, mening/o	membrane

Combining Form	Definition
myel/o	spinal cord, medulla, myelin
neur/o	nerve
phren/o	mind
psych/o	mind
radic/o, radicul/o	nerve root
vag/o	vagus nerve
ventricul/o	little belly, ventricle

nervous
NURR vuss

13.1 The _____ system is a complex part of the body that has been studied extensively, yet there is still much more to learn. It is composed of the brain, spinal cord, and nerves. Together, these important organs enable you to sense the world around you, integrate this information to form thoughts and memories, and control your body movements and many internal functions. The brain and spinal cord form the **central nervous system,** or **CNS,** and the nerves and ganglia form the **peripheral nervous system,** or **PNS.**

homeostasis

neuron

13.2 The nervous system maintains body stability, or _____, by monitoring changes in the body and initiating responses to those changes. It is able to perform this important function by its ability to perceive changes, or stimuli, and convert this information into nerve impulses. A nerve impulse begins when a nerve cell, or **neuron,** opens its membrane channels to sodium and potassium ions, resulting in a flow of these ions across the cell membrane. The flow causes a sudden change in electrical current, which flows along the _____ and is transmitted to other adjacent neurons. The result is an impulse that can travel very quickly along the nerves in your skin and elsewhere and onward to your spinal cord and brain. Neurons are supported by other cells of nervous tissue, known as **neuroglia,** which make up most of the brain and spinal cord.

13.3 Use the anatomy terms that appear in the left column to fill in the corresponding blanks in Figures 13.1■ and 13.2■.

1. **brain**
2. **gray**
3. **ganglion**
4. **nerve**

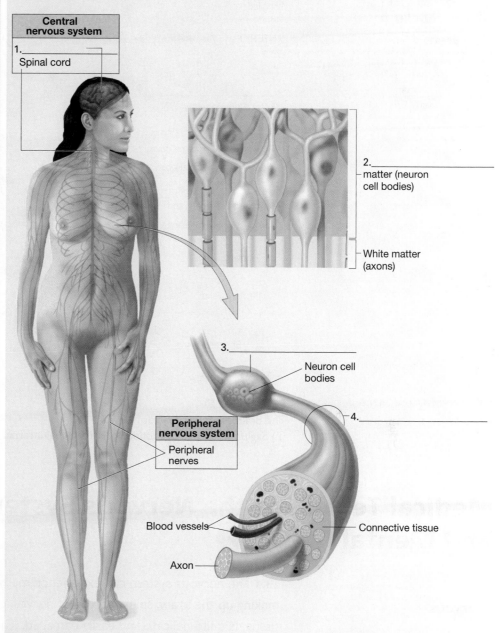

Central nervous system

1._____
Spinal cord

2._____
matter (neuron cell bodies)

White matter (axons)

3._____
Neuron cell bodies

4._____

Peripheral nervous system
Peripheral nerves

Blood vessels

Connective tissue

Axon

Figure 13.1 ■
Organization of the nervous system.

5. cerebral
6. left
7. cerebrum
8. cerebellum
9. stem

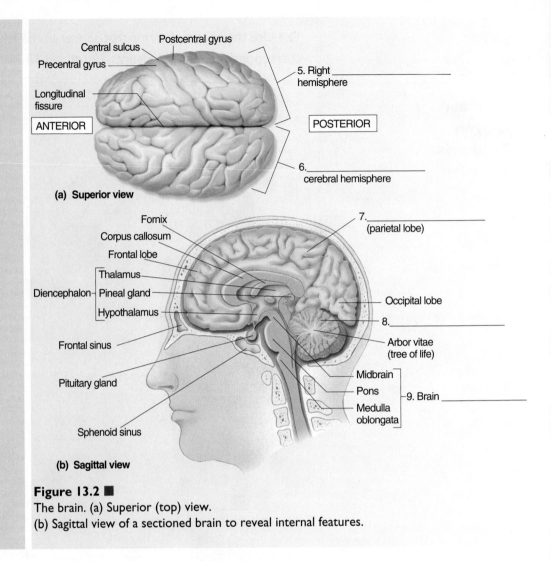

(a) **Superior view**

(b) **Sagittal view**

Figure 13.2 ■
The brain. (a) Superior (top) view.
(b) Sagittal view of a sectioned brain to reveal internal features.

Medical Terms for the Nervous System and Mental Health ▶▶▶▶▶

nervous

blood–brain barrier

13.4 The nervous system can experience many challenges to health. The tissue making up the brain, spinal cord, and nerves, called _____ tissue, is quite delicate and easily damaged. Therefore, it requires special protective features, such as bone, meninges, and cerebrospinal fluid (CSF). Protection from pathogens circulating in the bloodstream is further assisted by a barrier between brain fluids and the blood, known as the

_____-_____ _____,

which keeps most bacteria, harmful cells, and many toxins from entering the nervous system. Usually, the unwanted substances that successfully penetrate the blood–brain barrier are eliminated by special neuroglial cells in the brain, called microglia.

brain

stroke

13.5 Despite the measures protecting the brain and spinal cord, the nervous system may still experience infectious diseases, exposure to toxic substances, injury, and inherited conditions, any of which may lead to functional losses. For example, the most common affliction of the nervous system is stroke. Also known as cerebrovascular accident (CVA), it is a disruption of the normal flow of blood to the brain, resulting in the loss of _____ function that often proves fatal. According to the Centers for Disease Control (CDC), over 150,000 lives were lost in the United States from _____ in 2010, making it the third-most-common cause of death (behind heart disease and cancer).

study of

mind

13.6 The treatment of disorders affecting the nervous system is a relatively young branch of medicine known as **neurology** (noo RAHL oh jee). The combining form *neur/o* means "nerve," and the suffix *-logy* means "_____ ____" or "science of." Specialists within the broad field of neurology include **neurosurgeons** (NOO roh serj enz), whose medical practice focuses on brain or spinal cord surgery; **psychiatrists** (sye KYE ah trists), whose medical practice addresses mental illness; and **clinical psychologists** (sye KOL oh jists), who are mental health professionals trained in the treatment of behavioral disorders. The combining form *psych/o* means "_____."

13.7 In the following sections, you will study the prefixes, combining forms, and suffixes that combine to build the medical terms of the nervous system.

Signs and Symptoms of the Nervous System

Here are the word parts that specifically apply to the signs and symptoms of the nervous system that are covered in the following section. Note that the word parts are color-coded to help you identify them: prefixes are green, combining forms are red, and suffixes are blue.

Prefix	Definition
a-	without, absence of
hyper-	excessive, abnormally high, above
hypo-	deficient, abnormally low, below
par-	alongside, abnormal
poly-	excessive, over, many

Combining Form	Definition
cephal/o	head
esthesi/o	sensation
neur/o	nerve
phasi/o	to speak

Suffix	Definition
-algesia	pain
-algia	condition of pain
-asthenia	weakness
-ia	condition of

KEY TERMS A–Z

aphasia
ah FAY zee ah
a/phas/ia

13.8 The combining form *phasi/o* means "to speak," and the prefix *a-* means "without or absence of." Therefore, the inability to speak is known as _____. It is a clinical sign of a disease process causing the disability. The term is a constructed term composed of word parts. To highlight the word parts, aphasia can be written as ___/_____/____. It literally means "condition of without speaking."

cephalalgia
seff al AL jee ah

13.9 The clinical term for a **headache,** or a generalized pain in the region of the head, includes the combining form for head, *cephal/o,* and the suffix that means "condition of pain." The term is _____. It is a constructed term that can be written as cephal/algia and literally means "condition of head pain." There are several forms of cephalalgia, including muscle contraction (tension) headaches resulting from sustained muscle contractions often caused by tension; cluster headaches, in which the pain is felt on one side of the head in several areas; and migraine headaches, caused by circulatory disturbances and often accompanied by nausea.

convulsion
kon VUHL shun

13.10 A **convulsion** is a series of involuntary muscular spasms caused by an uncoordinated excitation of motor neurons that triggers muscle contraction. A _____ is a sign of a neurological disorder and is also called **seizure** (SEE zhur).

hyperalgesia
HIGH per al JEE zee ah

13.11 The symptom **hyperalgesia** is an excessive sensitivity to painful stimuli. The symptom **hypoalgesia** is a deficient sensitivity to normally painful stimuli. The constructed form of _____ is written hyper/algesia, and the term *hypoalgesia* is written hypo/algesia.

hyperesthesia
HIGH per ess THEE zee ah

13.12 The combining form *esthesi/o* means "sensation." When the prefix *hyper-* is included, a new term _____ is created that means an excessive sensitivity to a stimulus, such as touch, sound, or pain. This constructed term may be written as hyper/esthes/ia.

neuralgia
noo RAL jee ah

13.13 The suffix *-algia* means "condition of pain." A condition of pain in a nerve is a symptom known as _____ and can be written as neur/algia.

neurasthenia
noo ras THEE nee ah

13.14 The suffix *-asthenia* means "weakness." When the word root *neur* is included, the clinical term is spelled _____. The symptom of neurasthenia is a generalized experience of body fatigue, which is often associated with mental depression. Alternate terms sharing the same meaning include **chronic fatigue, fibromyalgia,** and **dysphoria.** The constructed form of *neurasthenia* is neur/asthenia.

paresthesia par ess THEE see ah	**13.15** The prefix *par-* means "alongside or abnormal." Combining it with the combining form for "sensation" forms the term _____. The symptom of **paresthesia** is an abnormal sensation of numbness and tingling caused by an injury to one or more nerves. It can be written as par/esthes/ia to identify its three word parts.
neuralgia noo RAL jee ah **polyneuralgia** pall ee noo RAL jee ah	**13.16** In Frame 13.13, you learned that _____ is a condition of pain in a nerve. A condition of pain in many nerves can be termed by adding the prefix that means "many," as in the clinical term _____. The term *polyneuralgia* is constructed of three word parts and can be written as poly/neur/algia.
syncope SIN ko pee	**13.17 Syncope** is a temporary loss of consciousness due to a sudden reduction of blood flow to the brain. _____ is often called "fainting." The term is a Greek word that means "a sudden loss of strength."

PRACTICE: Signs and Symptoms of the Nervous System

Linkup

Link the word parts in the list to create the terms that match the definitions. You may use word parts more than once. Remember to add combining vowels when needed—and that some terms do not use any combining vowel. The first one is completed as an example.

Prefix	Combining Form	Suffix
a-	asthen/o	-algia
hyper-	esthesi/o	-algesia
par-	neur/o	-ia
poly-	phasi/o	

Definition

1. the inability to speak

2. an extreme sensitivity to painful stimuli

3. pain in many nerves

4. an excessive sensitivity to a stimulus

5. generalized body fatigue and weakness

6. pain in a nerve

7. abnormal sensation of numbness and tingling caused by nerve injury

Term

1. *aphasia*

2. _____

3. _____

4. _____

5. _____

6. _____

7. _____

The Right Match

Match the term on the left with the correct definition on the right.

_____ 1. aphasia

_____ 2. cephalalgia

_____ 3. paresthesia

_____ 4. neuralgia

_____ 5. hyperesthesia

_____ 6. neurasthenia

_____ 7. convulsion

_____ 8. syncope

a. a series of involuntary muscle spasms

b. a vague condition of fatigue

c. excessive sensitivity to a stimulus

d. a headache

e. inability to speak

f. a sudden loss of consciousness

g. abnormal sensation of numbness

h. pain in a nerve

Diseases and Disorders of the Nervous System

Here are the word parts that specifically apply to the diseases and disorders of the nervous system, which are covered in the following section. Note that the word parts are color-coded to help you identify them: prefixes are green, combining forms are red, and suffixes are blue.

Prefix	Definition
a-	without, absence of
epi-	upon, over, above, on top
hemi-	half
intra-	within
mono-	one
para-	alongside or abnormal
poly-	excessive, over, many
quadri-	four

Combining Form	Definition
ather/o	fatty
aut/o	self
cephal/o	head
cerebell/o	little brain, cerebellum
cerebr/o	brain, cerebrum
crani/o	skull, cranium
embol/o	plug
encephal/o	brain
gli/o	glue
gnos/o	knowledge
hem/o	blood
hydr/o	water
later/o	side
mening/i, mening/o	membrane
my/o	muscle
myel/o	spinal cord, medulla, myelin
narc/o	numbness
neur/o	nerve
poli/o	gray
scler/o	hard
thromb/o	clot
vascul/o	little vessel
ventricul/o	little belly, ventricle

Suffix	Definition
-al	pertaining to
-ar	pertaining to
-cele	hernia, swelling, protrusion
-ia	condition of
-ic	pertaining to
-ion	process
-ism	condition or disease
-itis	inflammation
-lepsy	seizure
-malacia	softening
-oma	tumor
-osis	condition of
-pathy	disease
-plegia	paralysis
-rrhage	abnormal discharge
-troph	development
-us	pertaining to

KEY TERMS A–Z

agnosia
ahg NOH see ah

13.18 The combining form that means "knowledge" is *gnos/o*. The loss of the ability to interpret sensory information is a disorder known as _____, which is a constructed term that literally means "a condition without knowledge." It can be written as a/gnos/ia.

Alzheimer disease
ALTS high mer

13.19 Among some individuals over the age of 40 years, the brain undergoes gradual deterioration resulting in confusion, short-term memory loss, and restlessness. The disease is called _____ _____ and is abbreviated **AD**.

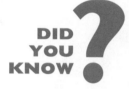 ▶▶▶▶▶ **Alzheimer Disease**

This disease is named after the German physician Dr. Alois Alzheimer, who, in 1906, was the first to draw the connection between the symptoms and the presence of abnormal clumps that form in the brains of patients who died of the disease. The clumps are now called amyloid plaques and neurofibrillary tangles in the cerebrum and are irreversible changes without a known cause or cure.

amyotrophic lateral sclerosis
ah my oh TROF ik * LAT er al * skleh ROH siss

13.20 A disease characterized by the progressive atrophy (loss) of muscle caused by hardening of nervous tissue on the lateral columns of the spinal cord is called **amyotrophic lateral sclerosis.** Also known as **Lou Gehrig disease** after the professional baseball player whose experience with this disease brought it to national attention in 1939, _____ _____ _____ is abbreviated **ALS**.
The term *amyotrophic* can be written as a/my/o/troph/ic and literally means "pertaining to without muscle development."

autism
AHW tizm

13.21 The Greek word *autos* means "self" or "same" and is the source of the combining form *aut/o*. The disease **autism** literally means "disease of self." _____ is a developmental disorder that varies in its severity with the patient, characterized by withdrawal from outward reality and impaired development in social conduct and communication. Children with autism often avoid eye contact with others and have perseverative behaviors such as rocking back and forth for long periods of time.

Bell palsy
behl * PAHL zee

13.22 In general, a **palsy** is a condition of muscular paralysis. In _____ _____, the patient suffers from paralysis of the face muscles on one side due to damage to the seventh cranial nerve.

cerebellitis
ser eh bell EYE tiss

13.23 An inflammation of the cerebellum is called _____. Symptoms of this disease include a loss of muscle coordination and equilibrium. This constructed term can be written as cerebell/itis.

cerebral aneurysm
seh REE bral * AN yoo rizm

13.24 An **aneurysm** is a circulatory problem caused by the weakened wall of a blood vessel, resulting in a bulge in the wall that is in danger of bursting. A _____ _____ affects arteries channeling blood to the brain, placing the brain at great risk of the damage that would result from a burst aneurysm (Figure 13.3■). A burst cerebral aneurysm is one major cause of stroke (Frame 13.28).

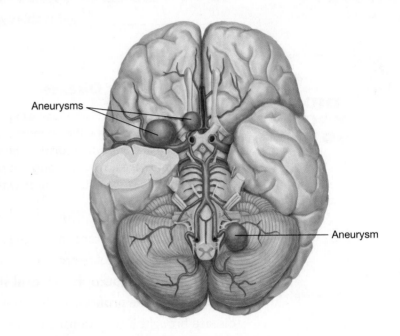

Aneurysms

Aneurysm

Figure 13.3 ■
Cerebral aneurysm. A cerebral aneurysm is the abnormal dilation of arteries supplying the brain, which is caused by a weakening of the arterial walls. In this illustration of the ventral side of the brain, three "berry" aneurysms are revealed as the ball-like swellings of the arteries in red.

cerebral atherosclerosis
seh REE bral *
ath er oh skleh ROH siss

cerebral embolism
seh REE bral * EM bol izm

13.25 The disease **cerebral atherosclerosis** affects arteries supplying the brain. The term contains six word parts, which are revealed by writing the term as cerebr/al ather/o/scler/osis. In _____ _____, the vessels gradually close due to the accumulation of fatty plaques, reducing the flow of blood to the brain. This disease also increases the risk of stroke (Frame 13.28), as atherosclerotic plaques have a tendency to break away and float downstream, causing plugs that lodge in blood vessels to cut off the blood supply completely during acute events. A moving blood clot in an artery of the brain is called a _____ _____ (seh REE bral * EM boh lizm). The condition of a stationary blood clot in an artery of the brain is known as **cerebral thrombosis** (seh REE bral * throm BOH siss).

cerebral hemorrhage
seh REE bral * HEM ohr ahj

13.26 Recall that the term **hemorrhage** means the loss of blood, or bleeding. A _____ _____ is the condition of bleeding from blood vessels associated with the cerebrum. The constructed form of this term is cerebr/al hem/o/rrhage.

cerebral palsy
seh REE bral * PAWL zee

13.27 A condition that appears at birth or shortly afterward as a partial muscle paralysis is called **cerebral palsy.** The paralysis of _____ _____ persists throughout life and is caused by a brain lesion present at birth or a brain defect that arose during development. Abbreviated **CP,** there is no treatment or cure.

cerebrovascular accident
seh REE broh VASS kyoo lar *
AKS ih dent

13.28 The clinical term for a **stroke** is **cerebrovascular accident** and is abbreviated **CVA** (Figure 13.4■). A _____ _____ occurs when the blood supply to the brain is reduced or cut off, resulting in the irreversible death of brain cells followed by losses of mental function or death. A CVA may be caused by emboli (moving blood clots), a thrombus (a lodged, stationary blood clot), or a hemorrhage (bleeding resulting from injured blood vessels or a burst aneurysm).

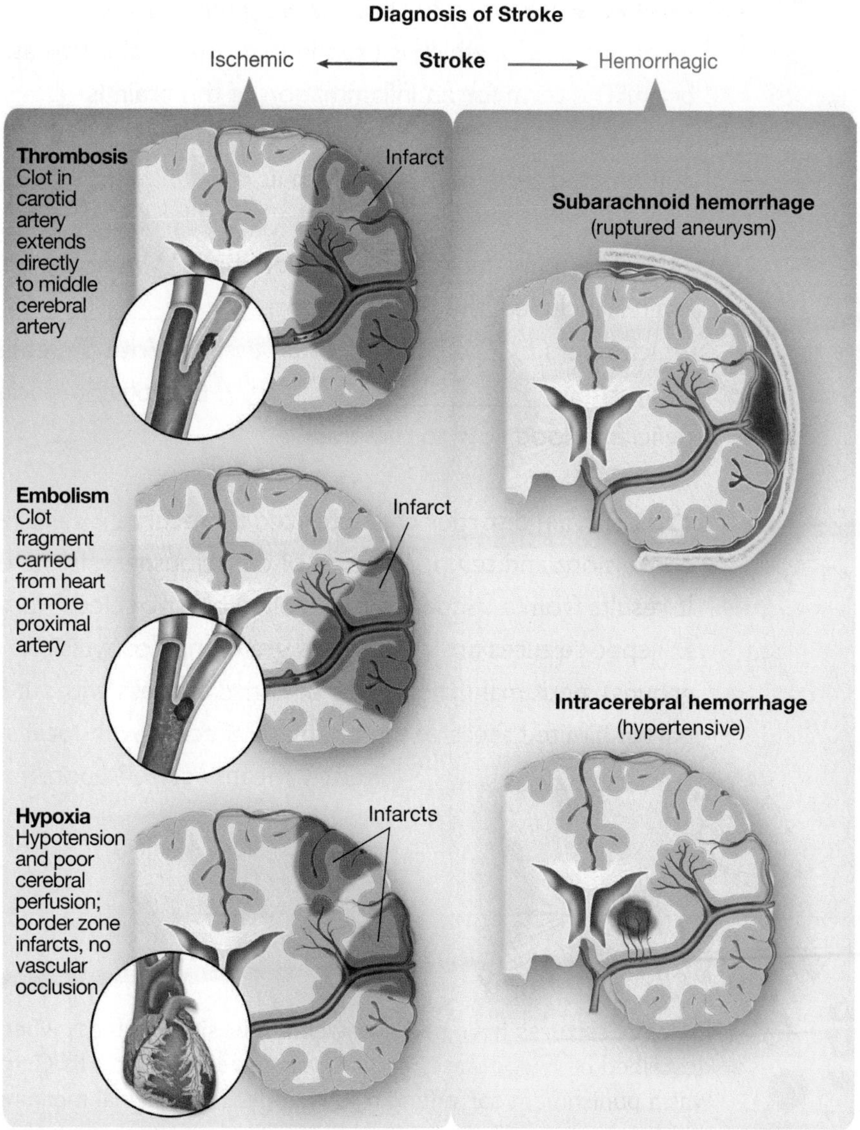

Figure 13.4 ■
Causes of cerebrovascular accident (CVA), or stroke.

coma KOH mah	**13.29** A **coma** is a general term describing several levels of abnormally decreased consciousness. The term _____ is derived from *koma*, the Greek word that means "deep sleep."
concussion kon CUSH uhn	**13.30** The Latin word that means "shaking" is *concussio*. This word has been used to create the medical term _____, which is an injury to soft tissue resulting from a blow or violent shaking. In a **cerebral concussion,** the cerebrum undergoes physical damage when it strikes against the inside wall of the cranium. A concussion is considered a minor injury, resulting in head pain and dizziness, and sometimes nausea. A more severe brain injury is called a **traumatic brain injury** (**TBI**), which often involves bleeding that can result in functional losses and death. Half of all TBIs in the United States are caused by motorcycle accidents.
encephalitis en seff ah LYE tiss	**13.31** A Greek word for brain is *encephalos,* providing us with the combining form, *encephal/o*, which is used in many medical terms associated with the brain. The term for an inflammation of the brain is _____. The condition of encephalitis is usually caused by bacterial or viral infection. The constructed term may be written as encephal/itis.
encephalomalacia en seff ah loh mah LAY she ah encephal/o/malacia	**13.32** The suffix *-malacia* means "softening." When the combining form for brain is included, the resulting term _____ is created, which refers to a softening of brain tissue. Write the constructed form of this term: _____/__/_____. Encephalomalacia is usually caused by deficient blood flow to the brain.
epilepsy EP ih lep see	**13.33** A brain disorder characterized by recurrent seizures, including convulsions and temporary loss of consciousness, is the disease **epilepsy.** It results from a sudden, uncontrolled burst of electrical activity in the brain. Epileptic seizures are classified as grand mal (convulsions affecting all muscle groups), petit mal (brief losses of consciousness without convulsions), or partial (limited areas of the brain are affected with local symptoms). The term _____ literally means "seized upon."

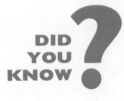

DID YOU KNOW

▶▶▶▶▶ Epilepsy

Epileptic seizures have been written about since 400 BC, when they were first described by Hippocrates in his book *Sacred Disease*. His Greek culture believed it was a punishment for offending the gods. The original meaning of the Greek word *epilepsia* is "seized upon by the gods." The misconception that epilepsy is divine punishment or a form of evil persisted until the late 19th century.

glioma
glee OH mah

13.34 A neoplasm (tumor) of glial cells is called a _____.
The term includes two word parts and can be written as gli/oma. A glioma becomes life threatening when it crowds out functional neurons (see Figure 13.5■).

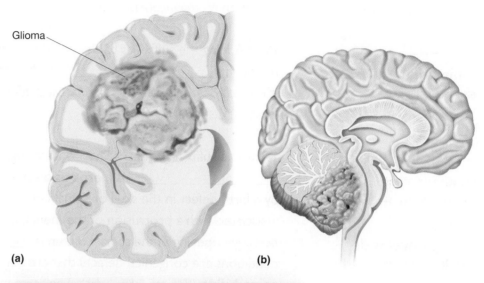

Glioma

(a)   (b)

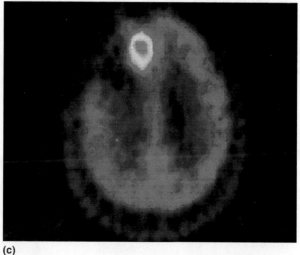

(c)

Figure 13.5 ■
Glioma. (a) Illustration of a large glioma (colored area) within the left cerebral hemisphere in a sectioned brain. Notice how the tumor crowds out normal brain tissue.
(b) A glioma may also press against the cerebellum and brain stem, causing a loss of motor function and reflexes.
(c) PET scan of a glioma within the frontal lobe. The red and yellow colors indicate that metabolic activity is very high, compared to normal nervous tissue in green and purple. This type of glioma is called a glioblastoma multiforme, which is a fast-growing tumor.
Source: Courtesy of Dr. Giovanni DiChiro and Dr. Ramesh Raman of the Neuroimaging Branch, National Institute of Neurological Disorders and Stroke, National Institutes of Health.

hydrocephalus
HIGH droh SEFF ah luss

13.35 The term **hydrocephalus** literally means "head water." This constructed term may be written as hydr/o/cephal/us. It is a congenital disease caused by an abnormally increased volume of cerebrospinal fluid (CSF) in the brain ventricles of a child before the cranial sutures have sealed, resulting in enlargement of the cranium and, in many cases, brain damage.
_____ can be surgically corrected by placement of a **CSF shunt** that drains the excess fluid.

meningioma

meh nin jee OH mah

13.36 The meninges are several layers of membranes surrounding the brain and spinal cord, which include the pia mater, arachnoid mater, and dura mater. The combining form *mening/i* means "membrane." Adding the suffix *-oma* forms the term _____, which is a benign tumor of the meninges usually arising from the arachnoid mater and occurring within the superior sagittal sinus on top of the brain. The constructed form of this term is written mening/i/oma.

meningitis

men in JYE tiss

13.37 Adding the suffix *-itis* to the word root that means "membrane" forms the term _____, which is an inflammation of the meninges. It is usually caused by a bacterial or viral infection. The constructed form is written mening/itis.

meningocele

men IN goh seel

meningomyelocele

men IN goh MYE eh loh seel

13.38 The suffix *-cele* means "hernia, swelling, or protrusion." A _____ is a protrusion of the meninges, usually caused by a birth defect in the skull or spinal column (see Figure 13.6■). A term associated with a protrusion of the meninges and spinal cord through a defective opening in the spinal column is _____. Both conditions are congenital defects that are part of the congenital disease called **spina bifida** (SPYE nah * BIF ih dah). The term *meningomyelocele* contains five word parts and can be written as mening/o/myel/o/cele.

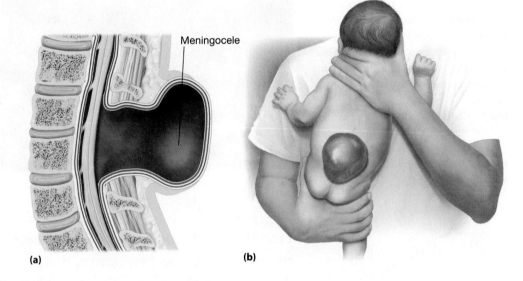

Figure 13.6 ■
Meningocele. (a) A meningocele is a herniation of the meninges, usually associated with the spinal cord. It is illustrated in this cross-sectional view of a portion of the vertebral column as the large swelling. When it occurs in a newborn, it is a congenital defect known as *spina bifida*. (b) Illustration of a child born with spina bifida, with a large meningocele.

Meningocele

(a)   (b)

multiple sclerosis

MULL tih pull * skleh ROH siss

13.39 A disease characterized by the deterioration of the myelin sheath covering axons within the brain is known as _____
_____, abbreviated **MS** (Figure 13.7■). It is a progressive disease without a known cause, diagnosed by episodes of localized functional losses that eventually lead to paralysis and death. It is believed to be an autoimmune disease, due to evidence showing the destruction of the myelin is caused by the body's immune response. Notice the term *sclerosis* contains two word parts, scler/osis, and means "condition of hard."

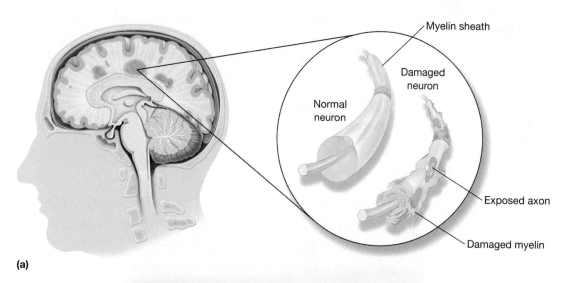

(a)

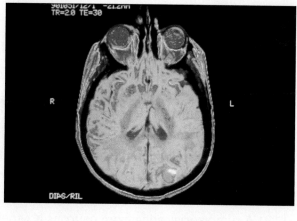

(b)

Figure 13.7 ■

Multiple sclerosis (MS). (a) A disease characterized by the gradual development of small areas of hardened (sclerotic) tissue in the cerebrum, it results in a gradual loss of brain function. The inset compares a normal neuron with a damaged neuron in the brain.

(b) MRI of the brain showing MS lesions in blue.

Source: Courtesy of Dr. Leon Kaufman, University of California, San Francisco, and the National Cancer Institute, National Institutes of Health.

myelitis
mye eh LYE tiss

13.40 The combining form that means "spinal cord" is *myel/o*, which is derived from the Greek word meaning "marrow," *myelos*. Inflammation of the spinal cord is called _____, which can also be written as myel/itis. It is usually caused by a bacterial infection spreading from the meninges to the spinal cord, and if not treated, it can result in muscle paralysis or sensory loss.

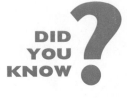

DID YOU KNOW?

▶▶▶▶▶ **myel/o**

The combining form *myel/o* has four different meanings: "bone marrow, spinal cord, medulla," and "myelin." The combining form is derived from the Greek word *myelos,* which means "middle." This derivative was used to describe a "middle" structure: the medulla of the brain is in the middle between the brain and spinal cord, marrow lies in the middle of a bone, and myelin is in the middle of a nerve cell. Over time, *myel/o* was assigned separate meanings whenever its use became accepted.

narcolepsy
NAR koh lep see

13.41 A sleep disorder characterized by sudden uncontrollable episodes of sleep, attacks of paralysis, and hypnagogic hallucinations (dreams intruding into the wakeful state) is called **narcolepsy.** _____ literally means "numb seizure."

neuritis
noo RYE tiss

polyneuritis
PALL ee noo RYE tiss

13.42 Inflammation of a nerve is called _____. It is usually caused by a bacterial or viral infection of the connective tissue coverings surrounding a nerve, although it may also result from physical injury to the nerve. In the condition _____, many nerves at once are inflamed. The term *polyneuritis* includes three word parts and can be written as poly/neur/itis. Polyneuritis may be an early sign of increased pressure within the cranium, called **intracranial** (*intra-* = "within"; crani/al = "pertaining to the cranium") **pressure.**

neuroma
noo ROH mah

13.43 A tumor originating from neurons is generally called a _____. This constructed term may be written as neur/oma.

neuropathy
noo ROH path ee

polyneuropathy
pall ee noo ROH path ee

13.44 A disease affecting any part of the nervous system, such as a cranial nerve, the brain, or the spinal cord, is known as a _____. When many parts are affected by the condition, the prefix *poly-* is added to change the term to _____. The four word parts of the term *polyneuropathy* can be shown as poly/neur/o/pathy.

paraplegia
pair ah PLEE jee ah

quadriplegia
qwad rih PLEE jee ah

13.45 The suffix -plegia means "paralysis," or the inability to contract muscles. In _____, muscles of the legs and lower body are paralyzed. Other forms of paralysis include **monoplegia** (mon oh PLEE jee ah), in which one limb is paralyzed; **hemiplegia** (hem ee PLEE jee ah), paralysis on one side of the body; and _____ (qwad rih PLEE jee ah), paralysis from the neck down including all four limbs. Note how the prefixes alter the meaning of the term: para- for "alongside," mono- for "one," hemi- for "half," and quadri- for "four."

Parkinson disease
PARK ihn son

13.46 A chronic degenerative disease of the brain characterized by tremors, rigidity, and shuffling gait is called **Parkinson disease.** The cause of _____ _____ is not yet known. It is also called **parkinsonism** and is abbreviated **PD.**

poliomyelitis
poh lee oh my eh LYE tiss

13.47 Caused by one of several viruses belonging to the family poliovirus, the disease **poliomyelitis** is characterized by inflammation of the gray matter of the spinal cord, often resulting in paralysis. _____ is commonly referred to as **polio.** A vaccine for this disease has been available since 1955; it thwarted a pandemic that was destroying many lives prior to that year.

rabies
RAE beez

13.48 Rabies is an acute, often fatal, infection of the central nervous system that is caused by a virus transmitted to humans by the bite of an infected animal. _____ was formerly called **hydrophobia** (hye droh PHO bee ah), which means "fear of water," after it was observed that one symptom of mental loss from the infection is a fear of water.

ventriculitis
vehn TRIK yoo LIE tiss

13.49 The condition of inflammation of the ventricles of the brain is known as _____. Its most common cause is a blockage of one of the channels that carry cerebrospinal fluid (CSF). The constructed form of this term is ventricul/itis. When it strikes an infant, it results in hydrocephalus (Frame 13.35).

PRACTICE: Diseases and Disorders of the Nervous System

Break the Chain

Analyze these medical terms:

    a) Separate each term into its word parts; each word part is labeled for you (**p** = prefix, **r** = root, **cf** = combining form, and **s** = suffix).

    b) For the Bonus Question, write the requested definition in the blank that follows.

The first set has been completed for you as an example.

1. a) agnosia

                                        a/gnos/ia
                                        p   r   s

    b) *Bonus Question:* What is the meaning of the suffix? *condition of* _____

2. a) cerebellitis   _____/_____
                                          r   s

    b) *Bonus Question:* What is the meaning of the word root? _____

3. a) encephalitis   _____/_____
                                          r   s

    b) *Bonus Question:* What is the meaning of the word root? _____

4. a) epilepsy   _____/_____
                                          p   s

    b) *Bonus Question:* What is the meaning of the suffix? _____

5. a) meningitis   _____/_____
                                          r   s

    b) *Bonus Question:* What is the meaning of the suffix? _____

6. a) paraplegia   _____/_____
                                          p   s

    b) *Bonus Question:* What is the meaning of the suffix? _____

7. a) neuroma   _____/_____
                                          r   s

    b) *Bonus Question:* What is the meaning of the suffix? _____

8. a) neuritis   _____/_____
                                          r   s

    b) *Bonus Question:* What is the definition of the word root? _____

The Right Match

Match the term on the left with the correct definition on the right.

_____ 1. encephalitis

_____ 2. coma

_____ 3. Alzheimer disease

_____ 4. epilepsy

_____ 5. Parkinson disease

_____ 6. amyotrophic lateral sclerosis

_____ 7. Bell palsy

_____ 8. autism

_____ 9. concussion

_____ 10. stroke

_____ 11. cerebral palsy

a. recurrent seizures

b. partial muscle paralysis caused by a brain defect

c. a disease characterized by paralysis of face muscles on one side

d. an injury to the brain resulting from a blow or violent shaking

e. decreased consciousness

f. a developmental disorder that varies in severity

g. a disease characterized by brain deterioration

h. a disease characterized by tremors and rigidity

i. a cerebrovascular accident

j. a disease characterized by progressive atrophy of muscle

k. inflammation of the brain

Treatments, Procedures, and Devices of the Nervous System

Here are the word parts that specifically apply to the treatments, procedures, and devices of the nervous system, which are covered in the following section. Note that the word parts are color-coded to help you identify them: prefixes are green, combining forms are red, and suffixes are blue.

Prefix	Definition
an-	without, absence of
epi-	upon, over, above, on top

Combining Form	Definition
angi/o	blood vessel
cerebr/o	brain, cerebrum
crani/o	skull, cranium
dur/o	hard
ech/o	sound
electr/o	electricity
encephal/o	brain
esthesi/o	sensation
gangli/o, ganglion/o	swelling, knot
myel/o	spinal cord, medulla, myelin
neur/o	nerve
psych/o	mind
radic/o	nerve root
rhiz/o	nerve root
tom/o	to cut
vag/o	vagus nerve

Suffix	Definition
-al	pertaining to
-algesia	pain
-ectomy	surgical excision, removal
-gram	a record or image
-graphy	recording process
-ia	condition of
-iatry	treatment, specialty
-ic	pertaining to
-ist	one who specializes
-logy	study or science of
-lysis	loosen, dissolve
-plasty	surgical repair
-rrhaphy	suturing
-tome	cutting instrument
-tomy	incision, to cut

KEY TERMS A–Z

analgesic
anne ahl JEE sik

13.50 Pain management is an important part of treating many forms of disease. The most common form of pain management is the use of **analgesics,** such as aspirin, ibuprofen, and acetaminophen. The term _____ means "pertaining to without pain." A form of analgesic used for severe pain is codeine and morphine. Because they are classified as opioid compounds, they are called **opioid** (OH pee oyd) **analgesics.**

anesthesia
anne ehs THEE zee ah

anesthetist
anne EHS the tist

13.51 The primary type of pain management that is used during surgical procedures is _____. The term may be written as an/esthes/ia and means "without the condition of sensation." The anesthetic is usually a blend of narcotics designed to drop the patient into unconsciousness quickly and as risk-free as possible. It may be administered by inhalation, injection, or drip through a catheter. Anesthesia is managed by a physician called an **anesthesiologist** (anne ehs THEE zee AHL oh jist) and is often administered by a trained specialist called an _____. A **nerve block anesthesia** is an injection made into a nerve to block the conduction of impulses between the nerve and the CNS.

cerebral angiography
ceh REE bral * anj ee OHG rah fee

13.52 A diagnostic procedure that reveals blood flow to the brain by X-ray photography is known as **cerebral angiography.** An example of a cerebral angiogram is provided in Figure 13.8■. The _____ _____ procedure is capable of identifying cerebral aneurysm (Frame 13.24) and cerebral thrombosis (Frame 13.25) and tracking the damage that might occur following a cerebral hemorrhage (Frame 13.26). This term may be separated into its word parts by writing it as cerebr/al angi/o/graphy.

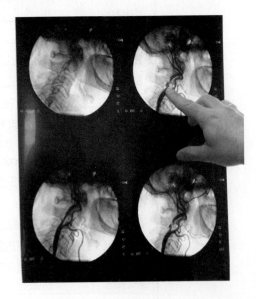

Figure 13.8 ■
Cerebral angiography. The four angiograms each reveal the distribution of blood vessels supplying the brain. The finger is pointing to a blockage in the major artery supplying the brain, called the internal carotid artery.
Source: © picsfive/Fotolia.

computed tomography
kom PYOO ted * toh MOG rah fee

13.53 A procedure involving the use of a computer to interpret a series of X-ray images and construct from them a three-dimensional view of the brain is known as **computed tomography.** Commonly called a **CT scan,** _____ _____ is particularly useful in diagnosing tumors, including gliomas (Frame 13.34).

craniectomy
kray nee EK toh mee

13.54 The surgical removal of part of the cranium is called _____. The term includes two word parts, which can be written as crani/ectomy. A craniectomy is usually performed to replace a fractured cranial bone.

craniotomy
kray nee OTT oh mee

13.55 In the slightly less major surgery called a **craniotomy,** an incision is made through the cranium to provide surgical access to the brain. The term _____ can be written as crani/o/tomy to reveal its three word parts. The surgical knife used to perform this operation is called a **craniotome** (crani/o/tome). A craniotomy is shown in Figure 13.9■.

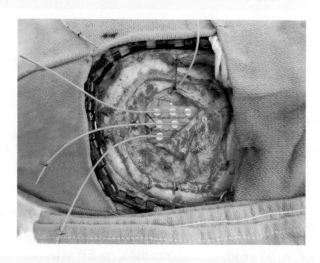

Figure 13.9 ■
Craniotomy. An area of the brain's surface is made accessible for additional procedures during a craniotomy, during which the cranium is penetrated. Electrodes have been placed onto the brain surface to monitor brain activity.
Source: Travis Hilliard/Shutterstock.

echoencephalography
ek oh en SEFF ah LOG rah fee

13.56 In the procedure **echoencephalography,** ultrasound (sound wave) technology is used to record brain structures in the search for abnormalities. _____ is abbreviated **EchoEG.** The term includes five word parts and can be written as ech/o/encephal/o/graphy.

effectual drug therapy

antidepressants

13.57 A general type of treatment to manage neurological disorders is known as **effectual drug therapy.** Examples of _____ _____ _____ include **antianxiety** medication that reduces patient anxiety levels, **anticonvulsants** that control convulsions occurring in diseases such as epilepsy, **antipyretics** that are effective against fever, _____ that combat depression, and **antipsychotics** that reduce hallucinations and confusion. Also, **tranquilizers** and **sedatives** are often used to calm agitated and anxious patients, whereas stronger **narcotics** produce stupor or induce sleep.

electroencephalography

ee LEK troh en SEFF ah LOG rah fee

electr/o/encephal/o/graphy

13.58 A diagnostic procedure that records electrical impulses of the brain to measure brain activity is called _____ and is abbreviated **EEG** (Figure 13.10■). Write the word part construction of this term: _____/__/_____/__/_____.

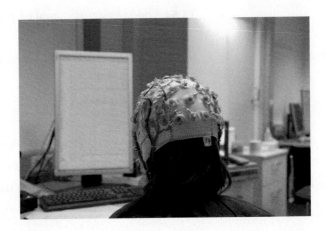

Figure 13.10 ■
Electroencephalography (EEG). To perform the EEG, electrodes attached to the patient's head pick up electrical signals and convey them to a computer for analysis and printing.
Source: © annedde/iStockphoto.com.

epidural

ep ih DUHR ahl

13.59 An **epidural** is the injection of a spinal block anesthetic into the epidural space external to the spinal cord. It is a common procedure to manage pain during painful childbirth labor or as an emergency procedure following severe trauma to the pelvic region. The term _____ is a constructed term that can be written as epi/dur/al and literally means "pertaining to on top of the dura (mater)."

evoked potential studies

13.60 A group of diagnostic tests that measures changes in brain waves during particular stimuli to determine brain function is known as **evoked potential studies,** or **EP studies.** _____ _____ _____ evaluate sight, hearing, and other senses.

ganglionectomy

GANG lee on EK toh mee

13.61 Surgical removal of a ganglion is known as _____, or **gangliectomy.** Both terms have only two word parts (ganglion/ectomy, gangli/ectomy).

lumbar puncture
LUM bar * PUNK shur

13.62 A **lumbar puncture** is the withdrawal (aspiration) of CSF from the subarachnoid space in the lumbar region of the spinal cord (Figure 13.11■). Abbreviated **LP,** a _____ _____ is performed to evaluate the composition of CSF. A lumbar puncture is commonly called a **spinal tap**.

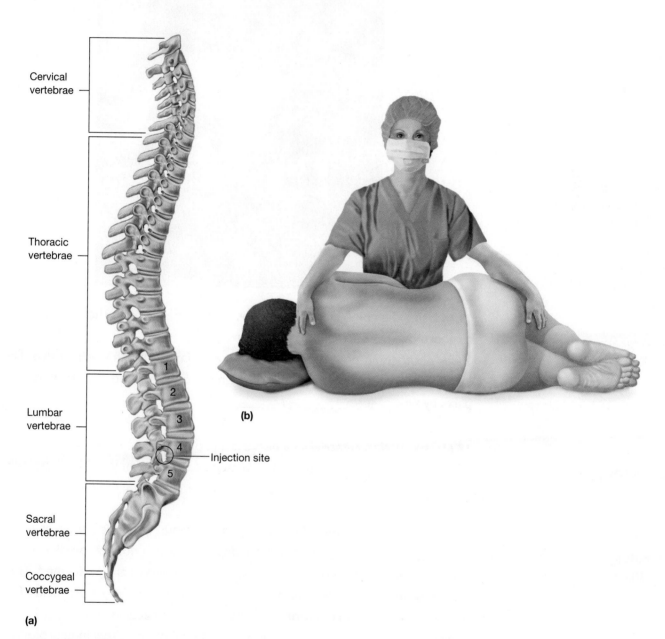

Cervical
vertebrae

Thoracic
vertebrae

Lumbar
vertebrae

1
2
3
4 — Injection site
5

(b)

Sacral
vertebrae

Coccygeal
vertebrae

(a)

Figure 13.11 ■

Lumbar puncture. Abbreviated LP, the lumbar puncture is a common procedure that withdraws cerebrospinal fluid from the lumbar region of the spinal canal for examination. Between vertebrae L4 and L5, the needle is pushed through the dura mater to enter the subarachnoid space and CSF circulation.
(a) Diagram of the vertebral column to illustrate the location where the needle is inserted for the LP procedure.
(b) Supporting the patient for a lumbar puncture.

magnetic resonance imaging

13.63 In the frequently used diagnostic procedure **magnetic resonance imaging,** powerful magnets are used to observe soft tissues in the body, including the brain. Abbreviated **MRI,** _____ _____ _____ is used to target brain tumors, brain trauma, MS, and other conditions (Figure 13.12■).

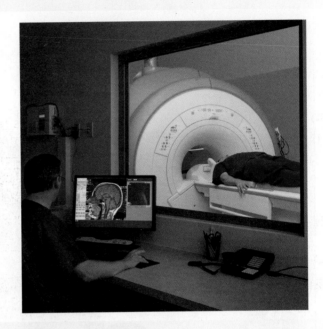

Figure 13.12 ■
Magnetic resonance imaging (MRI). The MRI lab includes the scanning instrument and a computer station. An MRI of the patient's brain is shown on the computer screen.
Source: © James Steidl/Fotolia.

myelogram
MY eh loh gram

myel/o/graphy

13.64 Using the combining form for spinal cord, *myell/o*, with the suffix for a record or image, *-gram*, forms the term _____. It is an X-ray photograph of the spinal cord following injection of a contrast dye. The procedure is called **myelography,** which can be separated into its word parts by writing it as _____/__/_____.

neurectomy
noo REK toh mee

13.65 The surgical removal of a nerve is a procedure known as _____. It can be written as neur/ectomy.

neurology
noo RAHL oh jee

neurologist
noo RAHL oh jist

13.66 The study and medical practice of the nervous system is known as _____. It is also the department of a hospital or clinic where medical procedures on the brain, spinal cord, and nerves are performed. The related term **neurologic** is an adjective associated with the general field of neurology, and a **neuroscientist** is one who participates in neurological research. A _____ is a physician who specializes in neurology, and a **neurosurgeon** is a surgical physician in neurology. The constructed term, *neurology*, can be written as neur/o/logy to reveal its three word parts.

neurolysis
noo RAHL ih siss

13.67 The procedure of separating a nerve by removing unwanted adhesions is known as **neurolysis.** _____ can be written as neur/o/lysis. The suffix *-lysis* means "loosen or dissolve."

neuroplasty NOO roh plass tee	**13.68** The suffix *-plasty* means "surgical repair." When adding the combining form for nerve, the term becomes _____. Thus, neuroplasty is the surgical repair of a nerve. Its three word parts may be shown as neur/o/plasty.
neurorrhaphy noo ROR ah fee	**13.69** The suffix *-rrhaphy* refers to a procedure involving sutures. When adding the combining form for nerve, the term becomes _____, or neur/o/rrhaphy. It means the suture of a nerve.
neurotomy noo ROT oh mee neur/o/tomy	**13.70** Recall that the suffix *-tomy* means "incision, to cut." Adding the combining form for nerve creates the term _____, which means incision into a nerve. Write the word part construction of this term: _____/__/_____.
positron emission tomography PAHZ ih tron * ee MISH un * toh MOG rah fee	**13.71** A scan using an injected radioactive chemical to provide a map of blood flow within the body that can be correlated to function is a computerized procedure known as _____ _____ _____. It is often called a **PET scan** and is a useful diagnostic procedure evaluating brain function.
psychiatry sigh KIGH ah tree	**13.72** The branch of medicine that addresses disorders of the brain resulting in mental, emotional, and behavioral disturbances is known as _____. The term may be written as psych/iatry, which means "treatment of the mind." A physician practicing in this field is a **psychiatrist,** who often uses **psychopharmacology,** or drug therapy targeting the brain, and **psychoanalysis,** or psychiatric therapy, to improve a patient's quality of life.
psychology sigh KALL oh jee **psychotherapy** SIGH koh THAIR ah pee	**13.73** In contrast to psychiatry, the field of _____ is not a medical specialty. It is the study of human behavior. The term *psychology* may be written as psych/o/logy, which means "study or science of the mind." However, a subdiscipline within this field, known as **clinical psychology,** uses applied psychology to treat patients suffering from behavioral disorders and emotional trauma. The technique used in treating behavioral and emotional issues is called _____.
radicotomy ray dih KOT oh mee	**13.74** Recall that the suffix *-tomy* means "incision, to cut." A surgical incision into a nerve root is called _____. It is also called **rhizotomy** because a nerve root has two combining forms, *radic/o* and *rhiz/o*.

reflex testing	**13.75 Reflex testing** is a series of diagnostic tests performed to observe the body's response to touch stimuli. _____ _____ is useful in assessing stroke, head trauma, birth defects, and other neurological challenges. The tests include **deep tendon reflexes (DTR)** involving percussion at the patellar tendon and elsewhere and Babinski reflex involving stimulation of the plantar surface of the foot.
vagotomy vae GOT oh mee	**13.76** The vagus nerve is a large cranial nerve passing from the brain stem into the thoracic and abdominal cavities. During a _____, several branches of the vagus nerve are severed to reduce acid secretion into the stomach in an effort to prevent the reoccurrence of peptic ulcer. The constructed form of this term is vag/o/tomy.

PRACTICE: Treatments, Procedures, and Devices of the Nervous System

Linkup

Link the word parts in the list to create the terms that match the definitions. You may use word parts more than once. Remember to add combining vowels when needed—and that some terms do not use any combining vowel.

Prefix	Combining Form	Suffix
an-	crani/o	-ectomy
	esthesi/o	-ia
	neur/o	-iatry
	psych/o	-logy
	vag/o	-rrhaphy
		-tomy

Definition   **Term**

1. the primary type of pain management that is used during surgical procedures   _____

2. surgical removal of part of the cranium   _____

3. the study and medical practice of the nervous system   _____

4. a procedure in which an incision is made through the cranium
    to provide surgical access to the brain   _____

5. suture of a nerve   _____

6. branch of medicine that addresses disorders of the brain
    that result in mental and emotional disturbances   _____

7. surgical severing of several branches of the vagus nerve
    to reduce acid secretion in the stomach   _____

8. the study of human behavior   _____

The Right Match

Match the term on the left with the correct definition on the right.

_____ 1. computed tomography

_____ 2. effectual drug therapy

_____ 3. reflex testing

_____ 4. sedative

_____ 5. analgesic

_____ 6. lumbar puncture

_____ 7. reflex testing

a. the withdrawal of CSF from the spinal cord

b. agent with a calming effect

c. treatment with medications to manage neurological disorders

d. deep tendon reflex and Babinski reflex

e. a procedure that constructs a 3-D view of the brain

f. series of tests that observe responses to touch stimuli

g. agent that relieves pain

Mental Health Diseases and Disorders

Here are the word parts that specifically apply to mental health diseases and disorders that are covered in the following section. Note that the word parts are color-coded to help you identify them: prefixes are green, combining forms are red, and suffixes are blue.

Prefix	Definition
bi-	two
dys-	bad, abnormal, painful, difficult

Combining Form	Definition
ment/o	mind
neur/o	nerve
phren/o	mind
psych/o	mind
schiz/o	to divide, split
somat/o	body

Suffix	Definition
-ia	condition of
-ic	pertaining to
-lexia	pertaining to a word or phrase
-mania	madness, frenzy
-osis	condition of
-pathy	disease
-phobia	fear

KEY TERMS A–Z

anxiety disorder
  ang ZIGH eh tee * dihs OR der

13.77 Anxiety is the apprehension of danger, filling a person with fear over the future. An _____ _____ occurs when this mental state dominates behavior. It is usually an acute response that includes restlessness, psychological tension, tachycardia, and shortness of breath.

attention deficit disorder

13.78 A neurological disorder characterized by short attention span and poor concentration is called **attention deficit disorder.** Abbreviated **ADD,** _____ _____ _____ is usually associated with school-age children but can also affect adults and makes learning very difficult. A similar disorder is **attention deficit hyperactivity disorder,** abbreviated **ADHD,** which has the added symptom of hyperactivity, or hyperkinesia.

bipolar disease
bigh POHL ar

13.79 Bipolar literally means "pertaining to two poles." The mental disorder called _____ _____ affects the cognitive functions of the cerebrum, causing alternating periods of high energy and mental confusion (known as mania, discussed in Frame 13.82) with low energy and mental depression (Figure 13.13■).

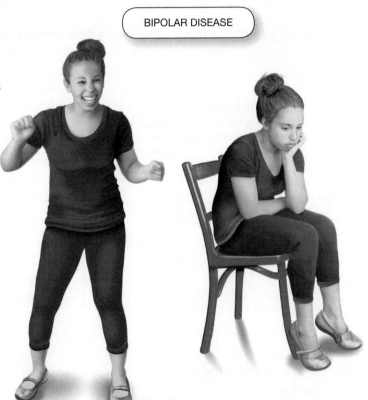

BIPOLAR DISEASE

MANIC

- Begins suddenly and escalates over several days
- Elevated mood
- Loud, rapid speech
- Grandiose statements
- Delusional thoughts
- Hyperactive

DEPRESSIVE

- Despairing
- Reduced, slow speech
- Reduced interest in pleasure
- Negative views
- Fatigue
- Loss of appetite
- Insomnia
- Suicidal thoughts

Figure 13.13 ■
Bipolar disease. The term *bipolar* means "pertaining to two poles." The individual with this form of mental disease cycles between the two extreme behaviors of high-energy mania and low-energy depression, each often lasting for days.

dementia
de MEN she ah

13.80 The Latin word that means *"not in the mind,"* **dementia,** is an impairment of mental function characterized by memory loss, disorientation, and confusion. _____ is usually associated with old age and sometimes accompanies Alzheimer disease (Frame 13.19).

dyslexia dihs LEKS ee ah	**13.81** Some individuals have a reading handicap that has a neurological cause, in which some letters and numbers are reversed in order by the brain. The condition is called **dyslexia.** _____ literally means "condition of difficult reading."
mania MAE nee ah	**13.82** The Greek word for madness or frenzy is _mania_. The clinical condition of _____ is an emotional disorder of abnormally high psychomotor activity, which includes excitement, a rapid movement of ideas, unstable attention, sleeplessness, and confusion between reality and imagination. Different forms of mania include the -mania suffix, such as **megalomania** (MEHG ah lo MAE nee ah), in which an individual believes oneself to be a person of great fame or wealth (_megalon_ means "great" in Greek), and **pyromania** (PIE roh MAE nee ah), which is an obsessive fascination with fire (_pyro_ in Latin means "fire").
neurosis noo ROH siss	**13.83** A **neurosis** is an emotional disorder involving a counterproductive way of dealing with mental stress. _____ is a constructed term with two word parts, which can be shown as neur/osis.
paranoia pahr ah NOY ah	**13.84** A person experiencing persistent delusions of persecution resulting in mistrust and combativeness suffers from **paranoia.** The term _____ is derived from a Greek word meaning "derangement, madness."
phobia FOE bee ah	**13.85** A **phobia** is an irrational, obsessive fear. Derived from the Greek word for fear, _phobos_, _____ is often used as a suffix (-_phobia_) when describing a particular fear. For example, fear of spiders is called **arachnophobia** because the root is from the Greek word _arachne_, which means "spider." Similarly, **agoraphobia** is the abnormal fear of public places (_agora_ means "meeting place" in Greek), **acrophobia** is the abnormal fear of heights (_acro_ means "peak" in Greek), and **phobophobia** is the fear of developing a phobia.
posttraumatic stress disorder	**13.86** Many individuals who have experienced a severe mental strain or emotional trauma, such as military combat or a physical assault, suffer from an acute condition that includes sleeplessness, anxiety, and paranoia. The condition is called _____ _____ _____ It is abbreviated **PTSD.**
psychopathy sy KOH path ee	**13.87 Psychopathy** is a general term for a mental or emotional disorder. _____ literally means "disease of the mind." Its word parts may be shown as psych/o/pathy.

psychosis sy KO siss	**13.88** An individual suffering from a gross distortion or disorganization of their mental capacity, emotional response, and capacity to recognize reality and relate to others may be diagnosed with the disease known as **psychosis.** The most common form of _____ is schizophrenia (Frame 13.90). The term can be written as psych/osis and literally means "condition of the mind."
psychosomatic SY koh soh MAT ik	**13.89** The term **psychosomatic** literally means "pertaining to mind and body." Its word parts can be shown as psych/o/somat/ic. It refers to the influence of the mind over bodily functions, especially disease. Among some people, their mind creates symptoms that suggest an illness when physical signs are absent. In others, a _____ illness can be a real physical illness resulting from mental anxiety, such as peptic ulcer and hypertension.
schizophrenia SKIZ oh FREHN ee ah schiz/o/phren/ia	**13.90** The most common form of psychosis is _____, which literally means "condition of split mind." It is characterized by delusions, hallucinations, and extensive withdrawal from other people and the outside world. There are many forms of schizophrenia, each type classified according to the experiences of the patient. It can be written to show its word parts: _____/__/_____/____.

PRACTICE: Mental Health Diseases and Disorders

The Right Match

Match the vocabulary term on the left with the correct definition on the right.

_____ 1. anxiety disorder

_____ 2. bipolar disease

_____ 3. dementia

_____ 4. posttraumatic stress disorder

_____ 5. paranoia

_____ 6. attention deficit disorder

a. a neurological disorder characterized by short attention span and poor concentration

b. a disorder that results from severe mental strain or emotional trauma

c. alternating periods of high energy and mental confusion (mania) with low energy and mental depression

d. persistent delusions of persecution that results in mistrust and combativeness

e. impairment of mental function characterized by memory loss, disorientation, and confusion

f. a disorder in which the mental state of apprehension and fear dominates behavior

Break the Chain

Analyze these medical terms:

   a) Separate each term into its word parts; each word part is labeled for you (**p** = prefix, **r** = root, **cf** = combining form, and **s** = suffix).

   b) For the Bonus Question, write the requested definition in the blank that follows.

1. a) dyslexia _____/_____
                        p   s

    b) *Bonus Question:* What is the definition of the prefix? _____

2. a) neurosis _____/_____
                        r   s

    b) *Bonus Question:* What is the definition of the word root? _____

3. a) psychopathy _____/___/_____
                            cf   s

    b) *Bonus Question:* What is the definition of the suffix? _____

4. a) psychosis _____/_____
                        r   s

    b) *Bonus Question:* What is the definition of the word root? _____

Abbreviations of the Nervous System and Mental Health

The abbreviations that are associated with the nervous system and mental health are summarized here. Study these abbreviations, and review them in the exercise that follows.

Abbreviation	Definition	Abbreviation	Definition
AD	Alzheimer disease	EchoEG	echoencephalography
ADD	attention deficit disorder	EEG	electroencephalography
ADHD	attention deficit hyperactivity disorder	EP	evoked potential
		LP	lumbar puncture
ALS	amyotrophic lateral sclerosis	MRI	magnetic resonance imaging
CNS	central nervous system	MS	multiple sclerosis
CP	cerebral palsy	PD	Parkinson disease
CSF	cerebrospinal fluid	PET	positron emission tomography
CT (CAT) scan	computed (axial) tomography scan	PNS	peripheral nervous system
		PTSD	posttraumatic stress disorder
CVA	cerebrovascular accident (stroke)	TBI	traumatic brain injury
DTR	deep tendon reflexes		

PRACTICE: Abbreviations

Fill in the blanks with the abbreviation or the complete medical term.

Abbreviation	Medical Term
1. _____	evoked potential
2. PET	_____
3. EEG	_____
4. _____	computed tomography scan
5. MRI	_____
6. _____	Parkinson disease
7. CP	_____
8. _____	echoencephalography
9. DTR	_____
10. _____	multiple sclerosis
11. CVA	_____
12. _____	Alzheimer disease
13. ALS	_____
14. _____	attention deficit disorder
15. ADHD	_____
16. _____	traumatic brain injury

▷▷▷▷ Chapter Review

Word Building

Construct medical terms from the following meanings. The first question has been completed for you as an example.

1. excessive sensitivity to painful stimuli   _____ *hyper*algesia

2. a pain in the head (headache)   _____algia

3. inflammation of the cerebellum   cerebell_____

4. a disease of blood vessels in the cerebrum   _____vascular disease

5. a tumor of neuroglial cells   gli_____

6. softening of brain tissue   encephalo_____

7. nervous system disease   neuro_____

8. excessive sensitivity to a stimulus   _____esthesia

9. inflammation of the brain   _____itis

10. protrusion of the meninges   meningo_____

11. literally a "condition of many hard" areas   _____sclerosis

12. inflammation of the spinal cord   _____itis

13. literally "nerve weakness"   neur_____

14. a tumor arising from nervous tissue   neur_____

15. pain in a nerve   neur_____

16. abnormal sensation of numbness   par_____

17. paralysis on one side of the body   _____plegia

18. inflammation of many nerves   poly_____

19. a disease of the mind   _____pathy

20. paralysis of all four limbs   _____plegia

21. abnormally increased volume of cerebrospinal fluid (CSF) hydro_____

22. excision of part of the skull   _____ectomy

23. incision into the skull   cranio_____

24. suture of a nerve   neuro_____

25. separating a nerve by removing adhesions   neuro_____

26. incision into a nerve   neuro_____

27. inflammation of the ventricles of the brain   ventricul_____

28. physician who specializes in neurology   _____logist

29. drug therapy that targets the brain   _____pharmacology

30. psychology technique used to treat behavioral issues   psycho_____

31. abnormally high psychomotor activity   _____ (do this one on your own!)

32. an irrational, obsessive fear   _____ (do this one on your own!)

▶▶▶▶ **Medical Report Exercises**

Melissa Tampico

Read the following medical report, then answer the questions that follow.

PGH

PEARSON GENERAL HOSPITAL

5500 University Avenue Metropolis, TX
Phone: (211) 594-4000 • Fax: (211) 594-4001

Medical Consultation: Neurology

Date: 10/11/2011

Patient: Melissa Tampico

Patient Complaint: Cephalalgia and neuralgia; polyneuritis on left upper limb and shoulder following automobile collision.

History: 19-year-old female, recently migrated from the Philippine Islands, with no prior history of medical concerns.

Family History: Father, 42-year-old, with Type 2 diabetes under dietary restrictions; mother, 40-year-old, with no neurological history.

Allergies: None

Physical Examination: Blood pressure elevated, 135/90, all other vitals normal. CT and MRI reveal subdural hemorrhage at 1.5 mm inferior to right squamosal suture.

Diagnosis: Traumatic brain injury with subdural hematoma of right temporal lobe.

Treatment: STAT craniotomy with insertion of shunt as needed to drain fluids; identify source of leakage and repair.

Jennifer Holland, M.D.

Jennifer Holland, M.D.

Photo Source: Ximagination/Shutterstock

Comprehension Questions

1. What patient complaint is an early indication of increasing intracranial pressure on the right side of the brain? _____

_____

_____

2. If the intracranial pressure is not relieved in time, what do you suppose might be the consequences to the patient?

_____

_____

3. Explain the meanings of the terms *neuralgia* and *cephalalgia*. _____

_____

_____

Case Study Questions

The following case study provides further discussion regarding the patient in the medical report. Fill in the blanks with the correct terms. Choose your answers from the following list of terms. (Note that some terms may be used more than once.)

analgesics	craniotomy	neuralgia
cephalalgia	intracranial	paresthesia
computed tomography	magnetic resonance imaging	polyneuritis

The patient, Melissa Tampico, was examined following an automobile collision. At the time of admittance she reported

symptoms of headache, or (a) _____, generalized pain in the nerves, or (b) _____,

of the right shoulder and upper arm. Physical examination showed an inflammation of multiple nerves, or

(c) _____, of the shoulder and upper arm. Anti-inflammatory medication and pain relievers, or

(d) _____, were prescribed for treatment. Two weeks after the first exam, the patient returned

with reported abnormal sensations along the left side of the body, or (e) _____. Following a

preliminary CT, or (f) _____ _____, scan, an MRI, or (g) _____

_____ _____ was ordered for a more complete evaluation. The MRI revealed

bleeding below the dura mater (subdural hemorrhage), which was increasing the (h) _____ (within the

cranium) pressure. An incision into the cranium, or (i) _____, was performed to stop the hemorrhage

and reduce the intracranial pressure. The patient made a complete recovery.

Jackson Parker

For a greater challenge, read the following medical report provided and answer the critical thinking questions that follow.

PEARSON GENERAL HOSPITAL

PGH

5500 University Avenue Metropolis, PA
Phone: (211) 594-4000 • Fax: (211) 594-4001

Medical Consultation: Neurology

Date: 06/15/2011

Patient: Jackson Parker

Patient Complaint: Mental confusion leading to attempted suicide.

History: 73-year-old male, diagnosed with chronic depression 8 years ago, history of drug use including amphetamines; veteran of Vietnam War.

Family History: Mother and father deceased, negative history of neurological disease.

Allergies: None

Physical Examination: Occasional grand mal seizures, aphasia, mental confusion, short-term memory loss, agnosia.

Diagnosis: Preliminary finding of PTSD. Pychosis resulting from encephalomalacia.

Treatment: Anticonvulsives to manage epilepsy; MRI to evaluate brain, followed by psychiatric evaluation and treatment.

Juan Menendez, M.D.

Juan Menendez, M.D.

Photo Source: Carme Balcells/Shutterstock

Comprehension Questions

1. What information provided by the history of the patient supports a preliminary diagnosis of PTSD? _____

_____

_____

2. What information did the MRI provide? _____

_____

_____

3. What is the meaning of the terms *aphasia* and *agnosia*? _____

_____

_____

Case Study Questions

The following case study provides further discussion regarding the patient in the medical report. Recall the terms from this chapter to fill in the blanks with the correct terms.

Jackson Parker, a 73-year-old patient, was admitted following an apparent attempted suicide, in which he

walked in front of a city bus on a busy street. The trauma of the accident triggered seizures, suggesting a

condition of (j) _____. Other symptoms included difficulty speaking, or (k) _____,

mental confusion, loss of short-term memory, and an abnormal sensation of numbness to many nerves, called

(l)_____ _____. It was determined that the patient suffered from AD, or

(m) _____ _____, in addition to the trauma injuries. Due to the accident trauma, the patient

was evaluated further with CT scans and MRI. The MRI identified a slow leakage of blood within the brain, or a

(n) _____ _____. A (o) _____ _____ was scheduled to confirm the finding,

which would reveal the status of blood vessels supplying the brain. However, before the test could be made, a stroke,

or (p) _____ _____, occurred. Psychological testing soon determined that the patient had

suffered a severe impairment of mental function, or (q) _____. The mental condition was diagnosed as

a (r) _____, due to the incapacitating nature of the mental state. MRIs later showed a softening of brain

tissue, known as (s) _____, had resulted.

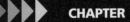

14

The Special Senses of Sight and Hearing

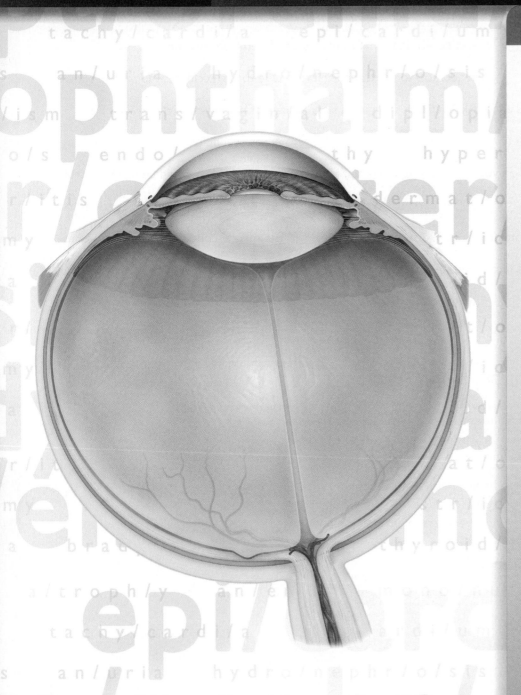

LEARNING OBJECTIVES

After completing this chapter, you will be able to:

1 Define and spell the word parts used to create terms for the special senses of sight and hearing.

2 Identify the major structures of sight and hearing.

3 Break down and define common medical terms used for symptoms, diseases, disorders, procedures, treatments, and devices associated with the special senses of sight and hearing.

4 Build medical terms from the word parts associated with the special senses of sight and hearing.

5 Pronounce and spell common medical terms associated with the special senses of sight and hearing.

Anatomy and Physiology Terms ▶▶▶▶▶

The following table provides the combining forms that specifically apply to the anatomy and physiology of the eyes and ears. Note that the combining forms are colored red to help you identify them when you see them again later in the chapter.

Combining Form	Definition	Combining Form	Definition
blephar/o	eyelid	opt/o	eye
conjunctiv/o	to bind together, conjunctiva	ot/o	ear
dacry/o	tear	retin/o	retina
ir/o	iris	rhin/o	nose
ocul/o	eye	scler/o	hard, sclera
ophthalm/o	eye		

sight	14.1 The special senses are a part of the nervous system that include sensory receptors, which are specialized neurons that respond to a change in the environment, called a stimulus. There are four special senses, each of which contains sensory receptors and supportive tissues. They are smell, or olfaction; taste, or gustation; _____, or vision; and hearing, or audition. In this chapter you will learn the medical terms of the two most important special senses, sight and hearing.
sensory receptors **ears**	14.2 The special sense of sight, or vision, is performed by the eyes, organs located in the orbits of the skull. Each eye contains _____ _____ sensitive to light, called photoreceptors, and supportive structures. The special sense of hearing, or audition, is centered within the _____, which contain sensory receptors that respond to mechanical vibrations. Also within the ears are receptors providing you with the sense of equilibrium.

1.   cornea
2.   lens
3.   retina
4.   sclera

14.3 Use the anatomy terms that appear in the left column to fill in the corresponding blanks in Figures 14.1■ and 14.2■.

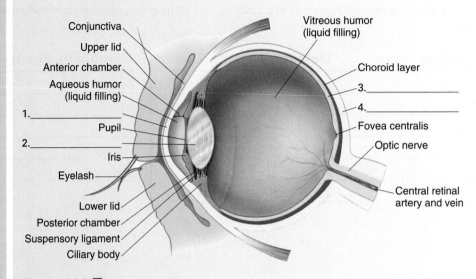

Conjunctiva
Upper lid
Anterior chamber
Aqueous humor (liquid filling)
1._____
Pupil
2._____
Iris
Eyelash
Lower lid
Posterior chamber
Suspensory ligament
Ciliary body

Vitreous humor (liquid filling)
Choroid layer
3._____
4._____
Fovea centralis
Optic nerve
Central retinal artery and vein

Figure 14.1 ■
The eye. Lateral view of a sectioned eyeball in its socket.

5.   malleus
6.   semicircular canals
7.   cochlea
8.   tympanic cavity
9.   tympanic membrane

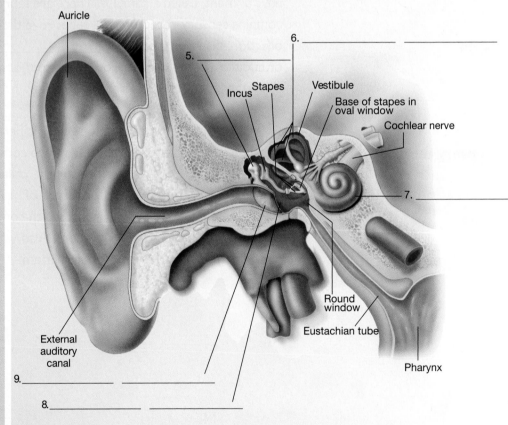

Auricle
5._____
6._____
Incus   Stapes   Vestibule
Base of stapes in oval window
Cochlear nerve
7._____
External auditory canal
Round window
Eustachian tube
Pharynx
9._____ _____
8._____ _____

Figure 14.2 ■
The ear. Lateral view of the ear region on one side of the head.

Medical Terms for the Special Senses of Sight and Hearing ▶▶▶▶▶

sight

retina

14.4 Because the eyes are partially exposed to the outside environment, they are subject to many forms of disease that can affect the sense of _____. Some diseases of the eye are inherited, whereas others may result from injury, infection, or old age. Diseases affecting other parts of the nervous system can also influence sight. For example, the optic nerve, the thalamus, and part of the occipital lobe of the cerebral cortex that interprets sight (called the visual cortex) all play important roles in the transmission and interpretation of impulses sent from the thin membrane of the eye containing photoreceptors, the _____. Consequently, a developmental defect, a lesion, or an injury affecting any of these parts can wreak havoc on the sense of sight.

hearing

equilibrium

14.5 Diseases of the ear may affect the functions of _____ or equilibrium or, in some cases, both. They include developmental defects, damage caused by infection and inflammation, and damage from injury. Hearing and equilibrium may also be challenged by tumors that block nerve impulse transmission to the brain and by diseases of the brain that affect the interpretation of sound or _____.

14.6 In the following sections, you will study the prefixes, combining forms, and suffixes that combine to build the medical terms of sight and hearing.

Signs and Symptoms of the Eyes and Sight

Here are the word parts that specifically apply to the signs and symptoms of the eyes that are covered in the following section. Note that the word parts are color-coded to help you identify them: combining forms are red, and suffixes are blue.

Combining Form	Definition
asthen/o	weakness
blephar/o	eyelid
cor/o	pupil
leuk/o	white
ophthalm/o	eye

Suffix	Definition
-algia	condition of pain
-ia	condition of
-itis	inflammation
-opia	condition of vision
-ptosis	drooping
-rrhagia	abnormal discharge

KEY TERMS A–Z

asthenopia
AHS then OH pee ah

14.7 The combining form asthen/o means "weakness," and the suffix -opia means "condition of vision." Therefore, a symptom of eye weakness, commonly referred to as "eyestrain," is known as _____. It is a short-term, or acute, symptom usually resulting from reading a computer screen or book without frequent breaks. The constructed form is written asthen/opia.

blepharoptosis
BLEF ah ropp TOH sis

14.8 The combining form for eyelid is blephar/o. In some people of senior age, the eyelid droops over the eye abnormally. Because the suffix -ptosis means "drooping," when it is added to the combining form for "eyelid" it forms the symptom _____. The word parts forming **blepharoptosis** can be shown as blephar/o/ptosis.

blepharitis
BLEF ah RYE tiss

14.9 A common symptom of an inflammation of an eyelid is called _____. If the inflammation or trauma damages the eyelid, it may be repaired in the procedure known as **blepharoplasty** (BLEF ah roh plass tee).

leukocoria
loo koh KOR ee ah

14.10 The pupil is the black opening through the iris that allows light to enter the posterior cavity of the eyeball. The abnormal appearance of a white film in the pupil is a sign of disease. It is called _____, which literally means "white in the pupil." The four word parts forming this term can be shown as leuk/o/cor/ia.

ophthalmalgia
off thal MAL jee ah

14.11 One combining form for eye is ophthalm/o. It is used to form many medical terms of the eye, which you are about to discover. In one of these, the suffix -algia is included and means "condition of pain." The symptom of eye pain is therefore called _____, which is pronounced off thal MAHL jee ah. It is a constructed term that can be written as ophthalm/algia.

ophthalmorrhagia

off thal moh RAHJ ee ah

14.12 A second medical term that includes the combining form *ophthalm/o* means "abnormal discharge of the eye." To build this term, the suffix for abnormal discharge, *-rrhagia*, is added. This term is _____, and is pronounced off THAL moh RAH jee ah. The constructed form is *ophthalm/o/rrhagia*.

PRACTICE: Signs and Symptoms of the Eyes and Sight

The Right Match

Match the term on the left with the correct definition on the right.

_____ 1. asthenopia

_____ 2. blepharoptosis

_____ 3. leukocoria

_____ 4. ophthalmalgia

_____ 5. ophthalmorrhagia

_____ 6. blepharitis

a. white in the pupil

b. abnormal discharge of the eye

c. inflammation of an eyelid

d. drooping of an eyelid

e. pain associated with an eye

f. eyestrain

Linkup

Link the word parts in the list to create the terms that match the definitions. You may use word parts more than once. Remember to add combining vowels when needed—and that some terms do not use any combining vowel. The first one is completed as an example.

Combining Form	Suffix
asthen/o	-algia
blephar/o	-ia
cor/o	-itis
leuk/o	-opia
ophthalm/o	-ptosis
	-rrhagia

Definition

1. white in the pupil

2. eyestrain

3. pain associated with an eye

4. abnormal discharge of an eye

5. drooping of an eyelid

6. inflammation of an eyelid

Term

leukocoria

_____

_____

_____

_____

_____

Diseases and Disorders of the Eyes and Sight

Here are the word parts that specifically apply to the diseases and disorders of the eyes, which are covered in the following section. Note that the word parts are color-coded to help you identify them: prefixes are green, combining forms are red, and suffixes are blue.

Prefix	Definition
a-	without, absence of
dipl-	double
hyper-	excessive, abnormally high, above

Combining Form	Definition
blephar/o	eyelid
conjunctiv/o	to bind together, conjunctiva
cyst/o	bladder, sac
dacry/o	tear
ir/o	iris
kerat/o	hard, cornea
lith/o	stone
ophthalm/o	eye
presby/o	old age
retin/o	retina
sinus/o	cavity
stigmat/o	point

Suffix	Definition
-iasis	condition of
-ism	condition or disease
-itis	inflammation
-malacia	softening
-opia	condition of vision
-pathy	disease
-plegia	paralysis

KEY TERMS A–Z

cataract
KAT ah rakt

14.13 The lens of the eye is normally transparent. In the condition known as **cataract,** transparency of the lens is reduced (Figure 14.3■). _____ formation is usually a normal part of the aging process. As you might guess, the common symptom of cataract is leukocoria, described in Frame 14.10.

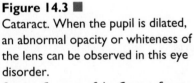

Figure 14.3 ■
Cataract. When the pupil is dilated, an abnormal opacity or whiteness of the lens can be observed in this eye disorder.
Source: Courtesy of the Centers for Disease Control.

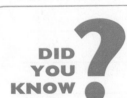 **▶▶▶▶ Cataract**

DID YOU KNOW?

The term *cataract* is from the Latin word that means "waterfall." It was an ancient belief that the gradual loss of vision was due to a veil that fell between the lens and the cornea, spilling over vision *like a waterfall.*

14.14 The conjunctiva is a thin membrane covering the anterior, exposed part of the eye and the inner eyelid. Bacteria may infect this membrane, causing inflammation known as _____. Commonly known as "pinkeye" because of the pink color of the sclera caused by the inflammation, itchy watery eyes and a crusty exudate are common signs (Figure 14.4■). The word part construction for this term can be written as conjunctiv/itis.

conjunctivitis
kon JUNK tih VYE tiss

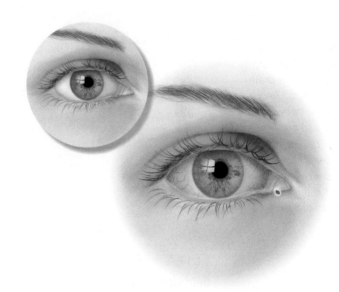

Figure 14.4 ■
Conjunctivitis, with the characteristic "pinkeye" appearance. A yellow crusty exudate is also common. The smaller inset image is a healthy eye, shown for comparison.

14.15 The lacrimal apparatus is a tear-forming gland with associated tubes and chambers, mainly located near the medial side of each eyeball. The combining form of lacrimal is *dacry/o*. The presence of rocky particles in the apparatus is a condition known as _____. It is a painful condition that often leads to inflammation of the lacrimal apparatus, known as _____. The word part construction of the term *dacryocystitis* can be written as dacry/o/cyst/itis. If the inflammation should pass into the adjacent sinuses, the condition becomes **dacryosinusitis** (DAK ree oh SYE nus EYE tiss).

dacryolithiasis
DAK ree oh lith EYE ah siss

dacryocystitis
DAK ree oh sist EYE tiss

14.16 A common cause of blindness is **detached retina.** It occurs when the retina tears away from the choroid layer of the eye. A _____ _____ can be caused by a severe blow to the head, high blood pressure, or old age.

detached retina

14.17 The condition of double vision is called **diplopia.** _____ may result from weakened extrinsic eye muscles, defects in the lens, or a condition of the brain.

diplopia
dih PLOH pee ah

glaucoma
  glaw KOH mah

14.18 In the disease of the eye known as **glaucoma,** a loss of vision occurs when the fluid pressure within the anterior chamber of the eyeball (called intraocular pressure) rises above normal. The rise of fluid pressure in _____ is often caused by a blockage in a small opening that normally drains the fluid (Figure 14.5■).

Figure 14.5 ■
Glaucoma. (a) A buildup of pressure within the eye cavities, often caused by a blockage of vessels that drain fluid, may damage the optic nerve at the back of the eyeball to result in a gradual loss of sight and blindness. (b) Glaucoma often causes reduced sight, such as the loss of the perimeter of a visual field as shown here.
Source: Courtesy of Kristen Oliver, Little Portraits Photography Studio.

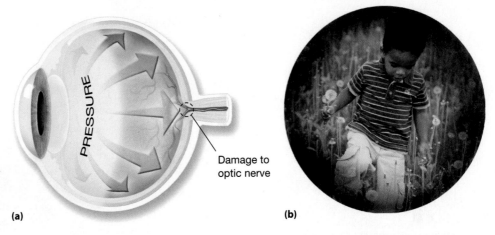

PRESSURE

Damage to optic nerve

(a) (b)

hordeolum
  hor DEE oh lum

14.19 A meibomian gland is a small gland in the eyelid that secretes lubricating fluid onto the conjunctiva. An infection of this gland produces a local swelling of the eyelid, known as a **hordeolum.** Also called a **sty,** the term _____ is derived from the Latin word, *hordeum,* which means "barley" (Figure 14.6■). A chronic form of this infection is often called a **chalazion** (kah LAY zee on), which is derived from *chalaza,* the Greek word that means "sty."

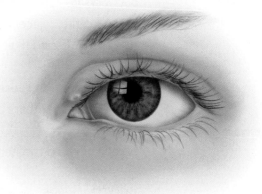

Figure 14.6 ■
Hordeolum (or sty).

iritis
eye RYE tiss

keratitis
kair aht EYE tiss

14.20 During a bacterial infection of the eye, parts of the eye may become inflamed. When the iris is affected, the condition is known as _____, and when the cornea becomes inflamed, it is called _____. The word part construction of the term *iritis* is written as ir/itis, and *keratitis* is kerat/itis.

macular degeneration

14.21 The macula lutea is a small area of the retina that contains a high density of photoreceptors, known as cone cells. Because of the high concentration of cone cells, it is the area of sharpest vision. Progressive deterioration of the macula lutea leads to a loss of visual focus and is called **macular degeneration** (Figure 14.7■). The abbreviated version of _____ _____ is **AMD** (age-related macular degeneration) because its most common cause is age.

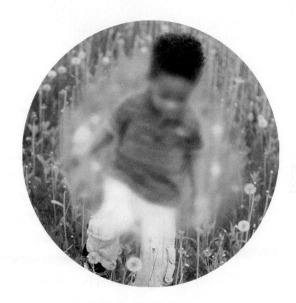

Figure 14.7 ■
Vision with macular degeneration is experienced with an inability to focus in the center of the visual field, as shown here.
Source: Courtesy of Kristen Oliver, Little Portraits Photography Studio.

ophthalmomalacia
off THAL moh mah LAY shee ah

ophthalmoplegia
off THAL moh PLEE jee ah

14.22 A frequently used combining form that means "eye" is *ophthalm/o*. In the term _____, the suffix *-malacia* is included to establish the meaning "softening of the eye." The word part construction of this term is written as ophthalm/o/malacia. Similarly, paralysis of the eye is termed _____ and is formed by adding the suffix that means "paralysis," which is *-plegia*. In this eye disease, the extrinsic eye muscles are unable to move the eyeball. Each of these eye conditions are forms of eye disease, or **ophthalmopathy** (OFF thalm MOH path ee).

retinopathy

ret in AH path ee

14.23 A general term for a disease of the retina is the term _____. The three word parts that form the term **retinopathy** can be written as retin/o/pathy. A common form of retinopathy occurs among people with diabetes mellitus, and is called **diabetic retinopathy** (Figure 14.8■).

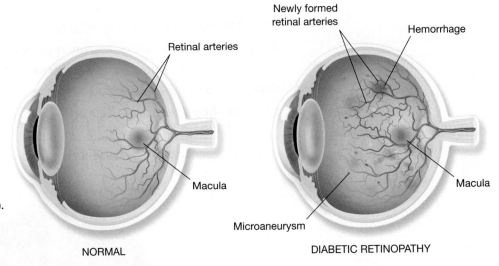

Newly formed
retinal arteries

Hemorrhage

Retinal arteries

Macula

Macula

Microaneurysm

NORMAL

DIABETIC RETINOPATHY

Figure 14.8 ■
Retinopathy. Illustration of a normal retina (left) and a diseased retina (right). The diseased retina exhibits changes common among people suffering from diabetes mellitus.

vision disorders

14.24 Conditions of the eye that result in a reduction of vision are generally called **vision disorders.** Often caused by defects in the lens, cornea, or shape of the eyeball, _____ _____ include nearsightedness, or **myopia** (mye OH pee ah); farsightedness, or **hyperopia** (HYE per oh pee ah); and **presbyopia** (PREZ bee oh pee ah), or reduction in vision due to age. **Emmetropia** (EM eh troh pee ah) is the normal condition of the eye, abbreviated **Em** (Figure 14.9■). Note that each of these terms includes the suffix -*opia*, which means "condition of vision." In the condition **astigmatism** (ah STIG mah tizm), the curvature of the eye is defective to produce blurred vision. It is abbreviated **Ast.**

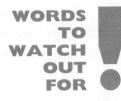

WORDS
TO
WATCH
OUT
FOR

▶▶▶▶▶ **Myopia**

You may recall from Chapter 6 that *my/o* is the combining form for muscle. It is derived from the Greek word for muscle, *myos*. However, in the word *myopia*, *my* is derived from the Greek word *myein*, which means "to shut." When followed by the suffix -*opia*, the term *myopia* translates into "condition of shut vision."

Emmetropia and Refractive Errors

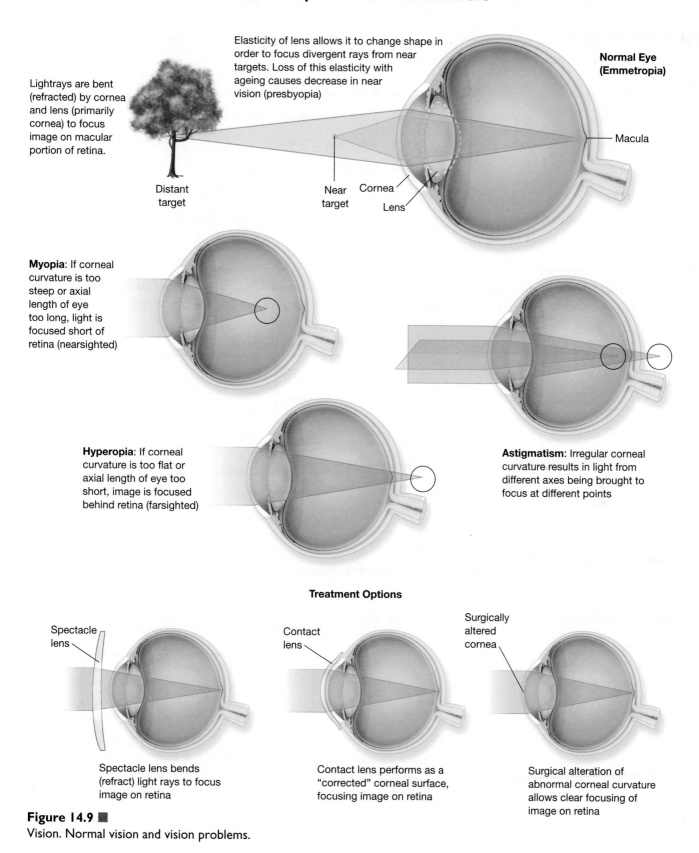

Elasticity of lens allows it to change shape in order to focus divergent rays from near targets. Loss of this elasticity with ageing causes decrease in near vision (presbyopia)

Normal Eye (Emmetropia)

Lightrays are bent (refracted) by cornea and lens (primarily cornea) to focus image on macular portion of retina.

Macula

Distant target

Near target

Cornea

Lens

Myopia: If corneal curvature is too steep or axial length of eye too long, light is focused short of retina (nearsighted)

Hyperopia: If corneal curvature is too flat or axial length of eye too short, image is focused behind retina (farsighted)

Astigmatism: Irregular corneal curvature results in light from different axes being brought to focus at different points

Treatment Options

Spectacle lens

Spectacle lens bends (refract) light rays to focus image on retina

Contact lens

Contact lens performs as a "corrected" corneal surface, focusing image on retina

Surgically altered cornea

Surgical alteration of abnormal corneal curvature allows clear focusing of image on retina

Figure 14.9 ■
Vision. Normal vision and vision problems.

PRACTICE: Diseases and Disorders of the Eyes and Sight

The Right Match

Match the vocabulary term on the left with the correct definition on the right.

_____ 1. glaucoma

_____ 2. cataract

_____ 3. macular degeneration

_____ 4. hordeolum

_____ 5. detached retina

_____ 6. ophthalmomalacia

   a. occurs when the retina tears away from the choroid layer

   b. progressive deterioration of the macula lutea

   c. softening of the eye

   d. loss of vision as a result of increased intraocular pressure

   e. a condition in which the transparency of the lens is reduced

   f. infection of the meibomian gland; also called a *sty*

Linkup

Link the word parts in the list to create the terms that match the definitions. You may use word parts more than once. Remember to add combining vowels when needed—and that some terms do not use any combining vowel.

Prefix	Combining Form	Suffix
a-	conjunctiv/o	-ism
dipl-	ir/o	-itis
	ophthalm/o	-opia
	retin/o	-pathy
	stigmat/o	

Definition	Term
1. bacterial infection of the conjunctiva	_____
2. double vision	_____
3. defective curvature of the eye that causes blurred vision	_____
4. inflammation of the iris	_____
5. disease of the retina	_____
6. eye disease	_____

Treatments, Procedures, and Devices of the Eyes and Sight

Here are the word parts that specifically apply to eye treatments, procedures, and devices that are covered in the following section. Note that the word parts are color-coded to help you identify them: prefixes are green, combining forms are red, and suffixes are blue.

Prefix	Definition	Combining Form	Definition	Suffix	Definition
intra-	within	cyst/o	bladder, sac	-ar	pertaining to
		dacry/o	tear	-logist	one who studies
		kerat/o	hard, cornea	-metrist	one who measures
		ocul/o	eye		
		opt/o	eye	-stomy	surgical creation of an opening
		radi/o	radius		
		rhin/o	nose	-tomy	incision, to cut

KEY TERMS A–Z

cataract extraction

14.25 During **cataract extraction,** a lens damaged by a cataract is surgically removed and replaced with a donor lens (Figure 14.10■). If a donor lens is not available for a _____ _____, an artificial **intraocular lens (IOL)** may be implanted.

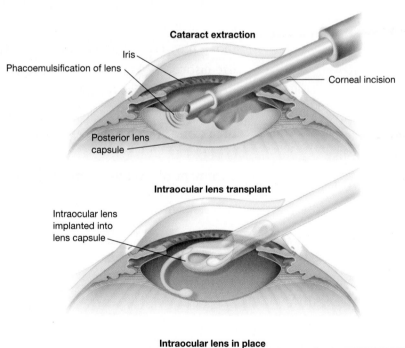

Cataract extraction

Phacoemulsification of lens — Iris

Corneal incision

Posterior lens capsule

Intraocular lens transplant

Intraocular lens implanted into lens capsule

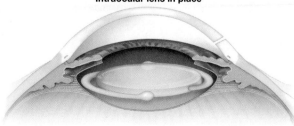

Intraocular lens in place

Figure 14.10 ■
Cataract extraction. The procedure involves a surgical removal of a cataract lens and its replacement with an artificial lens. The artificial lens is made of silicone and acrylic. Artificial lenses are called intraocular lenses.

corneal grafting	**14.26** The cornea is normally transparent, but may lose its transparency from exposure to ultraviolet light or become damaged from an injury. The most common treatment of corneal damage is **corneal grafting.** During a _____ _____, the injured cornea is removed and replaced by implantation of a donor or synthetic cornea.
dacryocystorhinostomy DAK ree oh SIS toh rye NOS toh mee	**14.27** To treat dacryocystitis, described in Frame 14.15, antibiotic eye drops are often used to defeat the bacterial infection. In some cases, a **dacryocystorhinostomy** may be needed. During a _____, a channel is surgically created between the nasal cavity and lacrimal sac to promote drainage. This term may be divided into its numerous word parts: dacry/o/cyst/o/rhin/o/stomy.
LASIK LAY sik	**14.28** The acronym for **laser-assisted in situ keratomileusis** is _____. It is the use of a laser to reshape the corneal tissue beneath the surface of the cornea to correct vision disorders, such as myopia, hyperopia, and astigmatism.
optometrist ahp TOM eh trist **ophthalmologist** off thal MAH loh jist	**14.29** Correcting vision disorders (Frame 14.24) is usually attempted by the use of **corrective lenses** or **contact lenses** following a vision examination by an **optometrist.** An _____ is a health professional (not a physician) trained to examine eyes to correct vision problems and eye disorders. As an alternative to using contact lenses for myopia, an **ophthalmologist** (off thal MAHL oh jist) may perform a **radial keratotomy** (RAY dee al * kair ah TOT oh mee), during which spokelike incisions are made into the cornea, which effectively flattens the cornea to correct for myopia. An _____ is a physician who specializes in the study and treatment of diseases associated with the eyes.

PRACTICE: Treatments, Procedures, and Devices of the Eyes and Sight

The Right Match

Match the vocabulary term on the left with the correct definition on the right.

_____ 1. cataract extraction

_____ 2. LASIK

_____ 3. radial keratotomy

_____ 4. corneal grafting

_____ 5. optometrist

_____ 6. ophthalmologist

a. removal and replacement of an injured cornea

b. a surgical correction for myopia in which incisions flatten the cornea

c. surgical removal and replacement of a lens damaged by a cataract

d. use of a laser to reshape the corneal tissue to correct vision

e. a physician specializing in the study and treatment of eye diseases

f. a health professional trained to examine eyes to correct vision problems

Break the Chain

Analyze these medical terms:

a) Separate each term into its word parts; each word part is labeled for you (**p** = prefix, **r** = root, **cf** = combining form, and **s** = suffix).

b) For the Bonus Question, write the requested definition in the blank that follows.

1. a) optometrist   opt/o/metrist
                              cf   s

   b) *Bonus Question:* What is the definition of the combining form? *eye* _____

2. a) dacryocystorhinostomy   _____/___/_____/___/_____/___/_____
                                    cf   cf   cf   s

   b) *Bonus Question:* What is the definition of the suffix? _____

3. a) ophthalmologist   _____/___/_____
                          cf   s

   b) *Bonus Question:* What is the definition of the combining form? _____

Signs and Symptoms of the Ears and Hearing

Here are the word parts that specifically apply to the signs and symptoms of the ears and hearing that are covered in the following section. Note that the word parts are color-coded to help you identify them: prefixes are green, combining forms are red, and suffixes are blue.

Prefix	Definition	Combining Form	Definition	Suffix	Definition
an-	without, absence of	ot/o	ear	-acusis	condition of hearing
hyper-	excessive, abnormally high, above			-algia	condition of pain
				-rrhagia	abnormal discharge
para-	alongside, abnormal			-rrhea	discharge

KEY WORDS A–Z

anacusis
AN ah KYOO siss

14.30 The suffix that means "condition of hearing" is -acusis. When the prefix an- is included, the constructed term _____ is created, which literally means "condition of absence of hearing" and refers to a total loss of hearing. It can be written as an/acusis.

hyperacusis
HIGH per ah KYOO siss

14.31 When the same suffix, -acusis, is used with the prefix that means "excessive, abnormally high, above," the term _____ is created, which literally means "condition of excessive hearing." It refers to a symptom of abnormally sensitive hearing. Replacing this prefix with another, para-, changes the meaning once again. The term **paracusis** (PAIR ah kyoo siss) is a symptom of partial loss of hearing.

otalgia
oh TAHL jee ah

14.32 The combining form that means "ear" is ot/o. When the suffix for a condition of pain, -algia, is included, the term _____ is created, which means "pain in the ear," or earache.

otorrhagia
oh toh RAJ ee ah

14.33 Another symptom of the ear using the combining form ot/o is **otorrhagia**. Because the meaning of the suffix -rrhagia is "abnormal discharge," the constructed term _____ means "abnormal ear discharge." The word parts are shown when the constructed form is written is ot/o/rrhagia.

otorrhea
oh toh REE ah

14.34 When the suffix -rrhea, which means "discharge," is added to the combining form for ear, the term _____ is created. This is a symptom of abnormal drainage (of pus) from the ear and can be written as ot/o/rrhea.

tinnitus
tinn EYE tuss

vertigo
VER tih go

14.35 Two common symptoms of the ears and hearing are not constructed of word parts. They are **tinnitus,** which is a ringing or buzzing sensation in the ears, and **vertigo,** which is a sensation of dizziness. _____ is from the Latin word *tinnio,* which means "jingling sound," and _____ is derived from the Latin word *vertigo,* which means "dizziness."

PRACTICE: Signs and Symptoms of the Ears and Hearing

The Right Match

Match the term on the left with the correct definition on the right.

_____ 1. anacusis

_____ 2. otalgia

_____ 3. hyperacusis

_____ 4. paracusis

_____ 5. otorrhagia

_____ 6. tinnitis

a. partial hearing loss

b. total hearing loss

c. abnormal discharge from the ear

d. pain in the ear, or earache

e. a ringing in the ears

f. overly sensitive hearing

Linkup

Link the word parts in the list to create the terms that match the definitions. You may use word parts more than once. Remember to add combining vowels when needed—and that some terms do not use any combining vowel. The first one is completed as an example.

Prefix	Combining Form	Suffix
an-	ot/o	-acusis
hyper-		-algia
para-		-rrhagia
		-rrhea

Definition

1. partial loss of hearing

2. abnormal drainage of pus from the ear

3. pain in the ear

4. bleeding from an ear

5. total hearing loss

6. overly sensitive hearing

Term

_____

_____

_____

_____

_____

_____

Diseases and Disorders of the Ears and Hearing

Here are the word parts that specifically apply to diseases and disorders of the ears and hearing, which are covered in the following section. Note that the word parts are color-coded to help you identify them: combining forms are red, and suffixes are blue.

Combining Form	Definition	Suffix	Definition
extern/o	exterior	-acusis	condition of hearing
mastoid/o	resembling a breast	-itis	inflammation
med/o	middle	-osis	condition of
ot/o	ear	-pathy	disease
presby/o	old age		
scler/o	hard, sclera		

KEY WORDS A–Z

mastoiditis
mas toyd EYE tiss

14.36 The term that literally means "inflammation of the part resembling a breast" is _____. The word part construction of this term is mastoid/itis. The mastoid process is an area of the temporal bone of the skull housing the middle and internal ear. Bacterial infections of the middle ear can travel into the mastoid area to produce mastoiditis, causing serious complications that can lead to impaired hearing or deafness.

Ménière disease
MEN yer

14.37 A chronic disease of the inner ear is known as **Ménière disease.** _____ _____ includes symptoms of vertigo, or dizziness, and tinnitus, a ringing in the ears (Frame 14.35).

otitis
oh TYE tiss

otitis media

14.38 The general term for inflammation of the ear is _____. In one form of this disease, the external auditory canal is involved causing local sensations of pain, and is called **otitis externa** (oh TYE tiss * eks TER nah). In another form, the middle ear is involved to cause local pain and a temporary loss of hearing. Known as _____ _____ (oh TYE tiss * MEE dee ah), it is relatively common among children, is caused by bacterial infection, and often requires antibiotic therapy (see Figure 14.11■). It is abbreviated **OM.** It has been estimated that 80% of all children will have contracted otitis media by their third birthday, and it is the most common cause of partial hearing loss. Both otitis externa and otitis media are **otopathies,** which literally means "diseases of the ear." The word part construction of the term otitis is ot/itis, and that of the term otopathy is _____/___/_____.

ot/o/pathy

Section through middle ear in otitis media

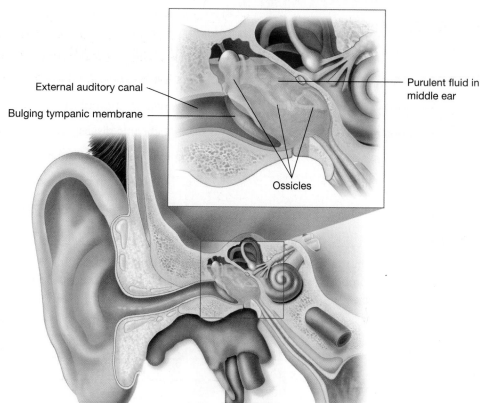

External auditory canal

Bulging tympanic membrane

Purulent fluid in middle ear

Ossicles

Figure 14.11 ■
Otitis media. This illustration shows an inflamed tympanic cavity, which is the most common source of ear pain in this infection. The eardrum may also become inflamed or bulge outward due to an accumulation of purulent fluid within the tympanic cavity.

otosclerosis
oh toh skler OH siss

14.39 An abnormal formation of bone within the ear, usually between the stapes and the oval window of the middle ear, is known as **otosclerosis**. The disease causes a progressive loss of hearing. Recall that the suffix -osis with the word root *scler* means "condition of hard." The term _____ includes four word parts, which can be shown by writing the word part construction as ot/o/scler/osis.

presbyacusis
pres bee a KYOO siss

14.40 A gradual loss of hearing with advancing age is a very common experience. The term for this disease combines the word root that means "old age," *presby*, with the suffix that means "condition of hearing," which you learned is -*acusis*. The resulting term is _____.

PRACTICE: Diseases and Disorders of the Ears and Hearing

The Right Match

Match the vocabulary term on the left with the correct definition on the right.

_____ 1. Ménière disease

_____ 2. presbyacusis

_____ 3. otitis media

_____ 4. otitis externa

_____ 5. mastoiditis

_____ 6. otopathy

a. any disease of the ear

b. inflammation of the middle ear

c. a chronic disease of the inner ear

d. inflammation of the mastoid area

e. inflammation of the external auditory canal

f. loss of hearing due to old age

Linkup

Link the word parts in the list to create the terms that match the definitions. You may use word parts more than once. Remember to add combining vowels when needed—and that some terms do not use any combining vowel.

Combining Form	Suffix
mastoid/o	-pathy
ot/o	-itis
scler/o	-osis

Definition

1. inflammation of the ear

2. an abnormal formation of bone within the ear

3. any disease of the ear

4. inflammation of the mastoid

Term

_____

_____

_____

_____

Treatments, Procedures, and Devices of the Ears and Hearing

Here are the word parts that specifically apply to ear treatments, procedures, and devices that are covered in the following section. Note that the word parts are color-coded to help you identify them: combining forms are red, and suffixes are blue.

Combining Form	Definition
audi/o	hearing
labyrinth/o	maze, inner ear
mastoid/o	resembling a breast
myring/o	membrane, eardrum
ot/o	ear
tympan/o	eardrum

Suffix	Definition
-ectomy	surgical excision, removal
-logist	one who studies
-logy	study or science of
-metry	measurement, process of measuring
-plasty	surgical repair
-scope	instrument used for viewing
-scopy	process of viewing
-tomy	incision, to cut

KEY WORDS A–Z

audiologist
aw dee AHL oh jist

audiometry
aw dee AH meh tree

14.41 The combining form *audi/o* means "hearing." The study of hearing disorders is a field of practice called **audiology.** One who specializes in hearing disorders and treatment is called an _____. The procedure involving the measurement of hearing is usually performed by an **audiologist,** and is called _____ (Figure 14.12■). The constructed form of the term *audiology* is written audi/o/logy, *audiologist* is audi/o/logist, and *audiometry* is audi/o/metry.

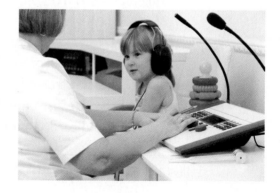

Figure 14.12 ■
Audiometry. The child in this photograph is undergoing a hearing test with an audiologist.
Source: Capifrutta/Shutterstock.

labyrinthectomy
lab ee rin THEK toh mee

14.42 In some severe cases of permanent hearing loss, the inner ear, or labyrinth, is surgically removed and replaced with a synthetic hearing device. The surgical removal of the inner ear is called _____. Its constructed form is written labyrinth/ectomy.

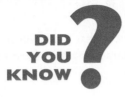

DID YOU KNOW ▶▶▶▶▶ **Labyrinth**

The combining form labyrinth/o is derived from the Greek word *labyrinth,* which means "a maze." It is believed to have originated from the ancient Lydian language that preceded the golden age of Greece. The term was used as the label for *the house of the double axe,* which was a maze designed to protect the inner sanctum of the throne room for Minos, the King of Crete. Over the years, the labyrinth became synonymous with the word *maze.* When early scientists first observed the twisting chambers of the inner ear, they were struck by its resemblance to a twisting maze, leading them to apply the term *labyrinth.*

mastoidectomy mas toyd EK toh mee **mastoidotomy** mas toyd AHT oh mee	**14.43** In some patients, it may become necessary to surgically remove part of the mastoid process of the temporal bone to treat severe mastoiditis (Frame 14.36). This procedure is called _____. The constructed form of this term is written mastoid/ectomy. The procedure is preceded by making an incision into the mastoid process in the procedure called _____. The constructed form of this term is mastoid/o/tomy.
myringoplasty mih RING oh plas tee **myringotomy** mih ring AH toh mee	**14.44** The combining form *myring/o* means "membrane." Because the eardrum is a membrane, this combining form may be used in terms in which the eardrum is described. Therefore, a surgical repair of the eardrum is called _____. Similarly, an incision into the eardrum is called _____. Both are constructed terms, and are written myring/o/plasty and myring/o/tomy.
ot/o/logy **otoscope** OH toh skope	**14.45** The medical field of ear disorders and their treatment is called **otology.** This constructed term may be written ___/__/_____ to show its word parts. The instrument that is used in a physical exam to view the ear canal and eardrum uses the same combining form and is called an _____. The exam procedure is called **otoscopy** (oh TOH skoh pee; Figure 14.13■).

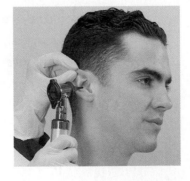

Figure 14.13 ■
An ear exam, or otoscopy, using an otoscope.
Source: Pearson Education

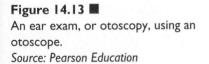

tympanometry
tim pan AH meh tree

tympanoplasty
tim PAN oh plass tee

14.46 You may recall that the eardrum is also called the tympanic membrane. This alternate term uses the combining form *tympan/o*, which means "eardrum." A procedure that evaluates the elasticity of the eardrum by measuring its movement includes this combining form in the word _____. Another term that uses this combining form describes the surgical repair of the eardrum, and is known as _____.

PRACTICE: Treatments, Procedures, and Devices of the Ears and Hearing

The Right Match

Match the vocabulary term on the left with the correct definition on the right.

_____ 1. mastoidectomy

_____ 2. otoscopy

_____ 3. tympanoplasty

_____ 4. labyrinthectomy

_____ 5. audiology

_____ 6. otology

a. physical examination of the ear canal and eardrum

b. the study of hearing disorders

c. surgical removal of part of the mastoid process

d. the medical field of ear disorders and treatment

e. surgical repair of the eardrum

f. surgical removal of the inner ear

Break the Chain

Analyze these medical terms:

a) Separate each term into its word parts; each word part is labeled for you (**p** = prefix, **r** = root, **cf** = combining form, and **s** = suffix).

b) For the Bonus Question, write the requested definition in the blank that follows.

1. a) otologist   _____/___/_____
                              cf   s

   b. *Bonus Question:* What is the definition of the combining form? _____

2. a) tympanometry   _____/___/_____
                              cf   s

   b) *Bonus Question:* What is the definition of the suffix?_____

3. a) myringoplasty   _____/___/_____
                              cf   s

   b) *Bonus Question:* What is the definition of the combining form? _____

Abbreviations of the Eyes and Ears

The abbreviations that are associated with the eyes and ears are summarized here. Study these abbreviations, and review them in the exercise that follows.

Abbreviation	Definition
AD	right ear; in Latin, *auris dexter*
AMD	age-related macular degeneration
AS	left ear; in Latin, *auris sinister*
AU	both ears; in Latin, *aures unitas*
Ast	astigmatism
Em	emmetropia
EENT	eye, ear, nose, and throat
ENT	ear, nose, and throat

Abbreviation	Definition
IOL	intraocular lens
LASIK	laser-assisted in situ keratomileusis
OD	right eye; in Latin, *oculus dexter*
OM	otitis media
OS	left eye; in Latin, *oculus sinister*
Oto	otology
OU	each eye; in Latin, *oculus uterque*
TM	tympanic membrane

PRACTICE: Abbreviations

Fill in the blanks with the abbreviation or the complete medical term.

Abbreviation	Medical Term
1. _____	otitis media
2. ENT	_____
3. _____	otology
4. AU	_____
5. _____	left ear
6. Em	_____
7. _____	intraocular membrane
8. AD	_____
9. _____	eye, ear, nose, and throat
10. TM	_____

Chapter Review

Word Building

Construct medical terms from the following meanings. The first question has been completed for you as an example.

1. inflammation of the cornea   kerat*itis*_____

2. a drooping eyelid   blepharo_____

3. a stone in the lacrimal apparatus   _____lithiasis

4. inflammation of the conjunctiva   conjunctiv_____

5. softening of the eye   _____malacia

6. paralysis of the eye   ophthalmo_____

7. a generalized disease of the retina   retino_____

8. a specialist who corrects vision disorders   _____metrist

9. inflammation of the lacrimal apparatus   _____itis

10. bleeding of the eye   ophthalmo_____

11. a symptom of white film in the cornea   _____cornea

12. inflammation of the middle ear   _____itis media

13. condition of pain in the ear   ot_____

14. abnormal formation of bone in the ear   oto_____

15. pus discharge from the external ear canal   oto_____

16. instrument of ear examination   _____scope

17. generalized disease of the ear   oto_____

18. a partial loss of hearing   para_____

▶▶▶▶ **Medical Report Exercises**

Salima Aziz _____

Read the following medical report, then answer the critical thinking questions that follow.

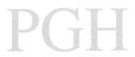

PEARSON GENERAL HOSPITAL

5500 University Avenue, Metropolis, TX
Phone: (211) 594-4000 • Fax: (211) 594-4001

Medical Consultation: Ophthalmology

Date: 10/15/2011

Patient: Salima Aziz

Patient Complaint: Right eye pain, crusty exudate, right eye pruritis and swelling that has spread to the left eye.

History: 16-year-old female with negative history for ophthalmology.

Family History: Unknown

Allergies: None

Physical Examination: Slight fever of 99.5°F, other vital signs normal. Right eyelid and OU with signs of inflammation and exudate.

Diagnosis: OU conjunctivitis, keratitis, and blepharitis.

Treatment: Antibiotic eyedrops with systemic antibiotic therapy; follow with office exam in two weeks.

Jana Abashiri, M.D.

Jana Abashiri, M.D.

Photo Source: Michael Jung/Shutterstock

Comprehension Questions

1. What patient complaints and evidence support the diagnosis of conjunctivitis?_____

_____

_____

2. Why would a treatment including antibiotics be prescribed for this ophthalmopathy?_____

_____

_____

3. What is the meaning of *OU ophthalmalgia*? _____

_____

_____

Case Study Questions

The following case study provides further discussion regarding the patient in the medical report. Fill in the blanks with the correct terms. Choose your answers from the following list of terms. (Note that some terms may be used more than once.)

conjunctivitis	keratitis	ophthalmalgia
blepharitis	ophthalmologist	OS

Salima Aziz, a 16-year-old female with no prior history of ophthalmic disease, complained to her parents of eye pain or

(a) _____ originating from the right eye and spreading to the left eye, or (b)_____ (abbreviation),

within a few days. She also noticed swelling of the eyelids, or (c) _____, with a crusty exudate, and her parents

became worried when they saw redness of the eye, suggesting the condition of (d) _____. Her parents

brought her to a physician specializing in eye care, called an (e) _____, immediately. During the eye exam,

the physician diagnosed inflammation of the right eyelid, inflammation of the conjunctiva, or (f) _____, and

inflammation of the cornea, or (g) _____, and identified the probable cause to be bacterial. As a result,

antibiotic eyedrops and systemic antibiotics were prescribed with follow-up visits scheduled.

Reggie Fletcher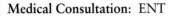

For a greater challenge, read the following medical report provided and answer the critical thinking questions that follow.

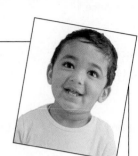

PGH PEARSON GENERAL HOSPITAL

5500 University Avenue, Metropolis, PA
Phone: (211) 594-4000 • Fax: (211) 594-4001

Medical Consultation: ENT

Date: 09/18/2011

Patient: Reggie Fletcher

Patient Complaint: Mother reports the child is pulling at the right ear, more crying and fussiness than usual, often relieved with acetaminophen, and failure to sleep through the night.

History: 2-year-old male child with no prior medical history in otology; all vaccinations up to date.

Family History: Mother and father free of related symptoms.

Allergies: None

Physical Examination: Child presents with fever 101.5°F; anxious with extreme sensitivity during exam; exam positive for AD myringitis; no loss of hearing evident.

Diagnosis: AD myringitis with possible otitis media.

Treatment: Treat with antibiotic eardrops with follow-up exam in 2 weeks for possible myringotomy with tympanic cavity drainage.

Judith N. VonTripp, M.D.

Judith N. VonTripp, M.D.

Photo Source: Ami Parikh/Shutterstock

Comprehension Questions

1. What evidence supports a diagnosis of AD myringitis with possible otitis media? _____

_____

_____

2. Why do you think a myringotomy may need to be performed if the child does not improve within 2 weeks? _____

_____

_____

Case Study Questions

The following case study provides further discussion regarding the patient in the medical report. Recall the terms from this chapter to fill in the blanks with the correct terms.

Reggie Fletcher, a 2-year-old male, was brought to the medical clinic after his behavior during the preceding several weeks indicated to his mother that he was experiencing ear pain, known as (h) _____, of the right ear, abbreviated (i) _____. His behavior included pulling or tugging at his right ear, an inability to sleep through the night, mild fever, and frequent fussiness. The general physician examined his ears using an (j) _____ and observed inflammation of the tympanic membrane, called (k) _____. Because this condition is often indicative of a potential infection within the middle ear, called (l) _____ _____, the physician referred the patient to (m) _____. Following an exam, the ear specialist, or (n) _____, determined a course of treatment to include antibiotic eardrops with follow-up exams to ensure the infection is defeated. Unfortunately, 2 weeks later the infection had spread into the tympanic cavity to produce the disease (o) _____ _____. The tympanic membrane was then surgically incised in a (p) _____ procedure and drainage tubes inserted into the tympanic cavity to drain the purulent fluids. One month after the patient had recovered, a hearing test, or (q) _____, was performed and found a 20% loss of hearing from the right ear.

15

The Endocrine System

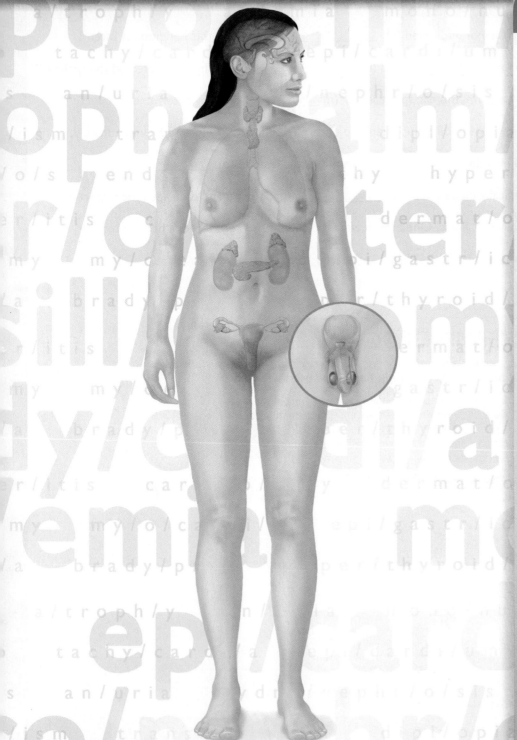

After completing this chapter, you will be able to:

1 Define and spell the word parts used to create terms for the endocrine system.

2 Identify the major organs of the endocrine system and describe their structure and function.

3 Break down and define common medical terms used for symptoms, diseases, disorders, procedures, treatments, and devices associated with the endocrine system.

4 Build medical terms from the word parts associated with the endocrine system.

5 Pronounce and spell common medical terms associated with the endocrine system.

Anatomy and Physiology Terms ▶▶▶▶▶

The following table provides the combining forms that specifically apply to the anatomy and physiology of the endocrine system. Note that the combining forms are colored red to help you identify them when you see them again later in the chapter.

Combining Form	Definition
aden/o	gland
adren/o	adrenal gland
crin/o	to secrete
gonad/o	sex gland
hormon/o	to set in motion
pancreat/o	sweetbread, pancreas
ren/o	kidney
thyr/o	shield, thyroid
thyroid/o	resembling a shield, thyroid

endocrine **gland** **gonads**	**15.1** The **endocrine** (EN doh krin) **system** works hand in hand with the nervous system to regulate body functions. The primary organs of the _____ system include the pituitary gland attached to the hypothalamus at the base of the brain, the thyroid _____ in the neck, the parathyroid glands embedded within the thyroid gland, the two adrenal glands located above each kidney, the pancreatic islets within the pancreas, and the _____, which include the ovaries of the female and testes of the male.
homeostasis **hormone**	**15.2** Like the nervous system, the endocrine system provides a method of control to keep the body functioning despite changing conditions in the environment. Thus, the primary role of the endocrine system is to manage _____, a state in which the body's equilibrium is maintained. Instead of regulating body activities with rapid nerve impulses, the endocrine organs secrete chemicals called **hormones** that are carried by the bloodstream. The result of _____ secretion is a change in cell functions, which alters body activities. When the endocrine system becomes deficient due to disease, the result is a homeostatic imbalance that often affects overall health.

15.3 Use the anatomy terms that appear in the left column to fill in the corresponding blanks in Figure 15.1■.

1. **gland**
2. **thyroid**
3. **adrenal**
4. **pancreas**
5. **testis**

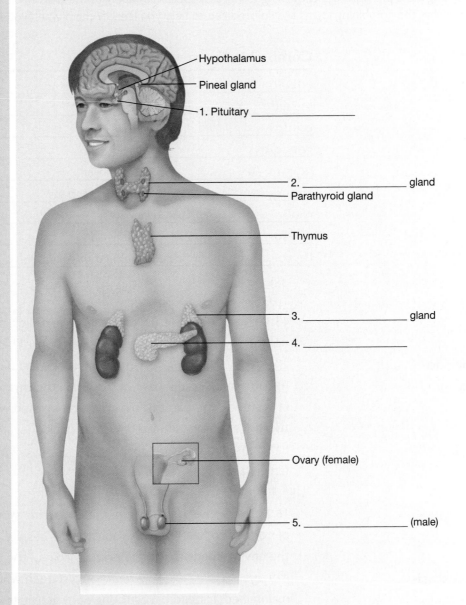

Hypothalamus

Pineal gland

1. Pituitary _____

2. _____ gland
Parathyroid gland

Thymus

3. _____ gland

4. _____

Ovary (female)

5. _____ (male)

Figure 15.1 ■
The endocrine glands of the endocrine system are distributed throughout the body.

Medical Terms for the Endocrine System ▶▶▶▶▶

hyposecretion	15.4 An array of disorders can occur when an endocrine gland fails to deliver the quantity of hormones needed to regulate body functions. In general, endocrine disease results from either abnormally high hormone production, called **hypersecretion,** or abnormally low hormone production, called _____. Either condition upsets the homeostatic balance of the body. Hypersecretion may arise due to an inherited disease or a tumor. Often, hyposecretion occurs if an endocrine gland suffers trauma due to an injury or infection, although it also may be caused by an inherited disorder or a tumor. Sometimes, an endocrine disorder includes an array of symptoms and involves multiple organs. This type of disease is generally known as a **syndrome.**
within **study** **science of**	15.5 The treatment of endocrine diseases is a focused discipline within medicine, called **endocrinology** (EN doh krin ALL oh jee). This is a constructed term that is written endo/crin/o/logy and includes the prefix endo- that means "_____," the combining form crin/o that means "to secrete," and the suffix -logy that means "_____ or _____ _____."
	15.6 In the following sections, you will study the prefixes, combining forms, and suffixes that combine to build the medical terms of the endocrine system.

Signs and Symptoms of the Endocrine System

Here are the word parts that specifically apply to the signs and symptoms of the endocrine system that are covered in the following section. Note that the word parts are color-coded to help you identify them: prefixes are green, combining forms are red, and suffixes are blue.

Prefix	Definition	Combining Form	Definition	Suffix	Definition
ex-	outside, away from	acid/o	a solution or substance with a pH less than 7	-ia	condition of
poly-	excessive, over, many			-ism	condition or disease
		acr/o	extremity	-megaly	abnormally large
		dips/o	thirst		
		hirsut/o	hairy	-osis	condition of
		ket/o	ketone	-s	plural
		ophthalm/o	eye	-uria	pertaining to urine, urination

KEY TERMS A–Z

acidosis
ass ih DOH siss

15.7 Recall that the suffix *-osis* means "condition of." The sign of excess acid in the body is therefore known as _____, and the constructed form of the term is acid/osis. It occurs when carbon dioxide, the primary waste product from cellular metabolism, accumulates in tissues (including blood) to form carbonic acid. Acidosis is a symptom of diabetes mellitus (Frame 15.21) and may also be caused by respiratory or kidney disorders.

15.8 A sign that includes enlargement of bone structure is known as **acromegaly.** The enlargement causes disfigurement, especially in the hands and face, and is a sign of hypersecretion of growth hormone (abbreviated **GH**) from the pituitary gland during adulthood (Figure 15.2■). _____ literally means "abnormally large extremity." It is a constructed term that is written acr/o/megaly.

acromegaly
ak roh MEG ah lee

Figure 15.2 ■
Acromegaly. Acromegaly is a metabolic disorder in which excessive amounts of growth hormone are secreted during adulthood, resulting in enlarged bones. The photographs show the same individual at ages 20, 30, and 40 years.
Source: Published in American Journal of Medicine, Vol 20, page 133, 1956, Dr. William H. Daughaday. Copyright Elsevier. With permission of Excerpta Media Inc.

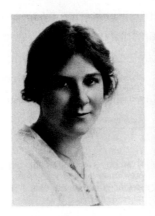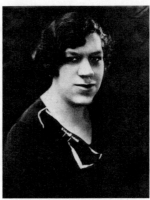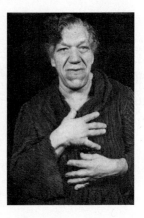

exophthalmos
eks off THAL mos

15.9 The abnormal protrusion of the eyes is known as **exophthalmos.** It is a classic symptom of excessive activity of the thyroid gland and literally means "outside eyes" (Figure 15.3■). _____ is a constructed term that is written as ex/ophthalm/o/s.

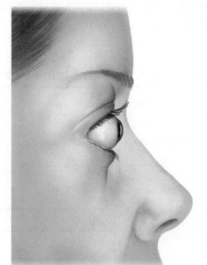

Figure 15.3 ■
Exophthalmos. The protrusion of the eyes is a common symptom of hyperthyroidism.

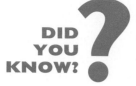

▶▶▶▶▶ **Thyroid**

The shape of the thyroid gland must have reminded the Greeks of a shield because the term is derived from the Greek word for this defensive warrior gear, *thyreos*.

goiter GOY ter	**15.10** A symptom of thyroid gland disease is a swelling on the anterior side of the neck in the location of the thyroid gland, known as a **goiter.** A _____ is an abnormal enlargement of the thyroid gland caused by a tumor, lack of iodine in the diet, or an infection.
hirsutism HER soot izm	**15.11** A symptom of excessive body hair in a masculine pattern is known as **hirsutism.** The term is derived from the Latin word *hirsutus,* which means "hairy." When _____ occurs in women, it is caused by the hypersecretion of androgens by the adrenal cortex. Excessive production of androgens in women may also lead to muscle and bone growth. The resulting pattern of masculinization is known as **adrenal virilism** (add REE nal * VIHR ill izm).
ketosis kee TOH siss **ketoacidosis** kee toh ah sih DOH siss	**15.12** A ketone body is a waste substance produced when cells are unable to metabolize carbohydrates. The condition called _____ is an excessive amount of ketone bodies in the blood and urine and is a symptom of unmanaged diabetes mellitus (Frame 15.21) and starvation. Because **ketosis** produces an acidic condition of the body, it is also known as **ketoacidosis** (KEE toh ass ih DOH siss). _____ contains four word parts and is written as ket/o/acid/osis.
polydipsia PALL ee DIP see ah	**15.13** The prefix *poly-* means "excessive, over, many." It is sometimes used to indicate an abnormally excessive amount. The combining form *dips/o* means "thirst." Thus, the symptom called _____ literally means "condition of excessive thirst." An abnormal state of excessive thirst occurs during certain disorders of the pituitary gland or the pancreas.
polyuria PALL ee YOO ree ah	**15.14** As you learned in Chapter 11, the term **polyuria** includes the prefix *poly-.* It is a symptom of pituitary gland disease that arises when the hormone **ADH** is not produced normally. It is also a symptom of unmanaged diabetes mellitus (Frame 15.21). _____ is the production of abnormally large volumes of urine.

PRACTICE: Signs and Symptoms of the Endocrine System

The Right Match

Match the term on the left with the correct definition on the right.

_____ 1. acidosis

_____ 2. ketosis

_____ 3. goiter

_____ 4. adrenal virilism

_____ 5. hirsutism

a. enlargement at the throat

b. a pattern of masculinization and hair distribution in women

c. excessive body hair

d. abnormal accumulation of waste materials that are acidic

e. excessive amount of ketone bodies in the blood and urine

Break the Chain

Analyze these medical terms:

a) Separate each term into its word parts; each word part is labeled for you (**p** = prefix, **r** = root, **cf** = combining form, and **s** = suffix).

b) For the Bonus Question, write the requested definition in the blank that follows.

The first set has been completed as an example.

1. a) *polydipsia*   *poly/dips/ia*
                                        p   r   s

   b) *Bonus Question:* What is the definition of the suffix? *condition of* _____

2. a) exophthalmos   _____/_____/___/_____
                                      p   cf   s

   b) *Bonus Question:* What is the definition of the combining form? _____

3. a) polyuria   _____/_____
                                      p   s

   b) *Bonus Question:* What is the definition of the suffix? _____

4. a) acromegaly   _____/___/_____
                                      cf   s

   b) *Bonus Question:* What is the definition of the combining form? _____

5. a) ketoacidosis   _____/___/_____/_____
                                      cf   r   s

   b) *Bonus Question:* What is the definition of the combining form? _____

Diseases and Disorders of the Endocrine System

Here are the word parts that specifically apply to the diseases and disorders of the endocrine system that are covered in the following section. Note that the word parts are color-coded to help you identify them: prefixes are green, combining forms are red, and suffixes are blue.

Prefix	Definition
endo-	within
hyper-	excessive, abnormally high, above
hypo-	deficient, abnormally low, below
para-	alongside, abnormal

Combining Form	Definition
aden/o	gland
adren/o	adrenal gland
calc/i, calc/o	calcium
carcin/o	cancer
crin/o	to secrete
glyc/o	sweet, sugar
gonad/o	sex gland
muc/o	mucus
pancreat/o	sweetbread, pancreas
thyr/o	shield, thyroid
thyroid/o	resembling a shield, thyroid

Suffix	Definition
-al	pertaining to
-emia	condition of blood
-ism	condition or disease
-itis	inflammation
-megaly	abnormally large
-oma	tumor
-osis	condition of
-pathy	disease
-penia	abnormal reduction in number, deficiency

KEY TERMS A–Z

adenitis
add en EYE tiss

adenopathy
add en OH path ee
aden/osis

15.15 A commonly used combining form that means "gland" is aden/o. When the suffix meaning "inflammation" is included, the term _____ is formed, which can be written in its constructed form as aden/itis. *Adenitis* is the general term for an inflammation of a gland. Similarly, the general term for a glandular disease is _____. Also, any disease of a gland is called an **adenosis** (add en OH siss). The constructed form of *adenopathy* is aden/o/pathy, and *adenosis* is _____/_____.

adenocarcinoma
ADD eh noh kar sih NOH mah

adenoma
ADD eh NOH mah

15.16 A malignant tumor that arises from epithelial tissue to form a glandular or glandlike pattern of cells is called an _____. As a constructed term with four word parts, it is written aden/o/carcin/oma. An adenocarcinoma is a life-threatening form of cancer. It often develops from a benign tumor of glandular cells, known as an _____. An adenoma may cause excess secretion by the affected gland.

adrenalitis
add REE nah LYE tiss

adrenomegaly
add ree noh MEG ah lee

15.17 Inflammation of the adrenal gland is a condition known as _____. It may result from tumor development or infection and is often revealed in women by the symptoms of adrenal virilism (Frame 15.11). This constructed term is written adren/al/itis. A similar disease in which one or both of the adrenal glands becomes enlarged is known as _____, which has three word parts and is written adren/o/megaly. Both adrenalitis and adrenomegaly are forms of **adrenopathy** (add ren AH path ee).

cretinism
KREE tin izm

15.18 A child suffering from the thyroid gland's inability to produce normal levels of growth hormone at birth may develop the condition called **cretinism.** A reduced mental development and physical growth occur in _____.

Cushing syndrome
KUSH ing * SIN drohm

15.19 A **syndrome** is a disease with an array of symptoms and involving multiple organs. A syndrome that is caused by excessive secretion of the hormone cortisol by the adrenal cortex, which affects many organs, is called **Cushing syndrome.** It is characterized by obesity, moon (round) face, hyperglycemia (Frame 15.25), and muscle weakness (Figure 15.4■). A common cause of _____ _____ is an adenoma (Frame 15.16) of the adrenal cortex.

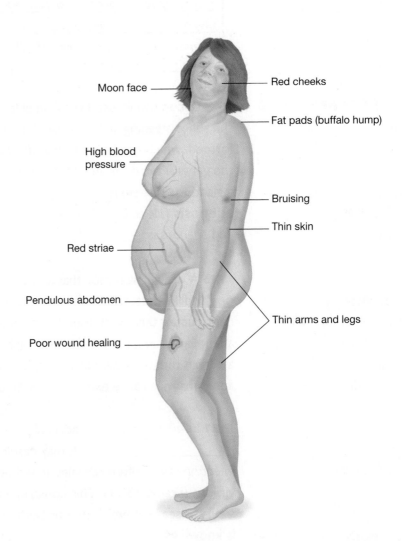

Moon face — Red cheeks

Fat pads (buffalo hump)

High blood pressure

Bruising

Thin skin

Red striae

Pendulous abdomen

Poor wound healing

Thin arms and legs

Figure 15.4 ■
Cushing syndrome. This syndrome includes the symptoms of obesity, moon face, hyperglycemia, and muscle weakness.

diabetes insipidus DYE ah BEE teez * in SIP ih duss	**15.20 Diabetes insipidus** (**DI**) is caused by hyposecretion of ADH by the pituitary gland. The disease _____ _____ is characterized by the symptoms of polydipsia (Frame 15.13) and polyuria (Frame 15.14).
diabetes mellitus DYE ah BEE teez * MELL ih tuss	**15.21** Although the term *diabetes* is shared by two diseases, the chronic disorder of carbohydrate metabolism known as **diabetes mellitus** has very little in common with diabetes insipidus (Frame 15.20; see the Did You Know? box to read why). Diabetes mellitus (**DM**) is a result of resistance of body cells to insulin, or a deficiency or complete lack of insulin production by cells of the pancreas. Two major forms of _____ _____ strike human health. Type 1, which is less common, usually requires hormone replacement therapy with insulin and appears during childhood or adolescence. The more common Type 2 usually appears during adulthood and is often associated with obesity (Figure 15.5■). Unlike Type 1, Type 2 can usually be managed with dietary restrictions and regular exercise, and it can be controlled with oral antidiabetic drugs. Common symptoms of both types include polydipsia (Frame 15.13), polyuria (Frame 15.14), and the abnormal presence of sugar in the urine (glycosuria). If unmanaged, diabetes mellitus causes large fluctuations in blood sugar levels, resulting in circulatory deficiencies that result in cerebrovascular disease leading to heart failure, kidney damage called **diabetic nephropathy** (DYE ah BET ik * nef ROHP ah thee) leading to kidney failure, and damage to the eyes
diabetic retinopathy DYE ah BET ik * ret in NOP ah thee	called _____ _____ that leads to blindness (see Figure 14.8 on page 450).

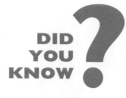

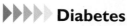

▶▶▶▶▶ Diabetes

The term *diabetes* is a Greek word that means "to pass through" or "to pass over." Another meaning is "siphon." The term was first used during the Middle Ages when a siphon was used by physicians to withdraw a sample of urine from a patient to test for an excess of sugar, which was often done by taste. The siphon "passed urine through" to a collection device. A sweet taste indicated sugar excess and a crude diagnosis of diabetes mellitus. The term *mellitus* is a Latin word that means "sweetened with honey." If the "taste test" did not indicate sweetness, but the patient still complained of excessive urination, the diagnosis was diabetes insipidus. As you might guess, the term *insipidus* is a Latin word that means "lacking flavor."

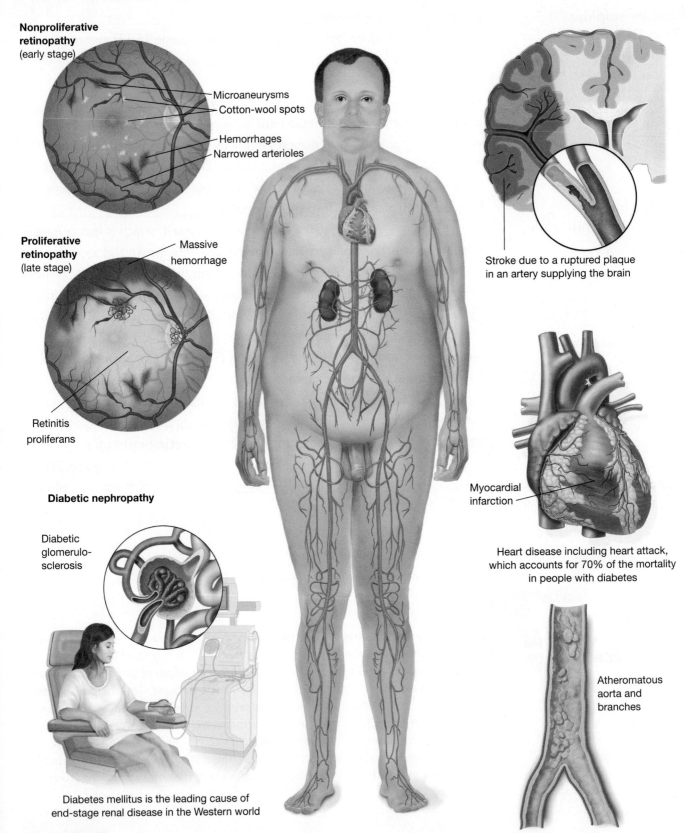

Diabetic retinopathy

Nonproliferative retinopathy (early stage)

- Microaneurysms
- Cotton-wool spots
- Hemorrhages
- Narrowed arterioles

Proliferative retinopathy (late stage)

Massive hemorrhage

Retinitis proliferans

Diabetic nephropathy

Diabetic glomerulo-sclerosis

Diabetes mellitus is the leading cause of end-stage renal disease in the Western world

Cerebrovascular disease

Stroke due to a ruptured plaque in an artery supplying the brain

Myocardial infarction

Heart disease including heart attack, which accounts for 70% of the mortality in people with diabetes

Atheromatous aorta and branches

Figure 15.5 ■

Diabetes mellitus. The metabolic disease diabetes mellitus, with symptoms of polydipsia, polyuria, and widely ranging blood sugar levels, produces many chronic complications if not managed carefully. They include an increased risk of blindness (diabetic retinopathy), kidney disease (diabetic nephropathy), and heart attack (cerebrovascular disease).

endocrinopathy
en doh krin OPP ah thee

15.22 The general term for a disease of the endocrine system is
_____. It is a constructed term with four word parts,
written as endo/crin/o/pathy. In most cases, endocrinopathy is the result of
either an excessive production of one or more hormones by an endocrine
gland or deficient production of one or more hormones. To identify which,
the prefixes *hyper-* ("excessive, abnormally high, above") and *hypo-* ("deficient,
abnormally low, below") are frequently used with the endocrine gland that is
diseased.

hyperadrenalism
HIGH per add REN al izm

hypoadrenalism
HIGH poh add REN al izm

15.23 Excessive activity of one or more adrenal glands is the disease called
_____. It is a constructed term written hyper/adren/al/ism.
In time, hyperadrenalism produces the symptoms that characterize Cushing
syndrome (Frame 15.19). The opposite disorder occurs when the adrenal
gland activity becomes abnormally reduced. Called _____,
it may lead to a chronic form called **Addison disease** if left untreated. The
constructed form of this term is written hypo/adren/al/ism.

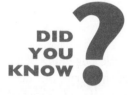 ▶▶▶▶▶ **Addison Disease**

In 1855, a series of signs and symptoms were connected for the first time into a
disease. They included "feeble heart action, anemia, irritability of the stomach, and
a peculiar change in the color of the skin." The syndrome was named to recognize
its discoverer, the English physician Thomas Addison, who correlated the symptoms and signs to a failure of the adrenal cortex.

hypercalcemia
HIGH per kal SEE mee ah

hypocalcemia
HIGH poh kal SEE mee ah

15.24 The suffix *-emia* means "condition of blood." When calcium
levels in the blood become abnormally high, the disease is known
as _____. The constructed form of this term is
hyper/calc/emia. The disease is a result of the abnormal release of calcium
from bones, which leads to softening of the bones if left untreated. It is caused
by excessive activity of the parathyroid glands. The condition of abnormally
low levels of calcium in the blood is called _____ and is also
called **calcipenia** (KAL sih PEE nee ah). It is caused by the abnormally low activity
of the parathyroid glands, which produce insufficient parathyroid hormone
(**PTH**). *Calcipenia* is a constructed term, written as calc/i/penia.

hypoglycemia
HIGH poh glye SEE mee ah

15.25 Another use of the suffix *-emia* is in the term **hyperglycemia,** which literally means "condition of blood excessive sugar." The constructed form of this term is hyper/glyc/emia. The chronic form of the disease often indicates the body may not be producing enough insulin or insulin receptor sites are resistant. It may lead to Type 2 diabetes mellitus (Frame 15.21). In the opposite condition, _____, blood sugar levels fall to abnormally low levels. It is caused by excessive insulin administration or excessive production by the pancreas and is often accompanied by headache, malaise (weakness), tremors, hunger, and anxiety. If left untreated, it can lead to coma and death.

hypoparathyroidism
HIGH poh pair ah THIGH royd izm
hypo/para/thyroid/ism

15.26 The excessive production of PTH by the parathyroid glands is a disorder known as **hyperparathyroidism.** This lengthy term contains four word parts: hyper/para/thyroid/ism. Usually caused by a tumor, it results in excessive calcium levels in the blood, or hypercalcemia (Frame 15.24). In the opposite condition called _____, PTH levels are reduced and the condition of hypocalcemia (Frame 15.24) occurs. The constructed form of this term is written 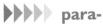____/____/_____/____.

WORDS TO WATCH OUT FOR ! ▶▶▶▶▶ **para-**

Note that the prefix *para-* doesn't always appear at the beginning of a term. In the term *hypoparathyroid,* it appears in the middle of the term. But don't let that confuse you: it is still a prefix, and it still means "alongside or abnormal."

hyperthyroidism
HIGH per THIGH royd izm

15.27 Excessive activity of the thyroid gland produces abnormally high levels of thyroid hormone in the disease _____, which accelerates metabolism. The constructed form of this term is hyper/thyroid/ism. Symptoms include exophthalmos (Frame 15.9), goiter (Frame 15.10), rapid heart rate, and weight loss. One form of chronic hyperthyroidism, called **Graves disease,** is believed to be an autoimmune disease. Another form, known as **thyrotoxicosis** (THIGH roh toks ih KOH siss), is an acute event that is triggered by infection or trauma and can become life threatening.

WORDS TO WATCH OUT FOR ! ▶▶▶▶▶ *hyper-* **or** *hypo-*?

The spelling of these two prefixes is very similar, but the difference in meaning is great. *Hyper-* means "excessive, abnormally high, above"; whereas *hypo-* means "deficient, abnormally low, below." An easy way to remember the difference is to think of the long o sound of the word "low," which matches the sound of the vowel in *hypo-*.

hypothyroidism
HIGH poh THIGH royd izm

15.28 When thyroid gland activity becomes deficient, thyroid hormone blood levels drop below normal in the disease called _____ (Figure 15.6■). The constructed form is written hypo/thyroid/ism. The symptoms of hypothyroidism include a slow heart rate, dry skin, low energy, and weight gain. In the chronic form of hypothyroidism known as **myxedema** (miks eh DEE mah), the subcutaneous layer beneath the skin becomes thick and hard, and the body retains water, aging the skin prematurely while puffing the face and thickening the tongue and hands. *Myxedema* literally means "swollen mucus."

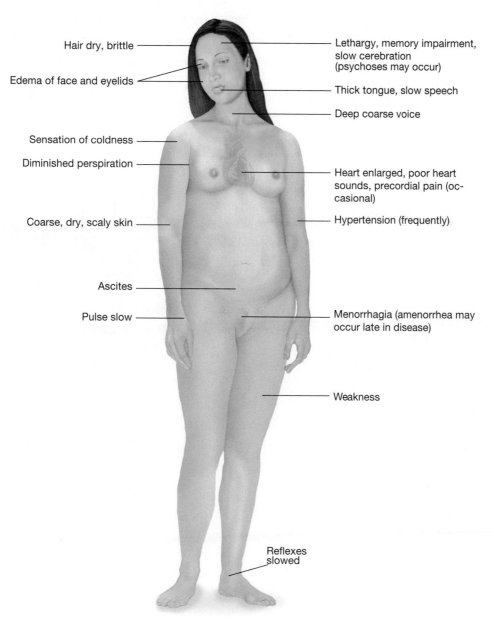

Hair dry, brittle

Edema of face and eyelids

Sensation of coldness

Diminished perspiration

Coarse, dry, scaly skin

Ascites

Pulse slow

Lethargy, memory impairment, slow cerebration (psychoses may occur)

Thick tongue, slow speech

Deep coarse voice

Heart enlarged, poor heart sounds, precordial pain (occasional)

Hypertension (frequently)

Menorrhagia (amenorrhea may occur late in disease)

Weakness

Reflexes slowed

Figure 15.6 ■
Hypothyroidism. Hyposecretion of the thyroid gland produces the symptoms that are illustrated.

hypogonadism
 HIGH poh GOH nad izm

hypo/gonad/ism

15.29 In the disease **hypogonadism,** abnormally low amounts of follicle-stimulating hormone (**FSH**) and luteinizing hormone (**LH**) are produced by the pituitary gland, which reduces the production of the sex hormones testosterone (produced by the male testes) and estrogen/progesterone (produced by the female ovaries). Also known as pituitary _____, it results in reduced sexual interest and reproductive capacity. If it occurs prior to puberty, the gonads (male testes and female ovaries) fail to develop. *Hypogonadism* is a constructed term, which is written as _____/_____/_____.

pancreatitis
 PAN kree ah TYE tiss

15.30 Inflammation of the pancreas is a disorder known as _____ (Figure 15.7■). It often results in a deficient production of insulin, which leads to hyperglycemia (Frame 15.25). Pancreatitis may be an acute reaction to infection or trauma, or a chronic condition resulting in progressive pancreatic failure, both of which can become life threatening. The term includes only two word parts: pancreat/itis.

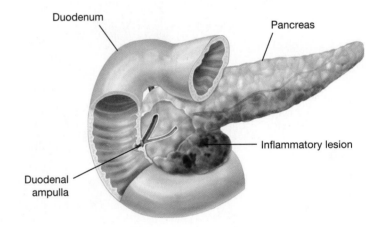

Duodenum

Pancreas

Inflammatory lesion

Duodenal ampulla

Figure 15.7 ■
Pancreatitis. Inflammation of the pancreas may be the result of a bacterial infection, trauma, or chronic disease such as cancer.

pituitary gigantism
pih TOO ih tair ee * JYE gant izm

15.31 Because the pituitary gland produces numerous hormones, a tumor or congenital defect of the pituitary can affect many body functions. In **pituitary dwarfism** (pih TOO ih tair ee * DWARF izm), the pituitary growth hormone is deficient at birth, resulting in short stature. An abnormally high production of pituitary growth hormone before adolescence results in _____ _____, and if it occurs after adolescence, it results in acromegaly (Frame 15.8). An illustration comparing dwarfism and gigantism is provided in Figure 15.8■.

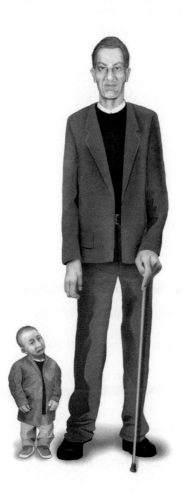

Figure 15.8 ■
Growth hormone disorders. Illustration of a pituitary giant and a pituitary dwarf, both adults of about the same age.

thyroiditis
THYE royd EYE tiss

15.32 Inflammation of the thyroid gland is called _____. The constructed form is thyroid/itis. Acute thyroiditis is usually caused by a local infection, whereas there are many forms of chronic thyroiditis that often lead to hyperthyroidism (Frame 15.27).

PRACTICE: Diseases and Disorders of the Endocrine System

Linkup

Link the word parts in the list to create the terms that match the definitions. You may use word parts more than once. Remember to add combining vowels when needed—and that some terms do not use any combining vowel. The first one is completed as an example.

Prefix	Combining Form	Suffix
hyper-	aden/o	-al
hypo-	adrenal/o	-emia
para-	calc/o	-ism
	carcin/o	-itis
	glyc/o	-oma
	pancreat/o	-pathy
	thyr/o	
	thyroid/o	

Definition

1. inflammation of a gland

2. glandular disease

3. malignant tumor that arises from epithelial tissue to form a glandular or glandlike pattern of cells

4. excessive activity of one or more adrenal glands

5. a disease that results from abnormally high levels of calcium in the blood

6. abnormally low blood sugar level

7. excessive production of parathyroid hormone by the parathyroid glands

8. a disease that results from abnormally low blood levels of thyroid hormone

9. inflammation of the pancreas

10. inflammation of the thyroid

Term

1. *adenitis*

2. _____

3. _____

4. _____

5. _____

6. _____

7. _____

8. _____

9. _____

10. _____

The Right Match

Match the term on the left with the correct definition on the right.

_____ 1. Addison disease

_____ 2. diabetic nephropathy

_____ 3. diabetes insipidus

_____ 4. pituitary gigantism

_____ 5. Cushing syndrome

_____ 6. Graves disease

_____ 7. diabetic retinopathy

_____ 8. diabetes mellitus

_____ 9. pituitary dwarfism

_____ 10. cretinism

a. caused by excessive secretion of adrenal cortex

b. a form of chronic hyperthyroidism; may be an autoimmune disease

c. chronic disorder of carbohydrate metabolism

d. kidney damage caused by diabetes mellitus

e. potentially vision-threatening damage to the eye in diabetics

f. caused by hyposecretion of adrenal cortex

g. short stature resulting from a deficiency in pituitary growth hormone

h. caused by hyposecretion of ADH by the pituitary

i. reduced mental development and physical growth that results from a lack of thyroid hormone at birth

j. results from an abnormally high production of pituitary growth hormone before adolescence

Treatments, Procedures, and Devices of the Endocrine System

Here are the word parts that specifically apply to the treatments, procedures, and devices of the endocrine system that are covered in the following section. Note that the word parts are color-coded to help you identify them: prefixes are green, combining forms are red, and suffixes are blue.

Prefix	Definition	Combining Form	Definition	Suffix	Definition
endo-	within	adren/o	adrenal gland	-al	pertaining to
para-	alongside, abnormal	crin/o	to secrete	-ectomy	surgical excision, removal
		thyr/o	shield, thyroid	-logist	one who studies
		thyroid/o	resembling a shield, thyroid	-logy	study or science of
				-oma	tumor
				-tomy	incision, to cut

KEY TERMS A–Z

adrenalectomy
add REE nal EK toh mee

15.33 A procedure involving the surgical excision, or removal, of one or both of the adrenal glands is known as **adrenalectomy.** The constructed form of this term is adren/al/ectomy. An _____ may become necessary if hormone therapy fails to correct hyperadrenalism (Frame 15.23).

endocrinologist

en doh krin ALL oh jist

15.34 You learned at the beginning of this chapter that the term *endocrine* literally means "to secrete within," and the field of medicine focusing on the study and treatment of endocrine disorders is called **endocrinology**. A physician specializing in this field is known as an _____. It is a constructed term written endo/crin/o/logist.

fasting blood sugar

15.35 Measuring blood sugar levels provides information about how well the body manages carbohydrate metabolism. In a procedure called

_____ _____ _____

(**FBS**), blood sugar levels are measured after a 12-hour fast. In a **postprandial blood sugar** (**PPBS**) exam, blood sugar levels are measured about 2 hours after a meal (postprandial means "after a meal"). In both tests, extreme variations in blood sugar or abnormally high glucose levels (hyperglycemia) are an indication of diabetes mellitus (Frame 15.21). A common method of testing blood sugar levels is shown in Figure 15.9■.

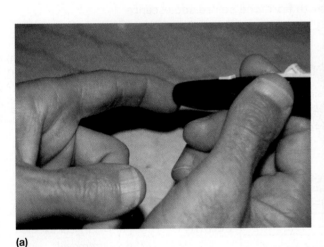
(a)

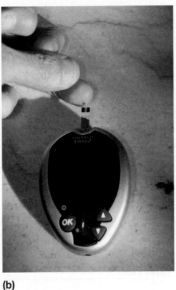
(b)

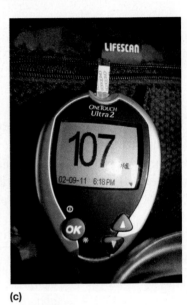
(c)

Figure 15.9 ■
Blood glucose measurement. A postprandial test may be self-administered. (a) A lance pierces the skin of a finger. (b) A small blood sample is gently squeezed onto a reagent strip. (c) The glucose meter will display the glucose concentration in the blood sample. A reading of 80 to 120 mg/dL is a normal range.
Source: Courtesy of Mala Kruss.

glucose tolerance test

15.36 A test that may be used to confirm a diagnosis of diabetes mellitus examines a patient's tolerance of glucose. Known as a

_____ _____ _____

(**GTT**), the patient is given glucose either orally or intravenously, then at timed intervals blood samples are taken and glucose levels measured and recorded. Large fluctuations of blood sugar confirm the diagnosis of diabetes mellitus.

hormone replacement therapy	**15.37** A failure of an endocrine gland to produce sufficient levels of a hormone, or hyposecretion, can have a serious impact on health. A common therapy to counteract hyposecretion is called **hormone replacement therapy** (**HRT**). Synthetic hormones or extracted hormones may be used in HRT. _____ _____ _____ may also be used following the surgical removal of an endocrine gland to restore homeostasis. It is an optional therapy for the treatment of symptoms associated with menopausal changes, although evidence suggests a slight risk of breast cancer with its use.
parathyroidectomy PAIR ah THIGH royd EK toh mee	**15.38** The surgical removal, or excision, of a parathyroid gland may be a treatment for parathyroid cancer, called **parathyroidoma,** or for hyperparathyroidism (Frame 15.26). The procedure is called _____ . The constructed form of this term is para/thyroid/ectomy.
radioactive iodine	**15.39** The producing cells of the thyroid gland use the element iodine as a necessary ingredient in forming thyroid hormones. One way in which thyroid function may be measured is to determine the amount of iodine taken into thyroid cells. In the diagnostic procedure known as **radioactive iodine uptake** (RAY dee oh AK tihv * EYE oh dyne * UP tayk), _____ _____ is used to track and measure its entry into thyroid gland cells with a scanning instrument. Abbreviated **RAIU,** a reduction of iodine uptake is an indication of deficient thyroid function.
radioiodine therapy RAY dee oh EYE oh dyne * THAIR ah pee	**15.40** Because the thyroid gland is the only organ of the body that uptakes iodine, an effective treatment against a thyroid tumor, or thyroidoma (Frame 15.41), is the use of radioactive iodine. Called _____ _____ , the radioactive iodine targets cells within the thyroid gland and destroys them.

thyroid scan
THIGH royd * skan

thyroidoma
THIGH royd OH mah

15.41 A procedure measuring thyroid function is called a **thyroid scan,** during which an image of the thyroid gland is obtained. The _____ _____ image is recorded with a scanning instrument following oral administration of a labeled substance, usually iodine (Figure 15.10■). Thyroid scans are usually employed to detect a thyroid tumor, known as a _____.

Figure 15.10 ■
Thyroid scan. The right image is the data from a thyroid scan, printed on a superimposed map of the thyroid gland from the patient, shown on the left with a goiter.

Goiter

thyroidectomy
THIGH royd EK toh mee

thyroidotomy
THIGH royd OTT oh mee

15.42 Recall the meaning of the suffix -*ectomy* is "surgical excision or removal." The surgical removal of the thyroid gland is therefore called _____. The constructed form is written thyroid/ectomy, and the procedure is illustrated in Figure 15.11■. Because the suffix -*tomy* means "incision, to cut," a _____ is a procedure in which the thyroid gland is surgically entered. This constructed term is written thyroid/o/tomy.

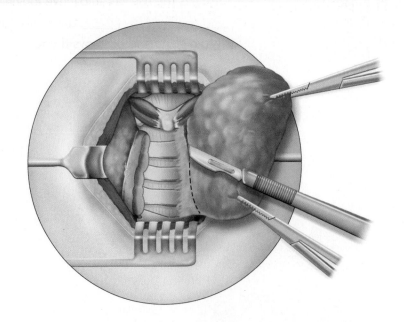

Figure 15.11 ■
Thyroidectomy. In this procedure, the thyroid gland is accessed by a vertical incision through the neck and removed.

thyroparathyroidectomy THIGH roh pair ah THIGH royd EK toh mee thyr/o/para/thyroid/ectomy	**15.43** In some cases, the parathyroid glands must be surgically removed with the thyroid gland. This procedure is called _____. Write the constructed form of this term: _____/___/_____/_____/_____.
thyroxine test THIGH rox een	**15.44** Thyroxine is one of several hormones produced by the thyroid gland. It regulates glucose metabolism and cell division in most cells of the body. A diagnostic test measuring thyroxine levels in the blood is simply called a _____ _____. It is often used as a diagnostic test for hyperthyroidism (Frame 15.27) or hypothyroidism (Frame 15.28).

PRACTICE: Treatments, Procedures, and Devices of the Endocrine System

The Right Match

Match the term on the left with the correct definition on the right.

_____ 1. fasting blood sugar

_____ 2. glucose tolerance test

_____ 3. hormone replacement therapy

_____ 4. radioactive iodine uptake

_____ 5. thyroid scan

_____ 6. thyroxine test

_____ 7. radioiodine therapy

a. synthetic or extracted hormones used to counteract hyposecretion

b. a procedure used to determine amount of iodine taken into thyroid cells

c. a test that examines a patient's tolerance of glucose

d. a procedure in which blood sugar levels are measured after a 12-hour fast

e. a diagnostic test that measures thyroxine levels in the blood

f. treatment for a thyroid tumor that targets cells within the thyroid gland and destroys them

g. a procedure that obtains an image of the thyroid to measure thyroid function

Break the Chain ———————————————————————————

Analyze these medical terms:

    a) Separate each term into its word parts; each word part is labeled for you (**p** = prefix, **r** = root, **cf** = combining form, and **s** = suffix).

    b) For the Bonus Question, write the requested definition in the blank that follows.

1. a) adrenalectomy   _____/_____/_____
                                                r   s   s

    b) *Bonus Question:* What is the definition of the **first** suffix? _____

2. a) endocrinology   _____/_____/___/_____
                                                p   cf   s

    b) *Bonus Question:* What is the definition of the combining form? _____

3. a) thyroidoma   _____/_____
                                              r   s

    b) *Bonus Question:* What is the definition of the suffix? _____

4. a) thyroidotomy   _____/___/_____
                                            cf   s

    b) *Bonus Question:* What is the definition of the suffix? _____

5. a) thyroparathyroidectomy   _____/___/_____/_____/_____
                                            cf   p   r   s

    b) *Bonus Question:* What is the definition of the suffix? _____

Abbreviations of the Endocrine System

The abbreviations that are associated with the endocrine system are summarized here. Study these abbreviations, and review them in the exercise that follows.

Abbreviation	Definition
ADH	antidiuretic hormone
DI	diabetes insipidus
DM	diabetes mellitus
FBS	fasting blood sugar
FSH	follicle-stimulating hormone
GH	growth hormone
GTT	glucose tolerance test
HRT	hormone replacement therapy
LH	luteinizing hormone
PPBS	postprandial blood sugar
PTH	parathyroid hormone
RAIU	radioactive iodine uptake

PRACTICE: Abbreviations

Fill in the blanks with the abbreviation or the complete medical term.

Abbreviation

1. GTT
2. _____
3. PPBS
4. _____
5. FBS
6. _____
7. DM

Medical Term

_____

radioactive iodine uptake

_____

diabetes insipidus

_____

hormone replacement therapy

_____

▶▶▶▶▶▶ Chapter Review

Word Building _____

Construct medical terms from the following meanings. The first question has been completed as an example.

1. inflammation of a gland   aden*itis*_____

2. excessive production of thyroid hormones   _____thyroidism

3. peripheral nerve damage during diabetes mellitus   diabetic neuro_____

4. inflammation of the adrenal gland   adrenal_____

5. disease of the endocrine system   _____pathy

6. excessive calcium levels in the blood   hyper_____

7. a tumor of the parathyroid gland   parathyroid_____

8. caused by too much GH in adulthood   pituitary gigant_____

9. abnormally reduced adrenal activity   _____adrenalism

10. excessive body hair   _____ism

11. deficient production of PTH   hypo_____

12. abnormally low blood sugar levels   hypo_____

13. acute form of hyperthyroidism triggered by infection or trauma   thyro_____

14. form of hypothyroidism that involves water retention and swelling   myx_____

15. caused by deficient FSH and LH that results in reduced reproductive capacity   _____gonadism

Medical Report Exercises

Anita Del Rio _____

Read the following medical report, then answer the questions that follow.

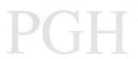 **PEARSON GENERAL HOSPITAL**

5500 University Avenue, Metropolis, UT
Phone: (211) 594-4000 • Fax: (211) 594-4001

Medical Consultation: Endocrinology

Date: 12/15/2011

Patient: Anita Del Rio

Patient Complaint: Malaise between meals, polydipsia, polyuria, cephalalgia, difficulty sleeping.

History: 13-year-old Hispanic female, 15 pounds underweight at 75 lbs. No blood tests recorded in file prior to visit.

Family History: Father 54-year-old with Type 1 DM, Mother 44-year-old with no medical file.

Allergies: None

Physical Examination: Vital signs normal. Blood test positive for ketone bodies and slight acidosis; FBS 220 confirmed with GTT; urinalysis high in glucose but otherwise clear.

Diagnosis: Diabetes mellitus Type 1.

Treatment: Treat as Type 1 DM with regular insulin injection and follow with FBS and GTT. Place on insulin regimen and enroll in DM management class with parent.

Jonathon McClary, M.D.

Jonathon McClary, M.D.

Photo Source: © Belinda Images/SuperStock

Comprehension Questions

1. What patient complaints are consistent with the signs? _____

_____

_____

2. Is the diagnosis temporary and capable of a cure with the prescribed treatment? _____

_____

_____

3. What are the meanings of the abbreviations FBS and GTT? _____

_____

_____

Case Study Questions

The following Case Study provides further discussion regarding the patient in the medical report. Fill in the blanks with the correct terms. Choose your answers from the following list of terms. (Note that some terms may be used more than once.)

acidosis	glucose	ketosis
endocrinology	hyperglycemia	polydipsia
fasting blood sugar	insulin	Type 1 diabetes

A 13-year-old patient, Anita Del Rio, was referred by her personal physician for an endocrinological evaluation in the

(a) _____ department, following a 4-week history of symptoms of energy loss between meals,

excessive thirst, or (b) _____, headache, polyuria (excessive urination), and sleeplessness.

A routine blood test had also been recorded by the physician and had shown ketone bodies in the blood, or

(c) _____, combined with a lowered blood pH, or (d) _____. Endocrinological

evaluation included an FBS, or (e) _____ _____ _____test,

followed by a (f) _____ tolerance test, and a urinalysis. The tests indicated the patient suffered

from excessive sugar levels in the blood, or (g) _____, that was due to a failure of islet beta cells

to produce proper levels of the hormone (h) _____. A diagnosis of (i) _____

_____ _____ was recorded. The patient was treated with regular insulin, trained

in self-glucose testing and insulin administration, and referred to a local educational program in diabetes management to

include her parents' participation.

Denaya Bellafonte _____

For a greater challenge, read the following medical report and answer the critical thinking questions that follow.

PGH   PEARSON GENERAL HOSPITAL

5500 University Avenue, Phone: (211) 594-4000
Metropolis, VA • Fax: (211) 594-4001

Medical Consultation: Endocrinology

Date: 12/29/2011

Patient: Denaya Bellafonte

Patient Complaint: Frequent headaches, loss of energy, weight gain, tenderness in the lower back, increased growth of body hair.

History: 30-year-old female with no prior surgeries, with two children aged 8 years and 11 years.

Family History: Father negative, mother with thyrotoxicosis who underwent thyroidectomy without complications at age 45, 3 years ago.

Allergies: None

Physical Examination: Vital signs normal. Cephalalgia, lethargy with loss of strength, obesity suggestive of Cushing syndrome, lumbar pain, increased hair growth suggestive of hirsutism, blood sugar elevated at 165mg/dL.

Diagnosis: Primary adrenopathy; later MRI identified the presence of a left adenoma as causative of lumbar pain and adrenal virilism.

Treatment: Biopsy of tumor indicated it is benign, and MRI indicated the tumor has damaged most of the left adrenal gland. Surgery to be scheduled in 2 weeks for left adrenalectomy with exploratory to ensure complete tumor removal.

Joseph Ryan, M.D.
_____
Joseph Ryan, M.D.

Photo Source: Karen Struthers/Shutterstock

Comprehension Questions

1. Why would a tumor of the adrenal gland lead to hirsutism in the patient?_____

   _____

   _____

2. What is the correlation between the patient's hyperglycemia and weight gain? _____

   _____

   _____

3. What is the meaning of the term *adrenopathy?*_____

   _____

   _____

Case Study Questions

The following case study provides further discussion regarding the patient in the medical report. Recall the terms from this chapter to fill in the blanks with the correct terms.

A 30-year-old patient, Denaya Bellafonte, was admitted for hospitalization following reports of symptoms that included frequent headaches, loss of energy, unexplained weight gain, and tenderness in the left lumbar region. More recently, increased body hair, or (j) _____, was an additional cause for concern. An early diagnosis was made of (k) _____, or an inflammation of the adrenals. Also, the attending physician believed that the lumbar pain could be explained by an abnormal enlargement of the adrenal glands, a condition known as (l) _____. In addition, the weight gain in the patient had produced a round "moon face" appearance that characterizes (m) _____ syndrome. This diagnosis also explained the elevated blood sugar levels, or (n) _____, combined with energy loss and muscle weakness. However, the actual cause remained a mystery until the patient's tender lumbar region was examined with MRI. This diagnostic tool revealed a tumor of the left adrenal gland. Apparently, the tumor had caused the adrenal cortex to hypersecrete male sex hormones known as (o) _____, which had caused the body hair, a sign of endocrine disease known as (p) _____. The tumor had also caused the hypersecretion of other adrenal cortex hormones, which led to the metabolic disturbance. A laparoscopic biopsy was performed, and the accompanying histology test confirmed the tumor was benign, and thereby called an (q) _____. Surgery was performed to remove the left adrenal gland, called a left (r) _____. Following the surgery the patient made a complete recovery with all symptoms abating within several weeks.

MEDICAL TERMINOLOGY INTERACTIVE

Medical Terminology Interactive is a premium online homework management system that includes a host of features to help you study. Registered users will find:

- Fun games and activities built within a virtual hospital
- Powerful tools that track and analyze your results—allowing you to create a personalized learning experience
- Videos, flashcards, and audio pronunciations to help enrich your progress
- Streaming video lesson presentations and self-paced learning modules

www.pearsonhighered.com/mti

Appendices ▶▶▶▶▶

Appendix A

Word Parts Glossary

The word parts that have been presented in this textbook are summarized with their definitions for quick reference. The chapter numbers correspond to the first chapter in which the word part is described. Prefixes are listed first, followed by combining forms and suffixes.

Prefix	Definition	Chapter
a-	without, absence of	1
ab-	away from	3
ad-	toward	3
ambi-	both	3
an-	without, absence of	3
ana-	up, toward	3
ante-	before	3
anti-	against, opposite of	1
bi-	two	3
brady-	slow	1
circum-	around	3
con-	with, together, jointly	1
contra-	counter, against	3
di-	double	3
dia-	through	3
dipl-	double	3
dis-	apart, away	3
dys-	bad, abnormal, painful, difficult	3
ec-	outside, out	3
ecto-	outside, out	3
en-	within, upon, on, over	11
endo-	within	1
ep-	upon, over, above, on top	3
epi-	upon, over, above, on top	1
eso-	inward	3
eu-	normal, good	3
ex-	outside, away from	3
exo-	outside, away from	3
extra-	outside	3
hemi-	half	3
heter-	different	3
hetero-	different	3

Prefix	Definition	Chapter
hyper-	excessive, abnormally high, above	3
hypo-	deficient, abnormally low, below	2
infer-	below	3
inter-	between	3
intra-	within	3
iso-	equal	7
macro-	large	3
mal-	bad	3
mega-	large, great	3
megalo-	large, great	3
meta-	after, change	3
micro-	small	1
mono-	one	3
multi-	many, more than once, numerous	3
neo-	new	1
nulli-	none	3
pan-	all	3
par-	alongside, abnormal	5
para-	alongside, abnormal	3
per-	through	4
peri-	around	3
poly-	excessive, over, many	2
post-	to follow after	3
pre-	to come before	1
primi-	first	3
pro-	before	4
pseudo-	false	3
quadri-	four	2
re-	back	10
semi-	half, partial	3
sub-	under, beneath, below	3
super-	above	3
supra-	above	3
sym-	together, joined	3
syn-	together, joined	2
tachy-	rapid, fast	3
tetra-	four	3
trans-	through, across, beyond	3
tri-	three	3
ultra-	beyond normal	3
uni-	one	3

Combining Form	Definition	Chapter
abdomin/o	abdomen	4
abort/o	miscarry	12
abras/o	to rub away	5
acid/o	a solution or substance with a pH less than 7	10
acr/o	extremity	15
actin/o	radiation	5
aden/o	gland	5
adren/o	adrenal gland	15
albin/o	white	5
albumin/o	albumin (a protein)	11
alveol/o	air sac, alveolus	9
amni/o	amnion	12
amnion/o	amnion	12
an/o	anus	10
andr/o	male	12
angi/o	blood vessel	8
ankyl/o	crooked	6
anter/o	front	4
aort/o	aorta	8
append/o	appendix	1
appendic/o	appendix	1
arter/o	artery	8
arteri/o	artery	8
arthr/o	joint	6
articul/o	joint	6
asthen/o	weakness	14
atel/o	incomplete	9
ather/o	fatty	8
atri/o	atrium	8
audi/o	hearing	14
aut/o	self	5
azot/o	urea, nitrogen	11
bacteri/o	bacteria	7
balan/o	glans penis	12
bi/o	life	1
bil/i	bile	10
blast/o	germ, bud, developing cell	7
blephar/o	eyelid	14
botul/o	sausage	7
brachi/o	arm	4
bronch/i	airway, bronchus	9

Combining Form	Definition	Chapter
bronch/o	airway, bronchus	9
burs/o	purse or sac, bursa	6
calc/i	calcium	15
calc/o	calcium	15
carcin/o	cancer	5
cardi/o	heart	1
carp/o	wrist	6
caud/o	tail	4
cec/o	blind intestine, cecum	10
cellul/o	little cell	5
cephal/o	head	4
cerebell/o	little brain, cerebellum	13
cerebr/o	brain, cerebrum	1
cervic/o	neck, cervix	4
cheil/o	lip	10
chol/e	bile, gall	10
cholecyst/o	gallbladder	10
choledoch/o	common bile duct	10
chondr/i	gristle, cartilage	4
chondr/o	gristle, cartilage	6
chori/o	membrane, chorion	12
chron/o	time	4
chym/o	juice	5
cirrh/o	orange	10
coccidioid/o	*Coccidioides immitis* (a fungus)	9
col/o	colon	10
colon/o	colon	10
colp/o	vagina	12
coni/o	dust	9
condyl/o	knuckle of a joint	6
conjunctiv/o	to bind together, conjunctiva	14
cor/o	pupil	14
coron/o	crown or circle, heart	8
cost/o	rib	6
cran/o	skull, cranium	4
crani/o	skull, cranium	4
crin/o	to secrete	15
crypt/o	hidden	5
cutane/o	skin	5
cyan/o	blue	5
cyes/o	pregnancy	12
cyesi/o	pregnancy	12
cyst/o	bladder, sac	9

Combining Form	Definition	Chapter
cyt/o	cell	2
dacry/o	tear	14
dent/o	teeth	10
derm/o	skin	1
dermat/o	skin	1
dilat/o	to widen	9
dips/o	thirst	15
dist/o	distant	4
diverticul/o	diverticulum	10
dors/o	back	4
duoden/o	twelve, duodenum	10
dur/o	hard	12
ech/o	sound	8
electr/o	electricity	1
embol/o	plug	8
embry/o	embryo	12
encephal/o	brain	1
enter/o	small intestine	1
epididym/o	epididymis	12
episi/o	vulva	12
erythr/o	red	7
esophag/e	gullet, esophagus	10
esophag/o	gullet, esophagus	10
esthesi/o	sensation	13
extern/o	exterior	14
fasci/o	fascia	6
fec/o	feces	10
femor/o	thigh, femur	4
fet/o	fetus	12
fibr/o	fiber	6
fibul/o	fibula	6
flux/o	flow	10
follicul/o	little follicle	5
fung/o	fungus	7
gangli/o	swelling, knot	13
ganglion/o	swelling, knot	13
gastr/o	stomach	1
gingiv/o	gums	10
gli/o	glue	13
globin/o	protein	7
glomerul/o	little ball, glomerulus	11
gloss/o	tongue	10
glott/o	opening into the windpipe	9

Combining Form	Definition	Chapter
gluc/o	sweet, sugar	11
glute/o	buttock	4
glyc/o	sweet, sugar	11
glycos/o	sweet, sugar	11
gnos/o	knowledge	13
gonad/o	sex gland	15
gravid/o	pregnancy	12
gravidar/o	pregnancy	12
gyn/o	woman	12
gynec/o	woman	12
halit/o	breath	10
hem/o	blood	1
hemat/o	blood	7
hepat/o	liver	1
hidr/o	sweat	5
hirsut/o	hairy	15
hom/o	same	4
home/o	same	4
hormon/o	to set in motion	15
hydr/o	water	7
hyster/o	uterus	1
iatr/o	physician	7
idi/o	individual	7
ile/o	to roll, ileum	10
ili/o	flank, hip, groin, ilium of the pelvis	4
immun/o	exempt, immunity	7
infer/o	below	4
inguin/o	groin	4
ir/o	iris	14
isch/o	hold back	8
ischi/o	haunch, hip joint, ischium	6
jejun/o	empty, jejunum	10
kerat/o	hard, cornea	5
ket/o	ketone	11
keton/o	ketone	11
kinesi/o	motion	6
kyph/o	hump	6
labyrinth/o	maze, inner ear	14
lact/o	milk	12
lamin/o	thin, lamina	6
lapar/o	abdomen	10
laryng/o	voice box, larynx	1
later/o	side	4

Combining Form	Definition	Chapter
lei/o	smooth	12
leuk/o	white	1
lingu/o	tongue	10
lip/o	fat	2
lith/o	stone	1
lob/o	round part, lobe	9
lord/o	bent forward	6
lumb/o	loin, lower back	4
lymph/o	clear water or fluid	7
mamm/o	breast	1
man/o	thin, scanty	8
mast/o	breast	1
mastoid/o	resembling a breast	14
maxim/o	biggest, highest	1
meat/o	opening, passage	11
med/o	middle	14
medi/o	middle	4
melan/o	black	5
men/o	month, menstruation	12
mening/i	membrane	13
mening/o	membrane	13
menisc/o	meniscus	6
menstru/o	month, menstruation	12
ment/o	mind	1
metr/i	uterus	12
metr/o	uterus	12
muc/o	mucus	9
muscul/o	muscle	1
my/o	muscle	6
myc/o	fungus	5
myel/o	bone marrow; spinal cord, medulla, myelin	6
myos/o	muscle	6
myring/o	membrane, eardrum	14
narc/o	numbness	13
nas/o	nose	9
nat/o	birth	1
necr/o	death	7
nephr/o	kidney	11
neur/o	nerve	1
noct/o	night	11
nosocom/o	hospital	7
nucle/o	kernel, nucleus	7
obstetr/o	midwife	12

Combining Form	Definition	Chapter
ocul/o	eye	14
olig/o	few in number	11
onych/o	nail	5
oophor/o	ovary	12
ophthalm/o	eye	14
opt/o	eye	14
or/o	mouth	10
orchi/o	testis	12
orchid/o	testis	12
orex/o	appetite	10
organ/o	tool	4
orth/o	straight	6
ost/o	bone	6
oste/o	bone	6
ot/o	ear	9
ovar/o	ovary	12
ox/i	oxygen	9
pancreat/o	sweetbread, pancreas	10
pariet/o	wall	6
parot/o	parotid gland	10
patell/o	patella	6
path/o	disease	1
pect/o	chest	8
pector/o	chest	8
ped/o	child	6
pedicul/o	body louse	5
pelv/o	bowl, basin	4
pen/o	penis	12
peps/o	digestion	10
pept/o	digestion	10
peritone/o	to stretch over, peritoneum	10
petr/o	stone	6
phag/o	eat, swallow	10
phalang/o	phalanges	6
pharyng/o	throat, pharynx	9
phasi/o	to speak	1
phleb/o	vein	8
phragm/o	partition	9
phragmat/o	partition	9
phren/o	mind	13
phys/o	growth	6
physi/o	nature	4
plasm/o	form	12

Combining Form	Definition	Chapter
pleur/o	pleura, rib	4
pneum/o	lung, air	9
pneumon/o	lung, air	9
poikil/o	irregular	7
poli/o	gray	13
polyp/o	small growth	10
por/o	hole	6
poster/o	back	4
presby/o	old age	14
proct/o	rectum or anus	1
prostat/o	prostate gland	12
protein/o	protein	11
proxim/o	near	4
pseud/o	false	12
psych/o	mind	1
pub/o	pubis	6
pulmon/o	lung	1
py/o	pus	9
pyel/o	renal pelvis	11
pylor/o	pylorus	10
radi/o	radius	6
radic/o	nerve root	13
radicul/o	nerve root	13
rect/o	rectum	10
ren/o	kidney	11
retin/o	retina	14
rhin/o	nose	1
rhiz/o	nerve root	13
rhythm/o	rhythm	8
rhytid/o	wrinkle	5
rrhythm/o	rhythm	8
sacr/o	sacred, sacrum	6
salping/o	trumpet	12
sarc/o	flesh, meat	6
schiz/o	to divide, split	13
scler/o	hard, sclera	5
scoli/o	curved	6
scop/o	viewing instrument	1
seb/o	sebum, oil	5
semin/o	seed, sperm	12
sept/o	putrefying; wall, partition	7
sial/o	saliva	10
sigm/o	the letter s, sigmoid colon	10

Combining Form	Definition	Chapter
sinus/o	cavity	9
skelet/o	skeleton	1
somat/o	body	13
son/o	sound	8
spadias/o	rip, tear	11
sperm/o	seed, sperm	12
spermat/o	seed, sperm	12
sphygm/o	pulse	8
sphyx/o	pulse	9
spir/o	breathe	9
splen/o	spleen	7
spondyl/o	vertebra	6
staphylococc/o	*Staphylococcus* (a bacterium)	7
steat/o	fat	10
sten/o	narrow	8
stern/o	chest, sternum	6
stigmat/o	point	14
stomat/o	mouth	10
streptococc/o	*Streptococcus* (a bacterium)	7
super/o	above	4
syn/o	connect	6
synov/o	synovial	6
synovi/o	synovial	6
tampon/o	plug	8
tars/o	tarsal bone	6
tax/o	reaction to a stimulus	6
ten/o	stretch, tendon	6
tendon/o	stretch, tendon	6
tens/o	pressure	8
test/o	testis, testicle	12
testicul/o	little testis, testicle	12
thorac/o	chest, thorax	4
thromb/o	clot	7
thym/o	wartlike, thymus gland	7
thyr/o	shield, thyroid	15
thyroid/o	resembling a shield, thyroid	15
toc/o	birth	12
tom/o	to cut	4
tonsill/o	almond, tonsil	1
tox/o	poison	7
trache/o	windpipe, trachea	9
trich/o	hair	5
troph/o	development	6

Combining Form	Definition	Chapter
tubercul/o	little swelling	9
tympan/o	eardrum	14
umbilic/o	navel, umbilicus	4
ur/o	urine	11
ureter/o	ureter	11
urethr/o	urethra	11
urin/o	urine	11
vag/o	vagus nerve	10
vagin/o	sheath, vagina	12
valvul/o	little valve	8
varic/o	dilated vein	8
vas/o	vessel	1
vascul/o	little vessel	8
ven/o	vein	8
ventr/o	belly	4
ventricul/o	little belly, ventricle	8
vertebr/o	vertebra	6
vesic/o	bladder	11
vesicul/o	small bag	12
volv/o	to roll	10
vulv/o	vulva	12
xer/o	dry	5
zo/o	animal, living	12

Suffix	Definition	Chapter
-a	singular	2
-ac	pertaining to	2
-acusis	condition of hearing	14
-ad	toward	2
-ade	process	8
-ae	plural	2
-al	pertaining to	1
-algesia	pain	13
-algia	condition of pain	2
-ar	pertaining to	2
-ary	pertaining to	1
-asthenia	weakness	2
-atresia	closure or absence of a normal body opening	2
-capnia	condition of carbon dioxide	9
-cele	hernia, swelling, protrusion	2

Suffix	Definition	Chapter
-centesis	surgical puncture	2
-clasia	break apart	2
-clasis	break apart	2
-clast	break apart	2
-crit	to separate	7
-cyesis	pregnancy	12
-desis	surgical fixation, fusion	2
-drome	run, running	2
-dynia	condition of pain	2
-ectasis	expansion, dilation	9
-ectomy	surgical excision, removal	1
-emesis	vomiting	2
-emetic	pertaining to vomiting	10
-emia	condition of blood	1
-genesis	origin, cause	6
-genic	pertaining to producing, forming	7
-gnosis	knowledge	4
-gram	a record or image	1
-graph	instrument for recording	2
-graphy	recording process	2
-hemia	condition of blood	2
-ia	condition of	1
-ial	pertaining to	7
-iasis	condition of	10
-iatry	treatment, specialty	1
-ic	pertaining to	1
-ician	one who practices	12
-ion	process	1
-ior	pertaining to	4
-ism	condition or disease	2
-ist	one who specializes	6
-itis	inflammation	1
-lepsy	seizure	13
-lexia	pertaining to a word or phrase	13
-logist	one who studies	1
-logous	pertaining to study	7
-logy	study or science of	1
-lysis	loosen, dissolve	3
-lytic	pertaining to loosen, dissolve	8
-malacia	softening	2
-mania	madness, frenzy	13
-megaly	abnormally large	7
-meter	measure, measuring instrument	2

Suffix	Definition	Chapter
-metrist	one who measures	14
-metry	measurement, process of measuring	2
-oid	resembling	9
-oma	tumor	2
-opia	condition of vision	14
-opsy	view of	2
-osis	condition of	2
-ous	pertaining to	2
-oxia	condition of oxygen	2
-pathy	disease	1
-penia	abnormal reduction in number, deficiency	2
-pexy	surgical fixation, suspension	2
-phagia	eating or swallowing	2
-phasia	speaking	1
-phil	loving, affinity for	2
-philia	loving, affinity for	1
-phobia	fear	2
-phonia	condition of sound or voice	9
-phylaxis	protection	2
-physis	growth	2
-plasia	formation, growth	2
-plasty	surgical repair	1
-plegia	paralysis	2
-pnea	breath	9
-practic	practice	2
-ptosis	drooping	6
-ptysis	to cough up	9
-rrhage	abnormal discharge	7
-rrhagia	abnormal discharge	2
-rrhagic	pertaining to abnormal discharge	7
-rrhaphy	suturing	2
-rrhea	discharge	2
-rrhexis	rupture	2
-s	plural	12
-salpinx	trumpet	12
-sclerosis	condition of hard	2
-scope	instrument used for viewing	1
-scopy	process of viewing	2
-sis	state of	8
-spasm	sudden, involuntary muscle contraction	2
-spasmodic	pertaining to a sudden, involuntary muscle contraction	10
-stasis	standing still	2

Suffix	Definition	Chapter
-staxis	dripping	9
-stomy	surgical creation of an opening	2
-therapy	treatment	7
-tic	pertaining to	6
-tome	cutting instrument	2
-tomy	incision, to cut	2
-tripsy	surgical crushing	2
-troph	development	13
-urea	urine	11
-uresis	urination	11
-uria	pertaining to urine, urination	11
-us	pertaining to	13
-y	process of	3

Appendix B

Abbreviations

The abbreviations from Chapters 1–15 are presented in alphabetical order. Additional abbreviations are also included to establish a complete listing of medical abbreviations. In each case, the abbreviations are presented in the form in which they are most common within the healthcare environment.

Abbreviation	Definition	Abbreviation	Definition
A	anterior	AMBS	American Medical Board of Specialists
A&P	auscultation and percussion	AMD	age-related macular degeneration
A&P repair	anterior and posterior colporrhaphy	AMI	acute myocardial infarction
A&P resection	abdominoperineal resection	AML	acute myelocytic leukemia
A&W	alive and well	amt	amount
AA	Alcoholics Anonymous	ant	anterior
ab	abortion	AODM	adult-onset (Type 2) diabetes mellitus
abd	abdomen	AP	anteroposterior
ABE	acute bacterial endocarditis	AP	angina pectoris
ABGs	arterial blood gases	ARDS	adult (acute) respiratory distress syndrome
ac	before meals	ARM	artificial rupture of membranes
ACL	anterior cruciate ligament	AS	left ear (in Latin, *auris sinister*)
ACTH	adrenocorticotropic hormone	AS	aortic stenosis
AD	right ear (in Latin, *auris dexter*)	as tol	as tolerated
AD	Alzheimer disease	ASA	aspirin (acetylsalicylic acid)
ad lib	as desired	ASCVD	arteriosclerotic cardiovascular disease
ADD	attention deficit disorder	ASD	atrial septal defect
Adeno-Ca	adenocarcinoma	ASHD	arteriosclerotic heart disease
ADH	antidiuretic hormone	Ast	astigmatism
ADHD	attention deficit hyperactivity disorder	AU	both ears (in Latin, *aures unitas*)
ADL	activities of daily living	AUL	acute undifferentiated leukemia
AED	automated external defibrillator	AV	atrioventricular
AFB	acid-fast bacilli	AVR	aortic valve replacement
Afib	atrial fibrillation	ax	axillary (armpit region)
AI	aortic insufficiency	BA	bronchial asthma
AIDS	acquired immunodeficiency syndrome	BBB	bundle branch block
AKA	above-knee amputation	BC	Bowman's capsule
alb	albumin	BCC	basal cell carcinoma
ALL	acute lymphocytic leukemia	BE	barium enema
ALS	amyotrophic lateral sclerosis	bid	twice a day
alt diem	alternate days	BK	below knee
alt hor	alternate hours	BKA	below-knee amputation
alt noct	alternate nights	BM	bowel movement
AMA	against medical advice	BOM	bilateral otitis media
AMA	American Medical Association	BP	blood pressure
amb	ambulatory		

Abbreviation	Definition	Abbreviation	Definition
BPH	benign prostatic hyperplasia	CLD	chronic liver disease
BR	bed rest	CLL	chronic lymphocytic leukemia
BRP	bathroom privileges	cm	centimeter
BS	blood sugar	CML	chronic myelogenous leukemia
BSO	bilateral salpingo-oophorectomy	CNS	central nervous system
BUN	blood urea nitrogen	CO	carbon monoxide
Bx	biopsy	CO_2	carbon dioxide
bx	biopsy	COLD	chronic obstructive lung disease
C	Celsius	cond	condition
C&S	stool culture and sensitivity	COPD	chronic obstructive pulmonary disease
c/o	complains of	CP	chest pain
Ca	calcium	CP	cerebral palsy
CA	cancer	CPAP	continuous positive airway pressure
CA-125	Cancer Antigen-125 Tumor Marker	CPK	creatine phosphokinase
CABG	coronary artery bypass graft	CPN	chronic pyelonephritis
CAD	coronary artery disease	CPR	cardiopulmonary resuscitation
cal	calorie	CRD	chronic respiratory disease
cap	capsule	creat	creatinine
CAPD	continuous ambulatory peritoneal dialysis	CRF	chronic renal failure
		CRNA	certified registered nurse-anesthetist
cath	catheter, catheterization	C-section	cesarean section
CBC	complete blood count	CSF	cerebrospinal fluid
CBR	complete bed rest	CT	calcitonin
CBS	chronic brain syndrome	CT (CAT) scan	computed (axial) tomography scan
cc	cubic centimeter	CTS	carpal tunnel syndrome
CC	colony count	Cu	copper
CCU	coronary care unit	CVA	cerebrovascular accident (stroke)
CDH	congenital dislocation of the hip	CVP	central venous pressure
CEA	carcinoma embryonic antigen	CXR	chest X-ray
CF	cystic fibrosis	D&C	dilation and curettage
CHB	complete heart block	D/S	dextrose in saline
CHD	coronary heart disease	D/W	dextrose in water
chemo	chemotherapy	DAT	diet as tolerated
CHF	congestive heart failure	DC	discontinued
CHO	carbohydrate	del	delivery
chol	cholesterol	DI	diabetes insipidus
CI	coronary insufficiency	DIC	diffuse intravascular coagulation
CIN	cervical intraepithelial neoplasia	diff	differential (blood count)
circ	circumcision	DJD	degenerative joint disease
CIS	carcinoma in situ	DLE	discoid lupus erythematosus
cl	clinic	DM	diabetes mellitus
Cl	chloride	DMD	Duchenne muscular dystrophy
cl liq	clear liquid	DNA	deoxyribonucleic acid

Abbreviation	Definition	Abbreviation	Definition
DO	physician specializing in osteopathy	FBD	fibrocystic breast disease
DOA	dead on arrival	FBS	fasting blood sugar
DOB	date of birth	Fe	iron
Dr	dram	FHT	fetal heart tones
DRE	digital rectal exam	flu	influenza
DRG	diagnosis-related group	FOBT	fetal occult blood test
DT	delirium tremens	FSH	follicle-stimulating hormone
DTR	deep tendon reflexes	FTT	failure to thrive
DVT	deep vein thrombosis	FUO	fever of undetermined origin
Dx	diagnosis	Fx	fracture
E	enema	g	gram
EBL	estimated blood loss	GB series	gallbladder series
ECG	electrocardiogram	GC	gonorrhea
ECHO	echocardiogram	GER	gerontology
EchoEG	echoencephalography	GERD	gastroesophageal reflux disease
ECT	electroconvulsive therapy	GH	growth hormone
ED	erectile dysfunction	GI	gastrointestinal
EDD	expected date of delivery	GSW	gunshot wound
EEG	electroencephalography	GTT	glucose tolerance test
EENT	eye, ear, nose, and throat	GU	genitourinary
EGD	esophagogastroduodenoscopy	GYN	gynecology
EKG	electrocardiogram	h	hour
Em	emmetropia	H	hypodermic
EMG	electromyography	H&H	hemoglobin and hematocrit
ENT	ear, nose, and throat	H&P	history and physical examination
EP	ectopic pregnancy	H_2O	water
EP	evoked potential	H_2O_2	hydrogen peroxide
ERCP	endoscopic retrograde cholangiopancreatography	HB	heart block
		HBV	hepatitis B virus
ERT	estrogen replacement therapy	HCl	hydrochloric acid
ESR	erythrocyte sedimentation rate	HCO_3	bicarbonate
ESRD	end-stage renal disease	HCT, Hct	hematocrit
ESWL	extracorporeal shock wave lithotripsy	HCVD	hypertensive cardiovascular disease
etio	etiology	HD	hemodialysis
EtOH	ethanol	Hg	mercury
EUS	endoscopic ultrasound	HGB, Hgb	hemoglobin
ex	external	HHD	hypertensive heart disease
F	Fahrenheit	HIV	human immunodeficiency virus
FACP	Fellow of the American College of Physicians	HNP	herniated nucleus pulposus; a herniated intervertbral disk
FACS	Fellow of the American College of Surgeons	HOB	head of bed
		HPV	human papillomavirus
FAS	fetal alcohol syndrome		

Abbreviation	Definition	Abbreviation	Definition
HRT	hormone replacement therapy	LGI	lower GI series
hs	hour of sleep	LH	luteinizing hormone
HSG	hysterosalpingogram	LI	lactose intolerance
HSV-2	herpes simplex virus type 2	LLL	left lower lobe (of lung)
ht	height	LLQ	left lower quadrant
HTN	hypertension	LMP	last menstrual period
Hx	history	LOC	loss of consciousness
hypo	hypodermic	LP	lumbar puncture
I&D	incision and drainage	LPN	licensed practical nurse
I&O	intake and output	LR	lactated Ringer's
IBD	inflammatory bowel disease	LTB	laryngotracheobronchitis
IBS	irritable bowel syndrome	LUL	left upper lobe
ICD	implantable cardioverter defibrillator	LUQ	left upper quadrant
ICU	intensive care unit	LV	left ventricle
IDC	infiltrating ductal carcinoma	LVN	licensed vocational nurse
IDDM	insulin-dependent diabetes mellitus	mcg	microgram
IHD	ischemic heart disease	MCH	mean corpuscular hemoglobin
IM	intramuscular	MCV	mean corpuscular volume
inf	inferior	MD	medical doctor
INR	international normalized ratio	MD	muscular dystrophy
IOL	intraocular lens	mEq	milliequivalent
IPPR	intermittent positive pressure breathing	Mets	metastasis
		MG	myasthenia gravis
irrig	irrigation	mg	milligram
isol	isolation	MI	myocardial infarction
IUD	intrauterine device	mL	milliliter
IV	intravenous	mm	millimeter
IVC	intravenous cholangiogram	MM	multiple myeloma
IVP	intravenous pyelogram	MOM	milk of magnesia
K	potassium	MR	may repeat
KCl	potassium chloride	MRA	magnetic resonance angiography
kg	kilogram	MRCP	magnetic resonance cholangiopancreatography
KUB	kidney, ureter, and bladder X-ray		
KVO	keep vein open	MRI	magnetic resonance imaging
L	liter	MRSA	methicillin-resistant *Staphylococcus aureus*
L&D	labor and delivery	MS	multiple sclerosis
LA	left atrium	MSH	melanocyte-stimulating hormone
lac	laceration	MVP	mitral valve prolapse
LAP	laparotomy	N&V	nausea and vomiting
LAS	lymphadenopathy syndrome	Na	sodium
LASIK	laser-assisted in situ keratomileusis	NA	nursing assistant
lat	lateral	NaCl	sodium chloride (salt)
LE	lupus erythematosus	NB	newborn

Abbreviation	Definition	Abbreviation	Definition
neuro	neurology	PD	Parkinson disease
NG	nasogastric	PDA	patent ductus arteriosus
NICU	neonatal intensive care unit	PDR	*Physician's Desk Reference*
NICU	neurology intensive care unit	PE	pulmonary embolism
NIDDM	noninsulin-dependent diabetes mellitus	PE	physical examination
		PED	pediatrics
NIVA	noninvasive vascular assessment	PEG	percutaneous endoscopic gastrostomy
noc	night	per	by
noct	night	PERRLA	pupils equal, round, reactive to light and accommodation
NPO	nothing by mouth		
NRDS	neonatal respiratory distress syndrome	PET	positron emission tomography
		PFT	pulmonary function test
NS	normal saline	PICC	peripherally inserted central catheter
NSAIDs	nonsteroidal anti-inflammatory drugs	PICU	pediatric intensive care unit
NSR	normal sinus rhythm	PID	pelvic inflammatory disease
NVS	neurovital signs	PIH	pregnancy-induced hypertension
O	objective	PKU	phenylketonuria
O_2	oxygen	PLT	platelet count
OA	osteoarthritis	PMS	premenstrual syndrome
OB	obstetrics	PNS	peripheral nervous system
OB/GYN	obstetrics/gynecology	po	postoperation
OD	right eye (in Latin, *oculus dexter*)	po	orally
OM	otitis media	post-op	postoperatively
OP	outpatient	PP	postpartum
Ophth	ophthalmic	PPBS	postprandial blood sugar
OR	operating room	PPD	purified protein derivative
ortho	orthopedics	pr	per rectum
OS	left eye (in Latin, *oculus sinister*)	PRBC	packed red blood cells
OSA	obstructive sleep apnea	pre-op	preoperation
OT	occupational therapy	PRK	photorefractive keratotomy
OT	oxytocin	PRL	prolactin
Oto	otology	prn	as needed
OU	each eye (in Latin, *oculus uterque*)	PSA	prostate-specific antigen
oz	ounce	pt	patient
P	phosphorus	PT	prothrombin time
PA	physician's assistant	PT	physical therapy
PA	posteroanterior	PTCA	percutaneous transluminal coronary angioplasty
PAC	premature atrial contractions		
Pap smear (test)	Papanicolaou smear (or test)	PTH	parathyroid hormone
PAT	paroxysmal atrial tachycardia	PTSD	posttraumatic stress disorder
pc	after meals	PTT	partial thromboplastin time
PCU	progressive care unit	PUL	percutaneous ultrasound lithotripsy
PCV	packed cell volume	PVC	premature ventricular contractions

Abbreviation	Definition	Abbreviation	Definition
PVD	peripheral vascular disease	SIDS	sudden infant death syndrome
Px	prognosis	SL	semilunar (pertaining to the heart valve)
q	every	SLE	systemic lupus erythematosus
qd	every day	SMR	submucous resection
qid	four times a day	SO	salpingo-oophorectomy
qn	every night	SPECT	single-photon emission computed tomography
qod	every other day		
qt	quart	SqCCa	squamous cell carcinoma
R	rectal	ss	one-half
R	right	SSE	soapsuds enema
RA	right atrium	St	stage (of cancer development)
RA	rheumatoid arthritis	staph	*Staphylococcus*
RAIU	radioactive iodine uptake	stat	immediately
RBC	red blood cell or red blood count	STI	sexually transmitted infection
RDS	respiratory distress syndrome	strep	*Streptococcus*
reg	regular	subq	subcutaneous
REM	rapid eye movement	sup	superior
resp	respiration	supp	suppository
RHD	rheumatic heart disease	surg	surgery
RK	radial keratotomy	SVD	spontaneous vaginal delivery
RLL	right lower lobe	T&A	tonsillectomy and adenoidectomy
RLQ	right lower quadrant	T_3	triiodothyronine
RN	registered nurse	T_4	thyroxine
ROM	range of motion	TAB	therapeutic abortion
RP	retrograde pyelogram	tab	tablet
RR	recovery room	TAH	total abdominal hysterectomy
rt	right	TAH/BSO	total abdominal hysterectomy/bilateral salpingo-oophorectomy
rt	routine		
RT	respiratory therapy	TAT	tetanus antitoxin
RUL	right upper lobe	TB	tuberculosis
RV	right ventricle	TBI	traumatic brain injury
Rx	prescription	TBSA	total body surface area
SA	sinoatrial	TCDB	turn, cough, deep breathe
SAB	spontaneous abortion	TCT	thrombin clotting time
SARS	severe acute respiratory syndrome	TEE	transesophageal echocardiogram
SBE	subacute bacterial endocarditis	temp	temperature
SBE	self breast examination	THA	total hip arthroplasty
sc	subcutaneous	THR	total hip replacement
SCA	sudden cardiac arrest	TIA	transient ischemic attack
SCI	spinal cord injury	tid	three times a day
SG	specific gravity	TKA	total knee arthroplasty
SHG	sonohistogram	TKR	total knee replacement
SICU	surgical intensive care unit	TM	tympanic membrane

Abbreviation	Definition	Abbreviation	Definition
TMJ	temporomandibular joint	UTI	urinary tract infection
TNM	tumor, node, metastasis	UV	ultraviolet
TPN	total parenteral nutrition	UVR	ultraviolet radiation
tr	tincture	VA	visual acuity
trach	tracheostomy	vag	vaginal
TSH	thyroid-stimulating hormone	VBAC	vaginal birth after cesarean section
TSS	toxic shock syndrome	VC	vital capacity
TUIP	transurethral incision of the prostate	VCUG	voiding cystourethrogram
TULIP	transurethral laser incision of the prostate	Vertebrae	
		C1 through C7	seven cervical vertebrae
TUMT	transurethral microwave thermotherapy	T1 through T12	twelve thoracic vertebrae
		L1 through L5	five lumbar vertebrae
TURP	transurethral resection of the prostate	VLAP	visual ablation of the prostate
TV	tidal volume	VPS	ventilation-perfusion scanning
TVH	total vaginal hysterectomy	V/Q scan	ventilation-perfusion scanning
TVS	transvaginal sonography	VS	vital signs
TWE	tapwater enema	VSD	ventricular septal defect
Tx	treatment	W/C	wheelchair
U	unit	WA	while awake
UA	urinalysis	WBC	white blood cell or white blood count
UGI	upper GI series		
UNG	ointment	wt	weight
UPPP	uvulopalatopharyngoplasty	XRT	radiation therapy
URI	upper respiratory infection		
US	ultrasound		

Appendix C

Pharmacology Terms

The major terms that are in common use in the field of pharmacology (preparation and dispensation of medications) are provided. The pronunciation guide and definition of each term is included.

absorption (ab SORP shun): the process of taking in, in which a drug moves into the body toward the target organ or tissue.

ACE inhibitor (AYSS * in HIB ih tor): angiotensin-converting enzyme inhibitor, a category of antihypertensive drugs that suppress the renin pathway to reduce blood pressure.

administration (ad min ih STRAY shun): providing a drug treatment to a patient.

adverse reaction (ad VERS * re AK shun): a harmful reaction to a drug that was administered at the proper dosage.

ampule (AM pyool): a sealed container containing a sterile solution to be used for injection.

analgesic (an al JEE zik): a compound that produces a reduced response to painful stimuli.

anesthetic (an ess THET ik): a compound that depresses neuronal function, resulting in a loss of the ability to perceive pain and other sensations.

antacid (ant ASS id): a substance that neutralizes or buffers an acid, usually taken orally to reduce hydrochloric acid in the stomach.

antianemic (an tee a NEE mik) agent: a drug that is used to treat or prevent anemia.

antianxiety (an tee ang ZI eh tee) agent: a drug that is used to treat anxiety such as fear, worry, or apprehension; usually a sedative or minor tranquilizer.

antiarrhythmic (an tee a RITH mik): a drug that is used to treat cardiac arrhythmia.

antibiotic (AN tee BYE ott ik): a chemical substance derived from a biological source (a mold or bacteria) that inhibits the growth of other microorganisms.

anticoagulant (AN tye koh AG yoo LANT): a drug that prevents or delays blood coagulation.

anticonvulsant (an tee kon VUL sant): a drug that reduces or prevents convulsive disorders, such as epilepsy.

antidepressant (an tee dee PRESS ant): a drug that counteracts depression.

antidiabetic (an tee DYE ah bet ik): a drug that reduces the amount of glucose in the blood; also called **hypoglycemic.**

antidiarrheal (an tee dye ah REE al): a drug that relieves the symptoms of diarrhea, usually by absorbing water from the large intestine and altering intestinal motility.

antidiuretic (an tee dye yoor EH tik): a drug that reduces the formation and excretion of urine.

antiemetic (an tee ee MET ik): a drug that is used to prevent or reduce nausea and vomiting.

antihistamine (an tih HISS tah meen): a class of drugs that suppress the action of histamines to counter the effects of inflammation.

antihormones (an te HOR mohnz): substances that inhibit or otherwise prevent the normal effects of certain hormones.

antihypertensive (an tee high per TEN sihv): a drug or treatment that reduces high blood pressure.

anti-inflammatory (an tee in FLAM a tor ee): a drug or treatment that reduces inflammation by acting on body function.

antimutagenic (an tee myoo tah JEN ik): a drug or treatment that reduces a substance's ability to form mutations in cells.

antineoplastic (an tee nee oh PLASS tik): a drug that is used to destroy or inhibit cancer cells, usually by inhibiting the synthesis of DNA.

antipsychotic (an tee sigh KOH tik): a drug that counteracts the symptoms of psychosis, such as schizophrenia and major behavioral disorders.

antiseptic (an tih SEP tik): a substance that prevents infection by inhibiting the growth of microorganisms.

antispasmodic (an tee spaz MOD ik): a drug or treatment that inhibits muscle contractions to relieve convulsions or spasms.

antitoxin (an tee TAHKS inn): an antibody that forms in response to antigenic poisonous substances. The antibody is often collected from its biological origin and concentrated for use in treatment against the antigenic toxin.

antitussive (an tee TUSS iv): a drug or treatment that relieves coughing.

bactericidal (bak teer ee SIGH dal): a drug or treatment that destroys bacteria.

barbiturate (barr BIHCH yoor aht): a derivative of barbituric acid, which acts as a depressant on the central nervous system. They are usually used as tranquilizers and hypnotics.

beta-blocker (BAY ta * block er): an agent that suppresses the rate and force of heart contractions by inhibition of beta-adrenergic receptors.

bioavailability (bye oh ah vayl ah BILL ih tee): the percentage of a drug that is available to the target organ or tissue.

biotoxin (bye oh TAHKS inn): any toxic substance formed in a living organism.

biotransformation (bye oh trans for MAY shun): the changes that occur to a chemical due to biological action within the body.

calcium channel blockers: a class of drugs that inhibit the movement of calcium ions into muscle cells, which thereby inhibits muscle contraction. They are useful in the treatment of heart disease that involves coronary spasms.

capsule (KAP suhl): a small container that is soluble in water, which is used for the oral administration of a dose of medication. It is abbreviated **cap.**

carcinogen (kar SIN oh jenn): any substance that causes cancer.

cardiotonic (kar dee oh TOHN ik): a substance that exerts a favorable effect on the action of the heart by increasing the force and efficiency of its contractions.

catabolic (kat ah BOHL ik): relating to catabolism, which is the metabolic breakdown of chemicals to produce energy in the form of ATP.

chemotherapy (KEE moh THAIR ah pee): treatment of disease by the use of chemical agents. The term is usually used to describe agents used in the treatment of cancer.

contraindication (kon trah in dih KAY shun): a symptom or circumstance that renders the administration of a drug to be inadvisable.

detoxify (dee TAHK sih fye): to diminish or remove the poisonous quality of a substance or pathogen.

disinfectant (diss in FEK tant): a chemical that destroys microorganisms and is thereby often used to sanitize objects and surfaces.

distribution (diss trih BYOO shun): the pattern of absorption of drug molecules by the body once the drug has been administered.

diuretic (dye yoor EH tik): a drug that increases the production of urine by decreasing water reabsorption within the kidneys. It is often prescribed to reduce water retention by the body, which reduces blood pressure, edema, and congestive heart failure.

dose: the quantity of a drug that is to be administered at one time.

drug: a therapeutic agent; any substance (other than food) that is used in the diagnosis, prevention, or treatment of a disease.

drug fast: microorganisms that become tolerant or resistant to an antimicrobial drug treatment.

drug clearance: the elimination of a drug from the body, usually through excretion by the kidneys, lungs, liver, or intestinal tract.

drug interactions: the modification of a drug that results from the drug interacting with itself or with other drugs, components of the diet, or other chemicals that are administered. The modification can be either desirable or undesirable.

effect: the biological effect of the administration of a particular drug. The effect may be **local** if it is confined to the site of administration, or **systemic** if the effect is more widespread.

enteral (ENT er ahl): administration of a drug by the oral route (by way of the intestines), as distinguished from parenteral. Enteral administration is the most common route.

Food and Drug Administration (FDA): the federal agency responsible for evaluation and regulation of pharmaceuticals in the United States. The FDA also enforces regulations dealing with the manufacture and distribution of food and cosmetics. The mission of the FDA is the protection of American citizens from the sale of impure or unhealthy substances.

formula (FOR myoo lah): a prescription that includes directions for the compounding of a medical preparation.

formulary (FOR myoo lahr ree): a compilation of drugs and other relevant information that is used as a reference library by health professionals to prescribe treatment.

genotoxic (jee noh TAHK sik): a substance that is capable of damaging DNA and therefore may cause mutation or cancer.

grain: a minute hard particle of any substance or a unit of weight equivalent to 1/60 of a dram (1/437.5 ounce).

gram: a unit of mass in the metric system, equivalent to 15.432 grains.

granule (GRAHN yool): a very small pill that is usually gelatin coated or sugar coated.

hormone (HOR mohn): a chemical substance, usually a protein or steroid, that is secreted by an endocrine gland and transported by the circulatory system throughout the body. Upon making physical contact with a target cell, the hormone enters the cell and induces changes in metabolism, growth rate, protein synthesis, or synthesis of other compounds. The changes the hormone induces can have profound effects on body function.

homeopathy (hoh mee OPP ah thee): a system of medical treatment centered on the theory that large doses of a certain drug given to a healthy person will produce conditions that are relieved by the same drug in small doses during a diseased state.

hypnotics (hip NOTT iks): drugs that depress central nervous system function, resulting in drowsiness. They are used as sedatives and to produce sleep.

immunodeficiency (IM yoo noh dee FISH ehn see): a condition resulting from defective immune mechanisms, characterized by a frequent and rapid onset of infectious diseases.

infusion (inn FYOO zhun): the introduction of a fluid (other than blood) directly into a vein.

inhalation (inn hah LAY shun): a treatment that involves breathing in of a spray or vapor. The medication, known as the inhalant, is absorbed through capillaries in the mucous membranes of the upper respiratory tract.

injection (inn JEHK shun): introduction of a substance into the body with the use of a hollow needle. The injection may be beneath the skin (**subcutaneous** or **hypodermic**), into muscular tissue (**intramuscular, or IM**), into a vein (**intravenous, or IV**), or into the rectum (**rectal**).

laxative (LAHKS ah tihv): a substance that promotes bowel movement without pain or violent action. Laxatives work by softening the stool (decreasing water reabsorption), increasing the bulk of the feces, or lubricating the intestinal wall.

muscle relaxant: a drug that reduces muscle contraction.

nonprescription drugs: drugs that are not required (by the FDA) to be sold with a medical prescription. They are also called **over-the-counter (OTC)** drugs.

nonsteroidal anti-inflammatory drugs: a class of drugs that reduce the symptoms of inflammation (swelling, redness, and pain) and are not steroidal compounds. It is abbreviated **NSAID.** The most common NSAID is aspirin (salicylic acid).

ointment (OYNT ment): a semisolid, medicated mixture that is topically (externally) applied.

oral (OR ahl): the mouth, the most common route of drug administration.

parenteral (pah RENT er ahl): introduction of medication through a route other than the oral (intestinal) or inhalation (lungs) routes. It involves injection that may be subcutaneous, intravenous, intramuscular, or rectal.

pharmacist (FARM ah sist): a health professional formally trained to formulate and dispense prescription drugs and other medications.

pharmacodynamic (farm ah koh dye NAM ik): relating to drug action.

pharmacology (farm ah KALL oh jee): the science of drugs and their sources, chemistry, action within the body, and uses.

pharmacotherapy (farm ah koh THAIR ah pee): the treatment of disease by means of drugs.

pharmacy (FARM ah see): the practice of preparing and dispensing drugs; also, a place where drugs are prepared and dispensed.

placebo (plah SEE boh): a neutral, ineffective substance that is identical to a known drug, which is administered to a patient for the suggestive effect or during blind testing.

potency (POH ten see): the pharmacological activity of a drug. It is used to determine the amount of a drug to be administered to cause the desired effect.

prescription (pree SKRIP shun): a written order for pharmacotherapy, provided by an authorized health professional.

routes of administration: the various ways in which a drug may be administered; the options include subcutaneous injection, intravenous injection, intramuscular injection, rectal injection, oral, vaginal, rectal, or topical.

sedative (SED ah tiv): an agent that reduces central nervous system activity, producing a calming, quieting effect that is usually used to treat anxiety.

side effects: a reaction by the body resulting from a treatment program that is a diversion from the desired effects. The reaction can be beyond the desired effect and is usually undesirable.

solution (suh LYOO shun): a chemical mixture that includes a dissolved substance (solute) in a liquid medium (solvent).

stimulant (STIHM yool ant): an agent that increases the rate of activity of a body function.

superscription (SOO per skrip shun): the beginning of a prescription, consisting of the command recipe "take."

suppository (suh POZ ih tor ee): a medication that is introduced into one of the body orifices (other than the mouth), such as rectum, vagina, or urethra. It is usually a solid mass that melts at body temperature.

suspension (suh SPEN shun): a mixture of solid particles in a liquid medium that do not dissolve. The solid particles are usually dispersed through the liquid by blending.

tablet (TAB let): a small solid that contains medication for oral administration. Tablets may be designed to be swallowed whole, chewed, or dissolved prior to administration.

topical (TAHP ih kuhl): administration of a drug onto the surface of the skin.

toxicity (tahk SISS ih tee): the state of being poisonous. It is the level at which a drug's concentration in the body produces serious adverse effects.

toxicology (TAHK sih KALL oh jee): the science of poisons, in which the source, chemical properties, and body responses to poisonous substances are studied.

trade name: the name provided to a drug by its manufacturer and commonly used by the health community to identify the drug.

tranquilizer (TRAN kwill eye zer): a drug that brings tranquility, or a calming effect, to the mind without depression. It is abbreviated **trank.**

transdermal (trans DERM al): administration of a drug topically to unbroken skin for its absorption into deeper tissues.

United States Pharmacopeia (FARM ah KOP ee ah): a reference text approved by the Federal Food, Drug, and Cosmetic Act containing specifications for drugs, such as chemical properties, uses, recommended dosage levels, contraindications, adverse side effects, and so forth It is abbreviated **USP.**

vasoconstrictor (vaz oh kon STRIK tor): a chemical that causes blood vessels to constrict, which reduces blood flow and elevates blood pressure. Also called **vasopressors.**

vasodilator (vaz oh DYE lay tor): a chemical that causes blood vessels to relax, resulting in dilation that increases blood flow and lowers blood pressure. Due to their effect, they are in common use for acute heart failure.

vitamin (VYE tah min): an organic compound that is required for normal function of cells. Most vitamins are produced by the body, but those that are not are known as **essential vitamins** and must be included in the diet.

Appendix D

Word Parts for Describing Color, Number, and Plurals

Combining Forms for Terms Describing Color

Combining Form	Meaning
albin/o	white
chlor/o	green
chrom/o	color
cirrh/o	orange
cyan/o	blue
erythr/o	red
jaund/o	yellow
leuk/o	white
melan/o	black
xanth/o	yellow

Prefixes for Terms Describing Numbers

Prefix	Meaning
mono-	one
uni-	one
bi-	two
di-	two
tri-	three
quadr-	four
tetra-	four

Singular Versus Plural Endings

Singular Endings	Plural Endings	Example: Singular	Example: Plural
-a	-ae	fistula	fistulae
-ax	-aces	hemothorax	hemothoraces
-ex	-ices	cortex	cortices
-is	-es	diagnosis	diagnoses
-ix	-ices	cicatrix	cicatrices
-ma	-mata	fibroma	fibromata
-on	-a	ganglion	ganglia
-um	-a	bacterium	bacteria
-us	-i	fungus	fungi
-y	-ies	episiotomy	episiotomies

Appendix E

Answers to Practice Exercises and Chapter Reviews

Chapter 1

Practice: The Programmed Learning Approach

The Right Match
1. e
2. c
3. d
4. b
5. a

Talking Shop
1. (provided in chapter)
2. c
3. j
4. e
5. l
6. b
7. d
8. g
9. k
10. h
11. a
12. i

Practice: Constructed and Nonconstructed Terms

The Right Match
1. b
2. c
3. d
4. a

Practice: The Word Parts

The Right Match
1. c
2. e
3. f
4. a
5. b
6. d

Practice: Forming Words from Word Parts

The Right Match
1. d
2. b
3. a
4. c

Break the Chain
1a. & 1b. (provided in chapter)
2a. appendic/itis
    r / s
2b. inflammation
3a. hepat/itis
    r / s
3b. liver
4a. neo/nat/o/logy
   p / r /cv/ s
4b. yes, *nat*

5a. mamm/o/plasty
   r /cv/ s
5b. surgical repair
6a. electr/o/cardi/o/gram
   r /cv/ r /cv/ s
6b. two combining forms
7a. pre/nat/al
   p / r / s
7b. before

Fill It In
1. (provided in chapter)
2. mammoplasties
3. pericardia
4. sarcomas
5. cardiopathies

Linkup
1. (provided in chapter)
2. neonatology
3. neuropathy
4. mastectomy
5. rhinoplasty
6. endoscope
7. mammogram
8. pathologist
9. hysterectomy

Chapter Review

Word Building
1. (provided in chapter)
2. tonsillectomy
3. salpingoplasty
4. dermatitis
5. rhinology
6. mental
7. neuropathy
8. hemophilia
9. laryngitis
10. dermatology
11. laryngoscope
12. biology
13. endocarditis
14. bradycardia
15. antibiotic
16. dermatoplasty
17. neurology
18. cerebral
19. gastrectomy
20. encephalitis
21. hysteroscope
22. mammoplasty
23. appendectomy
24. hepatic

Chapter 2

Practice: Suffix Introduction

The Right Match
1. g
2. b, d, h

3. e
4. c
5. f
6. b, d, h
7. a
8. i
9. b, d, h

Suffix Linkup
1. (provided in chapter)
2. thermometer
3. laparoscopy
4. gastritis

Practice: Suffixes That Indicate an Action or State

The Right Match
1. e
2. a
3. h
4. b
5. d
6. c
7. f
8. g

Suffix Linkup
1. syndrome
2. biopsy
3. hemophilia
4. dysphagia
5. homeostasis

Practice: Suffixes That Indicate a Condition or Disease

Suffix Linkup
1. rhinorrhagia
2. tenodynia
3. amniorrhexis
4. lipoma
5. calcipenia
6. anorexia
7. neoplasia
8. myasthenia
9. seborrhea
10. meningocele
11. gastritis

The Right Match
1. c
2. e, k
3. a
4. h
5. j
6. g
7. b
8. e, k
9. d
10. i
11. f

Practice: Suffixes That Indicate Location, Number, or a Quality

The Right Match
1. d
2. e
3. a
4. c
5. b

Suffix Linkup
1. cardiac
2. cervical
3. ocular
4. pulmonary
5. bacterial
6. cephalic
7. nervous
8. cephalad
9. polycythemia

Practice: Suffixes That Indicate a Medical Specialty

The Right Match
1. c
2. d
3. b
4. a

Suffix Linkup
1. audiologist
2. pathology
3. chiropractic
4. podiatry

Practice: Suffixes That Indicate a Procedure or Treatment

The Right Match
1. i
2. f
3. g
4. h
5. a
6. c
7. b
8. d
9. l
10. e
11. j
12. k

Suffix Linkup
1. thoracocentesis
2. osteoclasis
3. lithotripsy
4. craniotome
5. arthrodesis
6. angiogram
7. angiography
8. thermometer
9. ovulation

10. mastopexy
11. prophylaxis
12. gastroplasty
13. gastroscope
14. craniotomy

Chapter Review

Word Building
1. (provided in chapter)
2. nervous
3. syndrome
4. osteoclasis
5. lipoma
6. hemophilia
7. audiologist
8. pathology
9. hematemesis
10. dysphagia
11. prophylaxis
12. thoracocentesis
13. podiatry
14. cardiomalacia
15. lithotripsy
16. tenodynia
17. gastroplasty
18. anorexia
19. meningocele
20. hypoxia
21. gastroscope
22. cervical
23. chiropractic
24. arthrodesis
25. biopsy
26. myasthenia
27. thermometer
28. esophagitis
29. laparoscopy
30. aphasia
31. hypophysis
32. quadriplegia
33. arthralgia
34. calcipenia
35. neoplasia
36. rhinorrhagia
37. angiogram
38. angiography
39. hypodermic
40. homeostasis
41. hysteratresia
42. adenosis
43. embolism
44. seborrhea
45. arteriosclerosis
46. bronchospasm
47. cephalad
48. fistulae

Chapter 3

Prefix Introduction

The Right Match
1. b
2. c
3. d

4. e
5. a

Prefix Linkup
1. (provided in chapter)
2. metabolism
3. conjoined
4. aphasia

Practice: Prefixes That Indicate Number or Quantity

The Right Match
1. f
2. g
3. h
4. b
5. e
6. c
7. n
8. l
9. d
10. i or j
11. m
12. a
13. i or j
14. k

Prefix Linkup
1. monoplegia
2. nulligravida
3. ambidextrous
4. polyphagia
5. tricuspid
6. oligospermia

Practice: Prefixes That Indicate Location or Timing

The Right Match
1. e
2. j
3. g
4. h
5. a or r
6. d
7. k
8. b
9. o
10. q
11. n
12. c
13. p
14. f
15. m
16. i
17. t
18. l
19. a or r
20. u
21. s

Prefix Linkup
1. anatomy
2. abduction
3. ectopic
4. dialysis
5. exotropia

6. inferior
7. paracusis
8. subcutaneous
9. syndrome
10. antenatal or prenatal

Practice: Prefixes That Indicate a Specific Quality about a Term

The Right Match
1. h
2. g
3. o
4. j
5. n
6. k
7. m
8. p
9. e
10. b
11. c
12. f
13. a
14. d
15. i
16. l

Prefix Linkup
1. pseudocyesis
2. aseptic
3. neonate
4. bradycardia
5. circumcision
6. transsexual
7. dyslexia
8. hyperthyroidism
9. malabsorption
10. megalocyte
11. ultrasound

Chapter Review

Word Building
1. (provided in chapter)
2. anticonvulsive
3. metabolism
4. diplopia
5. hemiplegia
6. multipara
7. nullipara
8. pandemic
9. diplegia
10. polyarteritis
11. primipara
12. adduction
13. dialysis
14. dislocated
15. ectopic
16. intradermal
17. pericardium
18. syndrome
19. asymptomatic
20. asepsis
21. bradykinesia
22. circumcision
23. euthanasia

24. hypocalcemia
25. pseudocyesis
26. tachycardia
27. conjoined
28. contraception
29. ambidextrous
30. bifocal
31. monoplegia
32. quadriplegia
33. semiconscious
34. tripara
35. unipara
36. abduction
37. anatomy
38. prenatal
39. endogastric
40. epidermis
41. esotropia
42. exotropia
43. extracellular
44. inferior
45. intervertebral
46. paracusis
47. postpartum
48. subcutaneous
49. superior
50. anoxia
51. dyslexia
52. heterotropia
53. macrocephaly
54. malabsorption

Chapter 4

Practice: Anatomy and Physiology Word Root Introduction

The Right Match
1. g
2. f
3. h
4. c
5. j
6. b
7. a
8. i
9. e
10. d
11. s
12. o
13. r
14. t
15. q
16. k
17. l
18. m
19. p
20. n
21. aa
22. x
23. z
24. ac
25. ab
26. v

27. u
28. y
29. w

Word Root Linkup
1. physiology
2. abdominal
3. hypochondriac
4. pericardial
5. pelvic

Chapter Review
Word Building
1. (provided in chapter)
2. home/o/stasis
3. CT scan
4. chron/ic
5. path/o/logy
6. acute
7. transverse plane
8. abdomin/o/pelv/ic cavity
9. endo/scopy
10. sign
11. tissues
12. thorac/ic region
13. magnetic resonance imaging
14. epi/gastr/ic
15. pleur/al
16. sagittal plane
17. umbilic/al
18. infection
19. ana/tom/y
20. physi/o/logy
21. dors/al
22. ventr/al
23. super/ior
24. anter/ior
25. medi/al
26. infer/ior
27. hypo/gastr/ic
28. lumb/ar
29. peri/cardi/al
30. pelv/ic

Chapter 5
Practice: Signs and Symptoms of the Integumentary System
The Right Match
1. c
2. a
3. f
4. h
5. b
6. g
7. e
8. d
9. n
10. l
11. m
12. j
13. i
14. k
15. u
16. t

17. r
18. s
19. o
20. q
21. p

Practice: Diseases and Disorders of the Integumentary System
The Right Match
1. h
2. a
3. e
4. g
5. c
6. d
7. f
8. b

Break the Chain
1a. & 1b. (provided in chapter)
2a. melan/oma
2b. tumor
3a. onych/o/myc/osis
3b. fungus
4a. pedicul/osis
4b. condition of
5a. scler/o/derm/a
5b. hard
6a. trich/o/myc/osis
6b. hair
7a. cellul/itis
7b. inflammation
8a. leuk/o/derm/a
8b. skin

Practice: Treatments, Procedures, and Devices of the Integumentary System
The Right Match
1. e
2. a
3. b
4. c
5. d

Linkup
1. (provided in chapter)
2. rhytidectomy
3. dermatoplasty
4. dermatoautoplasty
5. dermatome

Practice: Abbreviations
1. bx or Bx
2. basal cell carcinoma
3. SLE
4. squamous cell carcinoma
5. TBSA

Chapter Review
Word Building
1. (provided in chapter)
2. cellulitis
3. onychopathy
4. onychomycosis
5. xeroderma
6. abrasion

7. folliculitis
8. trichopathy
9. impetigo
10. nevus
11. macule
12. emollient
13. dermatologist
14. keloid
15. onychocryptosis
16. actinic keratosis
17. leukoderma

Medical Report Exercises
Medical Report Comprehension Questions
1. The cicatrices on the skin are the result of scar tissue accumulation as the skin attempts to heal the vesicles and the damage caused by itching.
2. New scar tissue can be prevented or at least minimized by providing relief from the pruritus (itching sensation) and with anti-inflammatory medications such as topical ointments.
3. Antibiotic therapy is included to combat bacterial infection that may arise with rupturing of vesicles.

Case Study Questions
a. dermatology; b. dermatitis; c. actinic keratotis; d. vesicles; e. pruritus; f. ulcers; g. cicatrices; h. keloids; i. emollients

Medical Report Comprehension Questions
1. Prolonged activity in outdoor sports, during which exposure to the sun was common, supports the initial diagnosis.
2. A common word for nevus is mole.
3. Antibiotic therapy should be necessary. Antibiotics will not attack cancer cells, and the incision to remove the tumor is minor.

Case Study Questions
j. emollient; k. nevus; l. dermatologist; m. melanoma; n. bx or Bx; o. dermatoautoplasty; p. cicatrix

Chapter 6
Practice: Signs and Symptoms of the Skeletal and Muscular Systems
Break the Chain
1a. & 1b. (provided in chapter)

2a. a/tax/ia
2b. movement
3a. a/troph/y
3b. development
4a. brady/kines/ia
4b. slow
5a. dys/kines/ia
5b. motion
6a. dys/troph/y
6b. process of
7a. hyper/troph/y
7b. excessive
8a. my/algia
8b. muscle
9a. ten/o/dynia
9b. condition of pain

Practice: Diseases and Disorders of the Skeletal and Muscular Systems
The Right Match
1. i
2. e
3. a
4. b
5. c
6. h
7. j
8. f
9. g
10. d

Linkup
1. (provided in chapter)
2. polymyositis
3. lordosis
4. epicondylitis
5. arthritis
6. osteomalacia
7. bursitis
8. osteitis
9. bursolith
10. meniscitis
11. tenosynovitis

Practice: Treatments, Procedures, and Devices of the Skeletal and Muscular Systems
The Right Match
1. e
2. c
3. d
4. a
5. b
6. h
7. i
8. j
9. g
10. f

Break the Chain
1a. arthr/o/desis
1b. surgical fixation
2a. chondr/ectomy
2b. cartilage

3a. crani/o/tomy
3b. no
4a. lamin/ectomy
4b. excision
5a. electr/o/my/o/graphy
5b. muscle
6a. orth/o/tic/s
6b. straight
7a. oste/o/clasis
7b. break apart
8a. ten/o/my/o/plasty
8b. surgical repair
9a. oste/o/plasty
9b. bone

Practice: Abbreviations
1. SCI
2. total knee arthroplasty
3. RA
4. Duchenne's muscular dystrophy
5. HNP
6. electromyogram
7. ACL
8. total hip replacement
9. L1 through L5
10. carpal tunnel syndrome
11. ROM
12. osteoarthritis
13. TKR
14. the twelve thoracic vertebrae
15. DJD
16. temporomandibular joint disease
17. MG

Chapter Review
Word Building
1. (provided in chapter)
2. osteoporosis
3. paraplegia
4. scoliosis
5. tenosynovitis
6. arthrogram
7. meniscitis
8. arthrotomy
9. myasthenia
10. myocele
11. carpal tunnel syndrome
12. arthrolysis
13. Paget's disease
14. herniated disk
15. arthroplasty
16. tenodynia
17. bursolith
18. ankylosis
19. bradykinesia
20. decalcification
21. arthrodesis
22. degenerative joint disease
23. external fixation
24. fibromyalgia
25. myeloma
26. atrophy

Medical Report Exercises
Medical Report Comprehension Questions
1. Broken skin at right ankle and X-rays
2. To confirm the diagnosis
3. The ankle

Case Study Questions
a. compound; b. tendonitis; c. myalgia; d. myositis; e. polymyositis; f. Pott's; g. tendonitis

Medical Report Comprehension Questions
1. Osteoporosis and osteoarthritis.
2. Osteoarthritis.
3. Osteoporosis is a condition of abnormal loss of bone density that is a common result of aging, especially among women. The term literally means "condition of holes in bone."

Case Study Questions
h. dyskinesia; i. arthralgia; j. orthopedics; k. kyphosis; l. kyphosis; m. osteoporosis; n. osteoarthritis.

Chapter 7

Practice: Signs and Symptoms of the Blood and the Lymphatic System
The Right Match
1. d
2. a
3. i
4. g
5. b
6. c
7. f
8. e
9. h

Break the Chain
1a. & 1b. (provided in the chapter)
2a. thromb/o/penia
2b. clot
3a. leuk/o/penia
3b. abnormal reduction in
4a. hem/o/lysis
4b. loosen, dissolve
5a. leuk/o/cyt/o/penia
5b. white

Practice: Diseases and Disorders of the Blood and the Lymphatic System
The Right Match
1. b
2. c
3. h
4. g

5. a
6. d
7. f
8. e
9. j
10. i

Linkup
1. (provided in chapter)
2. thymoma
3. anemia
4. botulism
5. hematoma
6. iatrogenic
7. hemophilia
8. hemoglobinopathy
9. lymphadenitis
10. mononucleosis
11. hydrophobia

Practice: Treatments and Procedures of the Blood and the Lymphatic System
The Right Match
1. c
2. f
3. j
4. b
5. a
6. e
7. d
8. g
9. h
10. i

Break the Chain
1a. immun/o/therapy
1b. treatment
2a. splen/ectomy
2b. spleen
3a. lymph/aden/ectomy
3b. gland
4a. immun/o/logy
4b. exempt
5a. hom/o/logous
5b. same
6a. hemat/o/logy
6b. study of
7a. aut/o/logous
7b. self
8a. anti/bi/o/tic
8b. against
9a. hem/o/stasis
9b. standing still
10a. thromb/o/lysis
10b. loosen, dissolve

Practice: Abbreviations
1. AIDS
2. complete blood count
3. PLT
4. red blood cell or red blood count
5. HGB, Hgb
6. prothrombin time
7. PTT

8. white blood cell or white blood count
9. HCT, Hct
10. human immunodeficiency virus

Chapter Review
Word Building
1. (provided in chapter)
2. anisocytosis
3. dyscrasia
4. malaria
5. erythropenia
6. hemophilia
7. leukemia
8. macrocytosis
9. staphylococcemia
10. autoimmune disease
11. polycythemia
12. poikilocytosis
13. septicemia
14. anticoagulant
15. homologous transfusion
16. hematocrit
17. hemostasis
18. platelet count
19. Hodgkin's disease
20. lymphadenitis
21. diphtheria

Medical Report Exercises
Medical Report Comprehension Questions
1. Persistent mild fever and body aches, tenderness of the armpit and groin lymph nodes.
2. Antibiotics may fail if the bacterial strain is resistant to its effects.
3. *Staphylococcemia* means "condition of *Staphylococcus aureus* in the blood" and is commonly called a staph infection.

Case Study Questions
a. lymphadenitis; b. lymphoma; c. Hodgkin's disease; d. splenomegaly; e. differential count; f. infection; g. septicemia; h. staphylococcemia; i. antibiotic; j. immunodeficiency; k. immunotherapy

Medical Report Comprehension Questions
1. Dietary supplements were administered to see if the cause of the symptoms is pernicious anemia.
2. Aplastic anemia is abnormally low levels of red blood cells due to a reduction of red marrow function.

3. Poikilocytosis is the presence of teardrop-shaped red blood cells, and anisocytosis is a more generalized term describing red blood cells as having abnormal shapes.

Case Study Questions

l. dyscrasia; m. complete blood count; n. hematocrit; o. hemoglobin; p. anemia; q. iron deficiency; r. anisocytosis; s. poikilocytosis; t. aplastic; u. leukemia

Chapter 8

Practice: Signs and Symptoms of the Cardiovascular System

Break the Chain

1a. & 1b. (provided in the chapter)
2a. brady/card/ia
2b. heart
3a. cardi/o/dynia
3b. condition of pain
4a. cardi/o/genic
4b. pertaining to producing
5a. cyan/osis
5b. blue
6a. angi/o/spasm
6b. sudden, involuntary muscle spasm

The Right Match

1. f
2. e
3. g
4. a
5. d
6. h
7. c
8. b

Practice: Diseases and Disorders of the Cardiovascular System

Linkup

1. (provided in chapter)
2. cardiomyopathy
3. atherosclerosis
4. angioma
5. pericarditis
6. angiocarditis
7. varicosis
8. thrombosis
9. hypertension

The Right Match

1. e
2. k
3. i
4. f
5. g

6. a
7. d
8. b
9. j
10. c
11. h

Practice: Treatments, Procedures, and Devices of the Cardiovascular System

The Right Match

1. d
2. g
3. e
4. f
5. a
6. h
7. c
8. b
9. j
10. i

Break the Chain

1a. arteri/o/gram
1b. a record or image
2a. ech/o/cardi/o/graphy
2b. sound
3a. embol/ectomy
3b. a plug
4a. sphygm/o/man/o/metry
4b. process of measuring
5a. phleb/o/tom/ist
5b. vein
6a. electr/o/cardi/o/graphy
6b. recording process
7a. cardi/o/pulmon/ary resuscitat/ion
7b. lung
8a. end/arter/ectomy
8b. within
9a. valvul/o/plasty
9b. surgical repair

Practice: Abbreviations

1. CHF
2. atrial septal defect
3. CABG
4. myocardial infarction
5. PET
6. cardiopulmonary resuscitation
7. ASHD
8. atrioventricular
9. ECG, EKG
10. coronary artery disease
11. AED
12. right ventricle
13. VSD
14. mitral valve prolapse

Chapter Review

Word Building

1. (provided in chapter)
2. angiocarditis
3. angiostenosis

4. angioma
5. arteriosclerosis
6. bradycardia
7. cardiodynia
8. endarterectomy
9. cardiomegaly
10. endocarditis
11. dysrhythmia
12. hypertension
13. myocardial infarction
14. myocarditis
15. electrocardiography
16. phlebitis
17. angiogram
18. angioplasty
19. angioscopy
20. arteriotomy
21. auscultation
22. echocardiography

Medical Report Exercises

Medical Report Comprehension Questions

1. Mild chest pain that is not characteristic of angina pectoris.
2. The mild chest pain combined with the dental extractions suggests a bacterial infection that originated from the mouth.
3. Congestive heart failure

Case Study Questions

a. angina pectoris; b. cardiology; c. cardiologist; d. electrocardiography; e. stress ECHO; f. block; g. myocardial infarction; h. angiostenosis; i. atherosclerosis; j. cardiovalvulitis; k. valvuloplasty

Medical Report Comprehension Questions

1. The cause of the abdominal pain is angiospasm from the aortic aneurysm.
2. The aortogram provided the evidence for the diagnosis of aortic aneurysm.
3. An angioplasty is a surgical repair of a blood vessel. In this case, it is performed to repair the aortic aneurysm, probably by the insertion of a stent to reinforce the weakened blood vessel wall.

Case Study Questions

l. hypertension; m. aortogram; n. angiospasm; o. aneurysm; p. angioplasty; q. arteriotomy

Chapter 9

Practice: Signs and Symptoms of the Respiratory System

The Right Match

1. i
2. f
3. d
4. e
5. a
6. b
7. c
8. j
9. g
10. h
11. k

Break the Chain

1a. & 1b. (provided in the chapter)
2a. dys/phonia
2b. condition of sound or voice
3a. dys/pnea
3b. difficult
4a. epi/staxis
4b. dripping
5a. hyper/pnea
5b. breath
6a. laryng/o/spasm
6b. larynx

Practice: Diseases and Disorders of the Respiratory System

Linkup

1. (provided in chapter)
2. sinusitis
3. bronchiectasis
4. tracheostenosis
5. asphyxia
6. tonsillitis
7. bronchogenic carcinoma
8. pneumoconiosis
9. tuberculosis
10. legionellosis
11. pulmonary embolism

The Right Match

1. h
2. e
3. g
4. a
5. i
6. d
7. c
8. j
9. f
10. b

Practice: Treatments, Procedures, and Devices of the Respiratory System

The Right Match

1. j
2. f

3. g
4. c
5. b
6. e
7. i
8. d
9. h
10. a

Break the Chain

1a. trache/o/tomy
1b. incision or to cut
2a. thora/centesis
2b. chest, thorax
3a. pneumon/ectomy
3b. lung, air
4a. bronch/o/scopy
4b. process of viewing
5a. aden/oid/ectomy
5b. resembling
6a. bronch/o/dilat/ion
6b. process
7a. lob/ectomy
7b. round part, lobe
8a. rhin/o/plasty
8b. nose
9a. sept/o/plasty
9b. surgical repair

Practice: Abbreviations

1. LTB
2. TB
3. adult (or acute) respiratory distress syndrome
4. CXR
5. cardiopulmonary resuscitation
6. CF
7. upper respiratory infection

Chapter Review

Word Building
1. (provided in chapter)
2. anoxia
3. bronchitis
4. respiratory distress syndrome (or ARDS, or NRDS)
5. auscultation
6. hypoxia
7. dyspnea
8. hypercapnia
9. bronchiectasis
10. pneumoconiosis
11. bronchogenic carcinoma
12. cystic fibrosis
13. tracheitis
14. asphyxia
15. bronchogram
16. thoracentesis (or thoracocentesis)
17. oximetry

Medical Report Exercises

Medical Report Comprehension Questions
1. Dyspnea, thoracalgia, and malaise support the diagnosis of TB infection.
2. It is likely that the TB infection originated from exposure brought home by either of his parents.
3. TB is an abbreviation for tuberculosis, a bacterial infection of the lungs and other organs that often becomes chronic and severe if not managed aggressively with antibiotic therapy.

Case Study Questions
a. coryza (or acute rhinitis);
b. laryngotracheobronchitis;
c. bronchodilating; d. tuberculosis (TB); e. acid-fast;
f. tuberculosis; g. chest X-rays

Medical Report Comprehension Questions
1. Pneumonia causes symptoms of dyspnea and thoracalgia.
2. It is important to locate the source of the infection, such as the home or school, to prevent the further spread of the disease.
3. The source of the infection causing pneumonia is the fungus *Pneumocystis jiroveci*.

Case Study Questions
h. dyspnea; i. thoracalgia;
j. auscultation; k. pulse oximeter;
l. spirometer; m. hypoxemia;
n. pneumonia; o. acid-fast;
p. *Pneumocystis jiroveci*;
q. pneumonia

Chapter 10

Practice: Signs and Symptoms of the Digestive System

The Right Match
1. c
2. a
3. b
4. f
5. i
6. e
7. h
8. d
9. g

Break the Chain
1a. & 1b. (provided in the chapter)

2a. dys/peps/ia
2b. digestion
3a. gastr/o/dynia
3b. stomach
4a. hemat/emesis
4b. vomiting
5a. steat/o/rrhea
5b. fat
6a. hepat/o/megal/y
6b. liver

Practice: Diseases and Disorders of the Digestive System

The Right Match
1. i
2. j
3. n
4. c
5. k
6. l
7. e
8. a
9. h
10. b
11. g
12. f
13. o
14. r
15. p
16. m
17. d
18. q

Linkup
1. (provided in chapter)
2. glossitis
3. cholelithiasis
4. proctoptosis
5. hepatoma
6. gastromalacia
7. esophagitis
8. gastroenteritis
9. pancreatitis
10. dysentery
11. anorexia nervosa
12. polyposis

Practice: Treatments, Procedures, and Devices of the Digestive System

The Right Match
1. f
2. c
3. h
4. g
5. e
6. d
7. i
8. a
9. j
10. b

Break the Chain
1a. anti/emetic
1b. vomiting

2a. gloss/o/rrhaphy
2b. tongue
3a. sigmoid/o/scopy
3b. the letter S (sigmoid)
4a. hemorrhoid/ectomy
4b. surgical removal
5a. lapar/o/tomy
5b. abdomen, abdominal cavity
6a. pylor/o/plasty
6b. surgical repair
7a. anti/dia/rrhe/al
7b. against
8a. gingiv/ectomy
8b. gums
9a. vag/o/tomy
9b. incision

Practice: Abbreviations

1. barium enema
2. IBD
3. upper GI series
4. GERD
5. nausea and vomiting
6. UGI
7. irritable bowel syndrome
8. LGI
9. stool culture and sensitivity
10. GI
11. fecal occult blood test
12. EGD
13. lactose intolerance

Chapter Review

Word Building
1. (provided in chapter)
2. hepatomegaly
3. dysphagia
4. cheilitis
5. cholecystitis
6. cholelithiasis
7. colitis
8. colorectal cancer
9. enteritis
10. gastromalacia
11. diverticulosis
12. hepatoma
13. sialoadenitis
14. hemorrhoidectomy
15. colostomy
16. proctoscopy
17. laparoscopy
18. glossorrhaphy
19. polypectomy

Medical Report Exercises

Medical Report Comprehension Questions
1. Crohn disease
2. A laparoscopy confirmed the initial diagnosis of Crohn disease. Also, a colonoscopy revealed inflamed diverticula of the colon, and a barium enema revealed inflammation of the ileum.

3. A laparoscopy is a diagnostic procedure in which a modified endoscope, called a laparoscope, is inserted into the abdomen to observe and surgically correct a condition.

Case Study Questions
a. diarrhea; b. flatus; c. constipation; d. lactose intolerance; e. irritable bowel syndrome; f. Crohn disease; g. inflammatory bowel; h. barium enema; i. laparoscopy

Medical Report Comprehension Questions
1. The father is the more likely source of an inherited condition.
2. The temporary ileostomy provides an opening to the exterior for waste materials during healing of the colon and anus.
3. A hemicolectomy is a surgical excision of a part of the colon.

Case Study Questions
m. anorexia nervosa; n. colitis; o. colonoscopy; p. stool culture; q. cecum; r. diverticulosis; s.hemicolectomy; t. ileostomy; u. hemorrhoidectomy

Chapter 11
Practice: Signs and Symptoms of the Urinary System

The Right Match
1. g
2. c
3. i
4. f
5. b
6. e
7. a
8. h
9. d

Break the Chain
1a. & 1b. (provided in chapter)
2a. azot/emia
2b. urea, nitrogen
3a. dys/uria
3b. pertaining to urine or urination
4a. an/uresis
4b. without or absence of
5a. py/uria
5b. pus

Practice: Diseases and Disorders of the Urinary System

The Right Match
1. b

2. c
3. e
4. f
5. a
6. d
7. j
8. g
9. i
10. k
11. h
12. m
13. l

Linkup
1. (provided in chapter)
2. glomerulonephritis
3. pyelonephritis
4. nephrolithiasis
5. hydronephrosis
6. nephroma
7. pyelitis

Practice: Treatments, Procedures, and Devices of the Urinary System

Break the Chain
1a. cyst/o/graphy
1b. recording process
2a. cyst/o/lith/o/tomy
2b. incision or to cut
3a. lith/o/tripsy
3b. stone
4a. hem/o/dia/lysis
4b. through
5a. cyst/o/rrhaphy
5b. no
6a. nephr/o/lysis
6b. loosen or dissolve
7a. nephr/o/gram
7b. a record or image
8a. nephr/o/tom/o/graphy
8b. kidney
9a. ureter/o/stomy
9b. surgical creation of an opening

The Right Match
1. d
2. e
3. a
4. b
5. c
6. h
7. k
8. i
9. l
10. f
11. g
12. j

Practice: Abbreviations
1. urinalysis
2. RP
3. catheter, catheterization
4. VCUG
5. intravenous pyelogram
6. UTI
7. hemodialysis

Chapter Review
Word Building
1. (provided in chapter)
2. anuria
3. bacteriuria
4. cystolith
5. nephritis
6. hematuria
7. ureterocele
8. enuresis
9. nephrolithiasis
10. nephropexy
11. pyelostomy
12. urethroplasty
13. ureterotomy
14. cystogram
15. nephrography
16. intravenous pyelogram
17. nephroscope
18. blood urea nitrogen (BUN)
19. urinometer
20. urinalysis

Medical Report Exercises
Medical Report Comprehension Questions
1. Lumbar pain, malaise, hematuria, loss of appetite, generalized body aches
2. *Nephrotomography* literally means a "recording process of a cut kidney" and refers to a diagnostic procedure of observing the internal structure of a kidney using a series of X-rays. The term *nephrectomy* is the surgical procedure involving the removal of a kidney.
3. Dialysis is ordered prior to surgery to stabilize the patient's condition, which will reduce the surgical risk of death.

Case Study Questions
a. urinalysis; b. albuminuria; c. hematuria; d. nephrotomography; e. nephroscopy; f.nephromegaly; g. polycystic kidney disease; h. pyelonephritis; i. hemodialysis; j. renal transplant

Medical Report Comprehension Questions
1. Any condition associated with the left kidney could cause the symptoms of lumbar pain, dysuria, and nocturia, such as polycystic kidney disease, glomerulonephritis, etc.
2. It is unlikely that Type 2 DM contributed to the renal calculi, because DM

usually causes high urine flow rather than low flow.
3. *Renal calculi* is the presence of mineral deposits, or stones, within the renal pelvis that interfere with the flow of urine, and *pyelonephritis* is inflammation of the renal pelvis and kidney nephrons.

Medical Report Case Study
k. dysuria; l. nocturia; m. urinalysis; n. nephrolithiasis; o. urology; p. urologist; q. pyelogram; r. nephroscopy; s.lithotripsy

Chapter 12
Practice: Signs and Symptoms of the Male Reproductive System

The Right Match
1. d
2. a
3. b
4. e
5. c

Break the Chain
1a. & 1b. (provided in chapter)
2a. olig/o/sperm/ia
2b. little
3a. test/algia
3b. testis
4a. urethr/itis
4b. inflammation
5a. a/sperm/ia
5b. without or absence of

Practice: Diseases and Disorders of the Male Reproductive System

The Right Match
1. d
2. a
3. e
4. b
5. f
6. c

Linkup
1. (provided in chapter)
2. balanitis
3. epididymitis
4. hydrocele
5. varicocele

Practice: Treatments, Procedures, and Devices of the Male Reproductive System

The Right Match
1. c
2. a
3. e
4. b
5. d

Break the Chain
1a. vas/ectomy

1b. vas deferens
2a. hydr/o/cel/ectomy
2b. hernia, swelling, or protrusion
3a. orchid/o/pexy
3b. testis
4a. prostat/ectomy
4b. surgical removal
5a. vas/o/vas/o/stomy
5b. surgical creation of an opening

Practice: Signs and Symptoms of the Female Reproductive System

Linkup
1. amenorrhea
2. colpodynia
3. mastalgia
4. menorrhagia
5. hematosalpinx
6. oligomenorrhea

Practice: Diseases and Disorders of the Female Reproductive System

The Right Match
1. b
2. c
3. a
4. e
5. f
6. d
7. i
8. g
9. j
10. k
11. h

Break the Chain
1a. vulv/itis
1b. vulva
2a. salping/o/cele
2b. fallopian tube
3a. a/mast/ia
3b. breast
4a. endo/metr/i/osis
4b. within
5a. lei/o/my/oma
5b. smooth

Practice: Treatments, Procedures, and Devices of the Female Reproductive System

The Right Match
1. i
2. e
3. a
4. h
5. c
6. g
7. d
8. b
9. f

Linkup
1. vulvectomy
2. colpoplasty
3. gynecology
4. hysterectomy
5. colporrhaphy
6. hysteropexy
7. mammogram
8. oophorectomy
9. salpingectomy

Practice: Signs and Symptoms of Obstetrics

Break the Chain
1a. dys/toc/ia
1b. condition of
2a. hyper/emesis
2b. excessive
3a. pseud/o/cyesis
3b. false
4a. poly/hydr/amni/o/s
4b. amnion

Practice: Diseases and Disorders of Obstetrics

The Right Match
1. c
2. f
3. a
4. h
5. g
6. b
7. e
8. d

Practice: Treatments, Procedures, and Devices of Obstetrics

The Right Match
1. d
2. a
3. f
4. c
5. b
6. e

Linkup
1. amniocentesis
2. episiotomy
3. fetometry

Practice: Sexually Transmitted Infections (STIs)

The Right Match
1. c
2. i
3. f
4. h
5. a
6. b
7. e
8. g
9. d

Practice: Abbreviations
1. prostate-specific antigen
2. STI

3. human immunodeficiency virus
4. TURP
5. benign prostatic hyperplasia
6. AIDS
7. HBV
8. herpes simplex virus type 2
9. DRE
10. human papilloma virus
11. CIN
12. dilation and curettage
13. CIS
14. hormone replacement therapy
15. NRDS
16. premenstrual syndrome
17. TAB
18. toxic shock syndrome
19. PID
20. transvaginal sonography
21. GYN
22. biopsy
23. Pap smear
24. erectile dysfunction
25. FBD
26. obstetrics
27. C-section
28. obstetrics/gynecology
29. SAB
30. pregnancy-induced hypertension
31. FAS
32. infiltrating ductal carcinoma

Chapter Review

Word Building
1. (provided in chapter)
2. testicular carcinoma
3. priapism
4. phimosis
5. circumcision
6. hepatitis
7. orchidotomy (or orchiotomy)
8. cryptorchidism
9. oligospermia
10. orchitis
11. varicocele
12. amenorrhea
13. leukorrhea
14. mastalgia
15. menorrhagia
16. oligomenorrhea
17. endometriosis
18. cervicitis
19. hysteratresia
20. mastoptosis
21. vulvovaginitis
22. prolapsed uterus
23. salpingo-oophorectomy
24. episiotomy
25. hysteroscopy
26. mammography
27. pseudocyesis
28. abortion
29. abruptio placentae

Medical Report Exercises

Medical Report Comprehension Questions
1. Dysmenorrhea, menorrhagia are both consistent with evidences that point to CIS.
2. A Pap smear was performed to evaluate stages of cervical cell changes as an examination for CIS, which is characterized by cell changes.
3. *Dysmenorrhea* is abnormal pain during menstruation and *menorrhagia* is an abnormally heavy menstrual flow.

Case Study Questions
a. dysmenorrhea; b. menorrhagia; c. leukorrhea; d. dilation and curettage; e. Papanicolaou (Pap) smear; f. HPV (human papilloma virus); g. colposcopy; h. carcinoma in situ of the cervix; i. cervical conization

Medical Report Comprehension Questions
1. Testicular cancer is supported by sensitivity in the scrotal and genital region, palpable lump on lateral aspect of right testis, and positive biopsy for nonseminoma testicular cancer in both testes.
2. The gonorrhea infection was obtained through unprotected sex.
3. A bilateral orchidectomy is surgical excision of both testes, also called castration.

Case Study Questions
j. oligospermia; k. orchi-epididymitis; l. balanorrhea; m. gonorrhea; n. testicular; o. orchidectomy; p. infertile

Chapter 13

Practice: Signs and Symptoms of the Nervous System

Linkup
1. (provided in chapter)
2. hyperalgesia
3. polyneuralgia
4. hyperesthesia
5. neurasthenia
6. neuralgia
7. paresthesia

The Right Match
1. e
2. d
3. g
4. h
5. c

6. b
7. a
8. f

Practice: Diseases and Disorders of the Nervous System

Break the Chain
1a. & 1b. (provided in chapter)
2a. cerebell/itis
2b. little brain or cerebellum
3a. encephal/itis
3b. brain
4a. epi/lepsy
4b. seizure
5a. mening/itis
5b. inflammation
6a. para/plegia
6b. paralysis
7a. neur/oma
7b. tumor
8a. neur/itis
8b. nerve

The Right Match
1. k
2. e
3. g
4. a
5. h
6. j
7. c
8. f
9. d
10. i
11. b

Practice: Treatments, Procedures, and Devices of the Nervous System

Linkup
1. anesthesia
2. craniectomy
3. neurology
4. craniotomy
5. neurorrhaphy
6. psychiatry
7. vagotomy
8. psychology

The Right Match
1. e
2. c
3. d
4. b
5. g
6. a
7. f

Practice: Mental Health Diseases and Disorders

The Right Match
1. f
2. c
3. e

4. b
5. d
6. a

Break the Chain
1a. dys/lexia
1b. bad, abnormal, painful, or difficult
2a. neur/osis
2b. nerve
3a. psych/o/pathy
3b. disease
4a. psych/osis
4b. mind

Practice: Abbreviations

1. EP
2. positron emission tomography
3. electroencephalography
4. CT scan
5. magnetic resonance imaging
6. PD
7. cerebral palsy
8. EEG
9. deep tendon reflex
10. multiple sclerosis
11. cerebrovascular accident
12. AD
13. amyotrophic lateral sclerosis
14. ADD
15. attention deficit hyperactivity disorder
16. TBI

Chapter Review

Word Building
1. (provided in chapter)
2. cephalalgia
3. cerebellitis
4. cerebral vascular disease
5. glioma
6. encephalomalacia
7. neuropathy
8. hyperesthesia
9. encephalitis
10. meningocele
11. multiple sclerosis
12. myelitis
13. neurasthenia
14. neuroma
15. neuralgia
16. paresthesia
17. hemiplegia
18. polyneuritis
19. psychopathy
20. quadriplegia
21. hydrocephalus
22. craniectomy
23. craniotomy
24. neurorrhaphy

25. neurolysis
26. neurotomy
27. ventriculitis
28. neurologist
29. psychopharmacology
30. psychotherapy
31. mania
32. paranoia

Medical Report Exercises

Medical Report Comprehension Questions
1. The early sign is the polyneuritis reported on the left limb and shoulder, which indicates possible brain damage to the right side.
2. The primary possible consequence to the patient is brain damage to the right temporal lobe.
3. The term *neuralgia* means a "pain in a nerve," and *cephalalgia* means a "pain in the head," or headache.

Case Study Questions
a. cephalalgia; b. neuralgia; c. polyneuritis; d. analgesics; e. paresthesia; f. computed tomography; g. magnetic resonance imaging; h. intracranial; i. craniotomy

Medical Report Comprehension Questions
1. Veteran of Vietnam War with a history of drug use and chronic depression are indicators of PTSD.
2. The MRI revealed a slow leakage of blood within the brain.
3. The term *aphasia* means a "condition of without speech," and *agnosia* means a "condition of without knowledge."

Case Study Questions
j. epilepsy; k. dysphagia; l. paresthesia; m. Alzheimer disease; n. cerebral hemorrhage; o. cerebral angioscopy; p. cerebrovascular accident; q. psychopathy; r. psychosis; s. encephalomalacia

Chapter 14

Practice: Signs and Symptoms of the Eyes and Sight

The Right Match
1. f
2. d

3. a
4. e
5. b
6. c

Linkup
1. (provided in chapter)
2. asthenopia
3. ophthalmalgia
4. ophthalmorrhagia
5. blepharoptosis
6. blepharitis

Practice: Diseases and Disorders of the Eyes and Sight

The Right Match
1. d
2. e
3. b
4. f
5. a
6. c

Linkup
1. conjunctivitis
2. diplopia
3. astigmatism
4. iritis
5. retinopathy
6. ophthalmopathy

Practice: Treatments, Procedures, and Devices of the Eyes and Sight

The Right Match
1. c
2. d
3. b
4. a
5. f
6. e

Break the Chain
1a. & 1b. (provided in chapter)
2a. dacry/o/cyst/o/rhin/o/stomy
2b. surgical creation of an opening
3a. ophthalm/o/logist
3b. eye

Practice: Signs and Symptoms of the Ears and Hearing

The Right Match
1. b
2. d
3. f
4. a
5. c
6. e

Linkup
1. paracusis
2. otorrhea
3. otalgia
4. otorrhagia

5. anacusis
6. hyperacusis

Practice: Diseases and Disorders of the Ears and Hearing

The Right Match
1. c
2. f
3. b
4. e
5. d
6. a

Linkup
1. otitis
2. otosclerosis
3. otopathy
4. mastoiditis

Practice: Treatments, Procedures, and Devices of the Ears and Hearing

The Right Match
1. c
2. a
3. e
4. f
5. b
6. d

Break the Chain
1. a) ot/o/logist
1. b) ear
2. a) tympan/o/metry
2. b) measurement
3. a) myring/o/plasty
3. b) membrane, eardrum

Practice: Abbreviations
1. OM
2. ear, nose, & throat
3. Oto
4. both ears
5. AS
6. emmetropia
7. IOL
8. right ear
9. EENT
10. tympanic membrane

Chapter Review

Word Building
1. (provided in chapter)
2. blepharoptosis
3. dacryolithiasis
4. conjunctivitis
5. ophthalmomalacia
6. ophthalmoplegia
7. retinopathy
8. optometrist
9. dacryocystitis
10. ophthalmorrhagia
11. leukocoria
12. otitis media
13. otalgia

14. otosclerosis
15. otorrhea
16. otoscope
17. otopathy
18. paracusis

Medical Report Exercises

Medical Report Comprehension Questions
1. The diagnosis of conjunctivitis is supported by ophthalmalgia, inflammation, and exudates.
2. Antibiotics is the common form of treatment because conjunctivitis is usually caused by a bacterial infection.
3. The meaning of *OU ophthalmalgia* is "pain in each eye."

Case Study Questions
a. ophthalmalgia; b. OS; c. blepharitis; d. conjunctivitis; e. ophthalmologist; f. conjunctivitis; g. keratitis

Medical Report Comprehension Questions
1. In an infant, the evidences include pulling at the ear, crying and fussiness, possible fever, and difficulty sleeping.
2. The myringotomy is performed to drain fluids from the tympanic cavity to relieve the pressure caused by the infection.

Case Study Questions
h. otalgia; i. AD; j. otoscope; k. myringitis; l. otitis media; m. ear, nose, & throat; n. otologist; o. otitis media; p. myringotomy; q. audiometry

Chapter 15

Practice: Signs and Symptoms of the Endocrine System

The Right Match
1. d
2. e
3. a
4. b
5. c

Break the Chain
1a. & 1b. (provided in chapter)
2a. ex/ophthalm/o/s
2b. eye
3a. poly/uria
3b. pertaining to urine or urination
4a. acr/o/megaly
4b. extremity

5a. ket/o/acid/osis
5b. ketone

Practice: Diseases and Disorders of the Endocrine System

Linkup
1. (provided in chapter)
2. adenopathy
3. adenocarcinoma
4. hyperadrenalism
5. hypercalcemia
6. hypoglycemia
7. hyperparathyroidism
8. hypothyroidism
9. pancreatitis
10. thyroiditis

The Right Match
1. f
2. d
3. h
4. j
5. a
6. b
7. e
8. c
9. g
10. i

Practice: Treatments, Procedures, and Devices of the Endocrine System

The Right Match
1. d
2. c
3. a
4. b
5. g
6. e
7. f

Break the Chain
1a. adren/al/ectomy
1b. pertaining to
2a. endo/crin/o/logy
2b. to secrete
3a. thyroid/oma
3b. tumor
4a. thyroid/o/tomy
4b. incision or to cut
5a. thyr/o/para/thyr/oid/ectomy
5b. surgical excision or removal

Practice: Abbreviations
1. glucose tolerance test
2. RAIU
3. postprandial blood sugar
4. DI
5. fasting blood sugar
6. HRT
7. diabetes mellitus

Chapter Review

Word Building
1. (provided in chapter)

2. hyperthyroidism
3. diabetic neuropathy
4. adrenalitis
5. endocrinopathy
6. hypercalcemia
7. parathyroidoma
8. pituitary gigantism
9. hypoadrenalism
10. hirsutism
11. hypoparathyroidism
12. hypoglycemia
13. thyrotoxicosis
14. myxedema
15. hypogonadism

Medical Report Exercises

Medical Report Comprehension Questions
1. Malaise between meals, polydipsia, polyuria, cephalalgia
2. No, the diagnosis is lifelong and not presently curable.
3. FBS is fasting blood sugar, which refers to a blood test for glucose following an overnight fast (that is, before breakfast). GTT is glucose tolerance test, in which a patient is given a known amount of glucose and the blood is tested for it at timed intervals.

Case Study Questions
a. endocrinology; b. polydipsia; c. ketosis; d. acidosis; e. fasting blood sugar; f. glucose; g. hyperglycemia; h. insulin; i. Type I diabetes

Medical Report Comprehension Questions
1. A tumor of the adrenal gland often causes hypersecretion of androgens, which leads to excess body hair or hirsutism.
2. Hyperglycemia is related to weight gain because it is an excessive amount of sugar in the blood, which encourages the deposition of fat into tissues.
3. Adrenopathy is any pathologic condition of the adrenal glands.

Case Study Questions
j. hirsutism; k. adrenalitis; l. adrenomegaly; m. Cushing; n. hyperglycemia; o. androgens; p. hirsutism; q. adenoma; r. adrenalectomy

Glossary-Index ▶▶▶▶▶

Terms that appear in boldface are Key Terms from the chapters. Definitions are provided here for these terms.

Anti-impotence therapy, a collection of therapies that address erectile dysfunction, or ED, 356

Antianxiety medication, 423

Antibiotic therapy, a therapy against bacterial infections, 172

Antibiotics, substances with known toxicity to bacteria used as a therapy against bacterial infections, 102, 172

discovery of, 173

Anticoagulant, a chemical agent that reduces the clotting process in blood, 173

Anticonvulsants, 423

Antidepressants, 423

Antidiarrheal, 292

Antiemetic, a drug that prevents or stops the vomiting reflex, 292

Antihistamine, a therapeutic drug that inhibits the effects of histamines, 247

Antipsychotics, 423

Antipyretics, 423

Antiretroviral therapy, use of drugs to battle viruses, 173

Antispasmodic, a drug that reduces peristalsis activity in the GI tract, 292

Anuresis, the inability to pass urine, 311

Anuria, the production of less than 100 mL of urine per day, 311

Anxiety disorder, a mental disorder in which anxiety dominates a person's behavior, 429

Aorta, 190, 199

Aortic insufficiency (AI), a condition in which the semilunar valve fails to close completely during ventricular diastole causing blood to return to the left ventricle, which makes the left ventricle work harder; also called aortic regurgitation, 196

Aortic regurgitation, a condition in which the semilunar valve fails to close completely during ventricular diastole; also called aortic insufficiency (AI), 196

Aortic stenosis, narrowing of the aorta, reducing the flow of blood through this large vessel, which causes the left ventricle to work harder than normal, 196

Aortitis, inflammation of the aorta often caused by a bacterial infection, 196

Aortogram, the image resulting from aortography, a procedure that obtains an X-ray photograph, MRI, or CT scan image of the aorta, 208

Aortography, a procedure that obtains an X-ray photograph, MRI, or CT scan image of the aorta; image is called an aortogram, 208

Aphagia, inability to swallow, literally "without eating", 271

Aphasia, the inability to speak, 8, 24, 41, 408

Aphonia, the absence of voice, 229

Aplastic anemia, a type of anemia in which the red bone marrow fails to produce sufficient numbers of normal blood cells, 159

Apnea, a longer-than-normal pause between breaths, 229

Appendages, the limbs, which are attached to the trunk, and include the head, arms, and legs, 69

Appendectomy, surgical removal of the appendix, 292

Appendicitis, inflammation of the appendix, 276, 276f

Arachnophobia, fear of spiders, 431

ARDS. See **Adult (or acute) respiratory distress syndrome**

Arrhythmia, loss of the normal rhythm of the heart; also called dysrhythmia, 192

Arterial blood gases, clinical test to identify levels of oxygen and carbon dioxide in arterial blood, 247

Arteriogram, the image resulting from arteriography, a procedure that obtains an image of an artery, 208

Arteriography, a procedure that obtains an image of an artery that is called an arteriogram, 208

Arteriopathy, the general term for a disease of an artery, 196

Arterioplasty, a procedure performed to repair an injured artery, 208

Arteriorrhaphy, suturing the opening in an artery after surgical repair, 208

Arteriosclerosis, a disease in which an artery wall becomes thickened and loses its elasticity, resulting in a reduced flow of blood to tissues, 27, 196

Arteriosclerotic heart disease (ASHD), a condition in which the coronary arteries supplying the heart are damaged by arteriosclerosis, 196

Arteriotomy, an incision into an artery, 208

Artery, 189, 308

Arthralgia, joint pain, 25, 116

Arthritis, inflammation and degeneration of a joint, 121, 122f

Arthrocentesis, a procedure in which excess fluids are aspirated through a surgical puncture in the joint, 135, 135f

Arthrochondritis, inflammation of articular cartilage within synovial joints, 122

Arthroclasia, procedure in which an abnormally stiff joint is broken during surgery to increase range of motion, 136

Arthrodesis, surgical fixation (stabilization) of a joint, 136

Arthrogram, an X-ray image of a joint that is printed on a film, 136

Arthrolysis, a therapy in which a joint is loosened of its restrictions, 136

Arthroplasty, surgical repair of a joint, 136

Arthroscopic surgery, a surgery that involves a visual examination of a joint cavity and integrates fiber optics, live action photography, and computer enhancement, 137, 137f

Arthroscopy, an endoscopic visual examination of a joint cavity, 137

Arthrotomy, surgical incision into a joint, 137

Digital rectal examination (DRE), a physical exam that involves the insertion of a finger into the rectum to feel the size and shape of the prostate gland through the wall of the rectum, 356, 357*f*

Dilation and curettage (D&C), a common procedure that is used for both diagnostic and treatment purposes involving the widening of the cervical canal and scraping of the uterus lining, 375

Diphtheria, infectious disease resulting in acute inflammation with formation of a leathery membrane in the throat, 160, 160*f*, 161

Diplopia, a condition of double vision, 42, 447

Direct inguinal hernia, type of hernia that is a protrusion into the scrotal cavity in males, 284

Directional terms, words used to describe the relative location of the body or its parts, 65–66

Disease, a failure of homeostasis resulting in instability of health, 73, 270

Diskectomy, a surgery that involves the removal of the intervertebral disk, 138

Dislocation, 46

Disorders

Distal, 66*t*, 309

Diuresis, excessive discharge of urine, 312, 313

Diverticula, small pouches that form on the wall of the colon, often present without symptoms or with mild bowel discomfort known as diverticulosis, 279

Diverticulitis, condition of inflammation of diverticula, or small pouches on the wall of the colon, 279

Diverticulosis, presence of small pouches called diverticula on the wall of the colon, often without symptoms or with mild bowel discomfort, 279

DJD. *See* **Degenerative joint disease**

DMD. *See* **Duchenne muscular dystrophy**

DO. *See* **Osteopath**

Doppler sonography, an ultrasound procedure that evaluates blood flow through a blood vessel, 212

Dorsal, 66

Dorsal cavity, the body cavity on the posterior side of the body that includes the cranial cavity and vertebral cavity, 69

Down syndrome, 386

DRE. *See* **Digital rectal examination**

DTR. *See* **Deep tendon reflexes**

Duchenne muscular dystrophy (DMD), a condition that causes skeletal muscle degeneration with progressive muscle weakness and deterioration, 124

Duct, 309

Duodenal ulcer, ulcer, or erosion, in the wall of the duodenum of the small intestine, 280

Duodenum (of small intestine), 269

Dwarf, an individual with abnormally short limbs and stature, 120

Dyscrasia, any abnormal condition of the blood, 161

Dysentery, acute inflammation of the GI tract that is caused by bacteria, protozoa, or chemical irritants, 280

Dyskinesia, difficulty in movement, 117

Dyslexia, a reading handicap in which the brain reverses the order of some letters and numbers, 51, 431

Dysmenorrhea, abnormal pain during menstruation, 362

Dyspepsia, commonly called indigestion, it is accompanied by stomach or esophageal pain or discomfort, 272

Dysphagia, difficulty in swallowing, 24, 272

Dysphonia, hoarse voice, 230

Dysphoria, 408

Dysplasia, 366

Dyspnea, difficult breathing, 230, 238

Dysrhythmia, another term for arrhythmia, an abnormal heart rhythm, 192

Dystocia, difficult labor, 384

Dystrophy, a deformity that arises during development, 118

Dysuria, difficulty or pain during urination, 312

E

E. coli, 280

Ear, 440–69
  abbreviations of, 464
  diseases and disorders of, 458–59
  lateral view of, 442*f*
  medical report exercises, 466–69
  medical terms of, 443
  signs and symptoms of, 456–57
  treatments, procedures and devices of, 461–63

Ears, nose, and throat specialist (ENT), physician who specializes in treatment of upper respiratory tract disease; also called an otolaryngologist, 251

Eating, 270

Ecchymosis, condition caused by leaking blood vessels in the dermis, producing purplish patches of purpura, 94

ECG. See **Electrocardiogram**

Echocardiogram, recorded data resulting from echocardiography, an ultrasound procedure that directs sound waves through the heart to evaluate heart function, 213

Echocardiography, an ultrasound procedure that directs sound waves through the heart to evaluate heart function; recorded data is typically called an echocardiogram, 213

EchoEG. See **Echoencephalography**

Echoencephalography, a procedure that uses ultrasound technology to record brain structures, 423

Eclampsia, a condition of high blood pressure associated with a pregnancy that may worsen to cause convulsions and possibly coma and death, 387

Ectopic pregnancy, a pregnancy occurring outside the uterus, 46, 387, 387*f*

Eczema, a chronic form of dermatitis characterized by flakiness of the epidermis, 93, 93*f*

ED. See **Erectile dysfunction**

Edema, swelling due to leakage of fluid from the bloodstream into the interstitial space between body cells, 84, 161, 247

EEG. See **Electroencephalography**

Effectual drug therapy, a general type of treatment to manage neurological disorders, 423

EKG. See **Electrocardiogram**

Electrical bone stimulation, a procedure that applies electricity to stimulate the healing process of a fracture, 139

Electrocardiogram (ECG or EKG), recorded data resulting from electrocardiography, a procedure in which electrodes are pasted to the skin of the chest to detect and measure the electrical events of the heart conduction system, 213

Electrocardiography, a procedure in which electrodes are pasted to the skin of the chest to detect and measure the electrical events of the heart conduction system and used to evaluate heart function; the record or image of the data is called an electrocardiogram (ECG or EKG), 213

Electroencephalography (EEG), a diagnostic procedure that records electrical impulses of the brain to measure brain activity, 424, 424*f*

Electromyography, a procedure that provides electrical stimulation of a muscle and records and analyzes the contractions, 139

Em. See **Emmetropia**

Embolectomy, the surgical removal of a floating blood clot, or embolus, 214

Embolism, a blockage or occlusion caused by a blood clot or foreign particle (including air or fat), an embolus, that moves through the circulation, 26, 200, 243

Embolus, an abnormal particle or blood clot that moves along with the bloodstream, 200, 243

Emmetropia (Em), the normal condition of the eye, 450

Emollient, a chemical agent that softens or smoothes the skin, 102

Emphysema, chronic lung disease characterized by dyspnea, chronic cough, barrel chest, and chronic hypoxemia and hypercapnia, 238, 238*f*

Empyema, another term for pyothorax, or the presence of pus in the pleural cavity, 243

Encephalitis, inflammation of the brain, 414

Encephalomalacia, an abnormal softening of brain tissue, 414

Endarterectomy, the surgical removal of the inner lining of an artery to remove a fatty plaque, 214

Endocarditis, inflammation of the endocardium, 20, 200

Endocervicitis, a form of cervicitis that occurs when the inner lining of the cervix becomes inflamed, 367

Endocrine system, 64, 470–98
  abbreviations of, 493
  anatomy and physiology terms, 471–72
  diseases and disorders of, 477–85
  medical report exercises, 495–98
  medical terms for, 473
  signs and symptoms of, 473–75
  treatments, procedure, devices of, 487–91

Endocrinologist, a physician specializing in endocrinology, 488

Endocrinology, the field of medicine that focuses on the study and treatment of endocrine disorders, 473, 488

Endocrinopathy, a general term for disease of the endocrine system, 481

Endogastric procedure, 46*f*

Endometrial ablation, a procedure in which lasers, electricity, or heat is used to destroy the endometrium, 375

Endometrial cancer, a malignant tumor arising from the endometrial tissue lining the uterus, 368
  stages of, 368*f*